T0325460

Gastrointestinal Bleeding

Gastrointestinal Bleeding

EDITED BY

Joseph J.Y. Sung MD, PhD

Professor of Medicine
Chairman, Department of Medicine & Therapeutics
Director, Institute of Digestive Disease
The Chinese University of Hong Kong
Hong Kong, People's Republic of China

Ernst J. Kuipers MD

Department of Gastroenterology and Hepatology, and Internal Medicine
Erasmus MC University Medical Centre
Rotterdam, the Netherlands

Alan N. Barkun MD, CM, MSc

Division of Gastroenterology
McGill University and the McGill University Health Centre
Montreal, Canada

SECOND EDITION

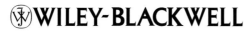

A John Wiley & Sons, Ltd., Publication

This edition first published 2012, © 2012 by Blackwell Publishing Ltd

Wiley-Blackwell is an imprint of John Wiley & Sons, formed by the merger of Wiley's global Scientific, Technical and Medical business with Blackwell Publishing.

Registered office: John Wiley & Sons, Ltd, The Atrium, Southern Gate, Chichester, West Sussex, PO19 8SQ, UK

Editorial offices: 9600 Garsington Road, Oxford, OX4 2DQ, UK
                     The Atrium, Southern Gate, Chichester, West Sussex, PO19 8SQ, UK
                     111 River Street, Hoboken, NJ 07030-5774, USA

For details of our global editorial offices, for customer services and for information about how to apply for permission to reuse the copyright material in this book please see our website at www.wiley.com/wiley-blackwell.

The right of the author to be identified as the author of this work has been asserted in accordance with the UK Copyright, Designs and Patents Act 1988.

Library of Congress Cataloging-in-Publication Data

Gastrointestinal bleeding / edited by Joseph J.Y. Sung, Ernst J. Kuipers, Alan N. Barkun. – 2nd ed.
      p. ; cm.
  Includes bibliographical references and index.
   ISBN 978-1-4051-9555-3 (hardback)
   I. Sung, Joseph J. Y. (Joseph Jao Yiu), 1959-   II. Kuipers, Ernst J.   III. Barkun, Alan.
   [DNLM: 1. Gastrointestinal Hemorrhage–diagnosis.   2. Gastrointestinal Hemorrhage–therapy.
WI 143]
   LC classification not assigned
   616.3′3–dc23
                                                                                    2011031413

A catalogue record for this book is available from the British Library.

Wiley also publishes its books in a variety of electronic formats. Some content that appears in print may not be available in electronic books.

Set in 9.5/13pt Meridien by Thomson Digital, Noida, India
Printed and bound in Singapore by Markono Print Media Pte Ltd

1   2012

Contents

List of Contributors

Disaya Chavalitdhamrong
CURE Digestive Diseases Research Center
David Geffen School of Medicine at UCLA
and Divisions of Digestive Diseases
UCLA Medical Center and West Los Angeles
VA Medical Center
Los Angeles, CA, USA

I. Lisanne Holster
Department of Gastroenterology
and Hepatology
Erasmus MC University Medical Center
Rotterdam, The Netherlands

Caroline M. den Hoed
Department of Gastroenterology
and Hepatology
Erasmus MC University Medical Center
Rotterdam, The Netherlands

Ana Ignjatovic
Wolfson Unit for Endoscopy
St Mark's Hospital, Imperial College London
London, UK

Vipul Jairath
NHS Blood and Transplant and Translational
Gastroenterology Unit
John Radcliffe Hospital
Oxford, UK

John T. Jenkins
Department of Colorectal Surgery
St Mark's Hospital, Imperial College London,
London, United Kingdom

Dennis M. Jensen
CURE Digestive Diseases Research Center
David Geffen School of Medicine at UCLA
and Divisions of Digestive Diseases
UCLA Medical Center and West Los Angeles
VA Medical Center
Los Angeles, CA, USA

Thomas O.G. Kovacs
CURE Digestive Diseases Research Center
David Geffen School of Medicine at UCLA
and Divisions of Digestive Diseases
UCLA Medical Center and West Los Angeles VA
Medical Center
Los Angeles, CA, USA

Larry H. Lai
Institute of Digestive Disease
The Chinese University of Hong Kong
Hong Kong, China

Johan F. Lange
Department of Surgery
Erasmus MC University Medical Centre
Rotterdam, the Netherlands

James Y.W. Lau
Institute of Digestive Disease
The Chinese University of Hong Kong
Hong Kong, China

Irene M. Mulder
Department of Surgery
Erasmus MC University Medical Centre
Rotterdam, the Netherlands

Brian P. Saunders
Department of Colorectal Surgery
St Mark's Hospital, Imperial College London,
London, United Kingdom

Ernest G. Seidman
McGill Center for IBD Research
Montreal General Hospital
Montreal, Canada

Daniela E. Serban
Pediatric Clinic II
Emergency Hospital for Children
University of Medicine and Pharmacy "Iuliu
Haţieganu"
Cluj-Napoca, Romania

CHAPTER 1

Gastrointestinal Bleeding: Presentation, Differential Diagnosis and Epidemiology

Joseph Sung

Institute of Digestive Disease, The Chinese University of Hong Kong, Hong Kong, China

Upper gastrointestinal bleeding (UGIB) represents a substantial clinical and economic burden, with reported incidence ranging from 48–160 cases per 100,000 adults per year (1–3). UGIB commonly presents with hematemesis and/or melena. In cases of severe UGIB, hematochezia (bright red or maroon colored blood per rectum) can be found. Depending on the speed of blood loss, hemodynamic status may be affected in different ways. In patients with severe blood loss in a short period of time, resting tachycardia (pulse > 100 beats per minute), hypotension (systolic blood pressure <100 mmHg) and postural drop in blood pressure (drop in systolic blood pressure of >20mmHg on standing) are evident, leading to dizziness and loss of consciousness in some cases. In patients with mild to modest blood loss over a longer duration of presentation, anemia, malaise and postural changes in pulse and blood pressure are common.

The incidence and prevalence of uncomplicated peptic ulcer have declined in recent years, largely due to the availability of treatments to eradicate *Helicobacter pylori* (*H. pylori*), and to the decreasing prevalence of *H. pylori* infection (4, 5). However, the use of acetylsalicylic acid (ASA) and other non-steroidal anti-inflammatory drugs (NSAIDs) that are associated with adverse gastrointestinal events is becoming more widespread. The mass vaccination against viral hepatitis B in newborns has also led to a decrease in cirrhosis and portal hypertension in high prevalence countries in Asia. As a result, the incidence of variceal hemorrhage due to viral hepatitis has declined, although alcoholic cirrhosis remains an important medical emergency.

Gastrointestinal Bleeding, Second Edition. Edited by Joseph J.Y. Sung, Ernst J. Kuipers and Alan N. Barkun. © 2012 Blackwell Publishing Ltd.
Published 2012 by Blackwell Publishing Ltd.

Table 1.1 Incidence of upper gastrointestinal hemorrhage associated with peptic ulcer disease.

Reference	Country	Study design	Timeframe	Hemorrhage Annual incidence (%)
Soplepmann et al. (11))	Estonia	Cohort study of consecutive new cases of peptic ulcer hemorrhage in secondary care.	1992–1993	0.057
Langman et al. (12)	England and Wales	Database review of admissions to secondary care.	1995	0.079 (age over 60 only)
Canoy et al. (39)	England	Database review of admissions to secondary care.	1996–1998	–
Higham et al. (40)	England	Database review of admissions to secondary care.	1996–1998	0.023
Paimela et al. (41)	Finland	Database review of admissions to secondary care.	1993–1997	0.043
van Leerdam et al. (2)	The Netherlands	Prospective cohort study of consecutive admissions to secondary care.	1993/4	DU: 0.013 (95% CI: 0.011–0.015)
				GU: 0.011 (95% CI: 0.009–0.013)
			2000	DU: 0.012 (95% CI: 0.010–0.014)
				GU: 0.010 (95% CI: 0.008–0.011)
Bardhan et al. (42)	England	Database review of admissions to secondary care.	1990–1994	0.021
			1995–2000	0.019
Ohmann et al. (43)	Germany	Prospective cohort study of admissions to secondary care.	2000	0.049
Ramsoekh et al. (44)	The Netherlands	Prospective cohort study of admissions to secondary care.	2000	0.022
Lassen et al. (5)	Denmark	Cohort study of admissions to secondary care.	1993	0.055 (95% CI: 0.049–0.062)
			2002	0.057 (95% CI: 0.051–0.064)
Kang et al. (45)	Scotland	Database review of admissions to secondary care.	2000–2002	0.022

CI: confidence interval; DU: duodenal ulcer; GU: gastric ulcer.

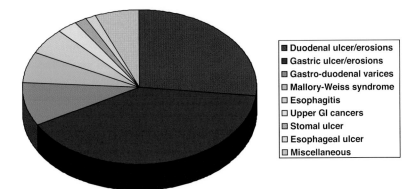

Duodenal ulcer/erosions
Gastric ulcer/erosions
Gastro-duodenal varices
Mallory-Weiss syndrome
Esophagitis
Upper GI cancers
Stomal ulcer
Esophageal ulcer
Miscellaneous

Figure 1.1 Common causes of upper gastrointestinal bleeding (Modified from Silverstein et al. (3) with permission from Elsevier.)

Causes of upper gastrointestinal bleeding

The most common causes of upper GI bleeding are depicted in large scale surveys (Table 1.1) (6, 7). Peptic ulcer disease usually constitutes slightly over 50% and esophagogastric varices 15–20% (Fig. 1.1). The other important conditions leading to UGIB include Mallory-Weiss tear, angiodysplasias and vascular ectasias, Dieulafoy's lesion, tumors of the upper gastrointestinal tract. In as many as 20% of patients, the diagnosis cannot be ascertained. On the other hand, in around 10% of patients, more than one source of bleeding may be identified.

Peptic ulcer and gastro-duodenal erosions

Both peptic ulcers and erosions are defined as a breach of the gastroduodenal mucosa as a result of peptic injuries. Differentiation of ulcers from erosions on endoscopic appearance is often based on the size (at least 5mm) and the presence of appreciable depth in ulcers. Both lesions are mainly caused by *Helicobacter pylori* infection and the use of non-steroidal anti-inflammatory drugs. With the wide use of aspirin and other anti-platelet agents as prophylaxis against coronary heart disease, cerebrovascular accident and prevention of cancer, the incidence of peptic ulcers related to these drugs are expected to rise. Stress related ulcers develop in patients who are hospitalized for major illness and life-threatening non-bleeding medical conditions. The risk of stress ulcer bleeding is probably higher in those who have respiratory failure and those with a bleeding diathesis. It has also been known that these patients have a higher mortality than those admitted to hospital with primary UGIB. The incidence varies widely in different countries and cohort studies. In recent years, however, evidence suggests that there is an increasing trend of peptic ulcer not related to *H. pylori* infection or NSAID, so-called non-HP non-NSAID ulcers (8). These patients are older and their risk of recurrent bleeding is higher and associated with higher mortality. The etiology behind this non-HP non-NASID ulcers remains unclear.

Bleeding from gastroduodenal ulcers stop in 90% of cases by the time patients arrive to hospital. However, recurrent bleeding occurs in 30–50% of cases if appropriate treatment is not given.

Incidence of peptic ulcer bleeding

A systematic review of upper gastrointestinal bleeding in 11 studies in Europe, reported on the incidence of complications associated with peptic ulcer extrapolated to the general population (Table 1.1) (9). Reported annual incidences of hemorrhage in the general population ranged from 0.019% (10) to 0.057% (11). A UK database study reported an annual incidence of 0.079% (12). However, this study was confined to individuals older than 60 years, and could therefore not be extrapolated to the population as a whole. Two national audits from the UK extended the analysis to include all causes of upper gastrointestinal hemorrhage and found a higher incidence. Blatchford and colleagues reported an annual incidence of 0.172% (95% CI: 0.165–0.180) in Scotland in 1992/1993 (13). Similarly, an audit performed during a four-month period in hospitals in the UK found an annual incidence of 0.103% (14). In this study, the annual incidence increased from 0.023% in individuals aged under 23 years to 0.485% in individuals aged over 75 years.

The few studies that have examined time trends in peptic ulcer hemorrhage reported no significant change in incidence over time. Bardhan and colleagues observed only a slight decrease in the annual incidence of hemorrhage in the UK, from 0.021% during 1990–1994 to 0.019% during 1995–2000 (10). Van Leerdam and colleagues similarly reported a statistically non-significant decrease in the incidence of both gastric and duodenal ulcer hemorrhage from 1993/4 to 2000 (2). However, Lassen and colleagues reported a slight increase in the annual incidence of hemorrhage in Denmark, from 0.055% in 1993 (95% CI: 0.049–0.062) to 0.057% in 2002 (5). Taha and colleagues studied the incidence of all upper gastrointestinal hemorrhage in individuals taking ASA 75 mg/day in Scotland (15). The annual incidence increased from 0.015% in 1996 to 0.018% in 1999 and 0.027% in 2002.

Mortality of peptic ulcer disease

Mortality after peptic ulcer hemorrhage ranges from 1.7% to 10.8%, depending on the reported series and the average mortality is 8.8%.

Increasing age, comorbid illness, hemodynamic shock on presentation, recurrent bleeding and need for surgery are important predictors of mortality in peptic ulcers bleeding after therapeutic endoscopy (16). Furthermore, delay in treatment for over 24 hours may be an important management issue. Recently, two studies from the US indicated that patients admitted after hours exhibited a higher mortality; although observational studies, the authors suggested this association may be related to lower rates of early intervention (17, 18).

However, not all cases of mortality are related to uncontrolled hemorrhage. In a single-center audit from Hong Kong which included 10,428 cases of confirmed peptic ulcer bleeding, only 25% of patients died from bleeding-related cause (e.g. uncontrolled bleeding, died on surgery, post-surgical complication endoscopy related complications, and death within 48 hours after endoscopy) (19). Comorbid illnesses such as cardiac, pulmonary, or cerebrovascular diseases, multi-organ failure or sepsis, and terminal malignancy constituted the majority of causes of death in this series. Therefore, the management of patients with peptic ulcer bleeding should not be focusing only on the control of hemorrhage. It is important to provide supportive care and management of patients' cardiopulmonary conditions. Drugs such as antiplatelet agents and anticoagulants which might be related to the development of peptic ulcer bleeding are often discontinued during UGIB. The early resumption of these drugs should be considered, balancing the risks and benefits of these treatments (20).

Sonnenberg studied mortality data from non-European countries including Argentina, Australia, Chile, Hong Kong, Japan, Mexico, Singapore and Taiwan (21) (Fig. 1.2). The age-standardized death rates in individual countries were tracked from 1971 to 2004. In all countries, there was a decline in gastric and duodenal ulcer mortality. The risk of dying from gastric and duodenal ulcer increased in consecutive generations born between the mid- and end of the nineteenth century and decreased in all subsequent generations. The peak mortality of gastric and duodenal ulcers occurred at the turn of the last century (Fig. 1.1). This decline in mortality which preceded the advent of endoscopic and pharmacological treatment is attributed to the decline in *H. pylori* infection. The bell shaped peak of ulcer occurrence among consecutive generations born between 1850 and 1950 is related to the interaction between a declining *H. pylori* infection and an advancing age of patients from these countries. In Europe, The data from the past 50–80 years show striking similarity (22) (Fig. 1.3). The risk of dying from gastric and duodenal ulcers increased among consecutive generations born during the second half of the nineteenth century until shortly before the turn of the twentieth century and then decreased in all subsequent generations. The time trends of gastric ulcer incidence preceded those of

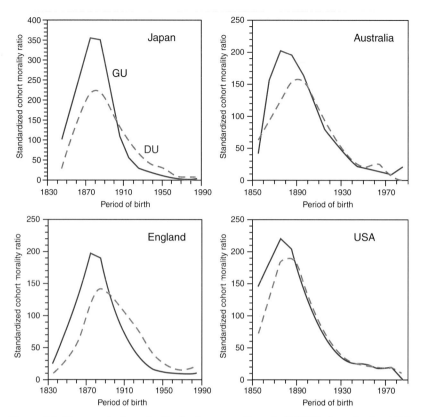

Figure 1.2 Time trends of standardized cohort mortality ratio (SCMR) of gastric ulcer (GU) and duodenal ulcer (DU) from Japan, Australia, US and UK (Reproduced from Sonnenberg (21) with permission from Wiley-Blackwell.)

duodenal ulcer by 10–30 years. The increase in consumption of NSAID and introduction of potent anti-secretory medications have not affected the long-term downward trends of ulcer mortality. The birth-cohort pattern is the most predominant factor influencing the temporal change of peptic ulcer mortality, probably related to *H. pylori* carriage rate.

Gastroesophageal varices

Gastroesophageal varices are often, but not always, the result of portal hypertension. Bleeding from gastroesophageal varices is now widely accepted as a phenomenon of "explosion" instead of "erosion." Varices develop usually when portal pressure builds up to above 20 mmHg and with a hepatic venous pressure gradient exceeding 12 mmHg, it is associated with a greater risk of continued or recurrent bleeding (23). Thus the risk of

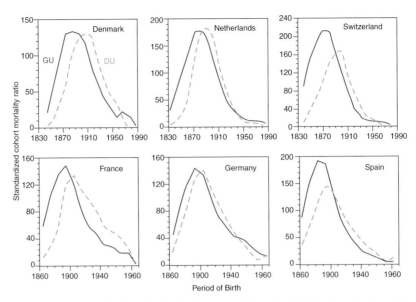

Figure 1.3 Time trends of standardized cohort mortality ratio (SCMR) of gastric ulcer (GU) and duodenal ulcer (DU) from European countries (Reproduced from Sonnenberg (21) with permission from Wiley-Blackwell.)

hemorrhage is related to the size of the varices, wall thickness and intra-variceal pressure. Several groups have confirmed that variceal size is the most important prognostic factor for variceal bleeding (24, 25). Red color signs, which include cherry-red spots and red wale markings, are also associated with more advanced grades of varices and a higher risk of hemorrhage. These signs are thought to represent focal weakness or "blowouts" in the variceal wall. Fibrin clots or "white nipple signs" are occasionally seen over the variceal columns which have recently bled. Beside the gross appearance of varices, patients with decompensated cirrhosis definitely fare worse than those with compensated liver function. Portal vein thrombosis is another poor prognostic indicator. The risk of bleeding from varices is related to the Child-Pugh score, not just because of more severe portal hypertension, but also because of other factors such as nutritional deficiency, coagulopathy and increased fibrinolysis in advanced liver disease. Recently, an association between bacterial infection and failure to control bleeding has been observed and a causal relationship implicated (26). Prophylactic antibiotic administration to cirrhotics with variceal bleeding results in reduced morbidity and mortality when infection is brought under control (27). A diurnal periodicity of variceal bleeding has also been observed. Bleeding episodes occur more frequently in the early morning and late evening, probably as a result of hyperdynamic blood flow in the portal system after meals.

Varices in direct continuity with the esophagus along the lesser and greater curves of the stomach are called gastroesophageal varices (GOV) types 1 and 2 respectively. Isolated gastric varices in the fundus (IGV1) occur less frequently than GOVs (10% vs 90%) but cause bleeding more often than either GOVs or isolated gastric varices at other loci in the stomach (IGV2).

Several prognostic indices have been developed to predict which patients with esophageal varices are likely to bleeding (28). Some of these are based on clinical parameters, others combined with endoscopic features, and the rest use a combination of endoscopic features, biochemical parameters and echo-Doppler ultrasound findings. The most widely used index is still the North Italian Endoscopic Club Index (NIEC Index) (24). This index is based on (1) severity of liver disease (Child-Pugh class), (2) size of varices and (3) presence of red markings on the varices. Based on this scoring system, cirrhotic patients are classified into one of six possible risk classes, each with a prediction rate of bleeding. The NIEC index has been prospectively validated in independent series. Yet, with the best prognostic index, one only predicts less than 40% of subsequent variceal bleeding. Obviously, many factors predisposing to variceal bleeding remain unknown.

Most variceal bleeding temporarily stops by the time patient arrives hospital. Without proper treatment, however, recurrent bleeding occurs in 30–40% within the next two to three days and up to 60% within one week (29). The risk of recurrent bleeding is presumably related to changes in hemodynamics of the portal system including an increase in portocollateral resistance after hypotension, increased splanchnic blood flow stimulated by blood in the gut, and an increase in portal venous pressure as a result of overzealous volume expansion during resuscitation. After the index bleeding, mortality is highest in the first five days and returns to baseline levels by three to four months (29). This is the critical time window for optimal treatment to improve survival of variceal bleeders. Complications related to bleeding and the treatment of bleeding substantially contribute to the mortality such as sepsis, hepatic encephalopathy, renal failure, and aspiration.

Mallory-Weiss syndrome

Mallory-Weiss Syndrome is a longitudinal mucosal laceration in the distal esophagus and proximal stomach. Although initially considered a rare cause of upper GI bleeding, the condition is being diagnosed more frequently and now accounts for 3–14% of patients presenting with UGIB (30). The prognosis of the condition is generally good, with only 5% of patients presenting with hemodynamic instability, and a small proportion with hematochezia. Mallory-Weiss syndrome can co-exist with other bleeding lesions, such as ulcers or varices, which could have caused the bleeding when esophageal mucosa is further damaged in vomiting. A transient increase in the pressure gradient between the intrathoracic and intragastric portion of the gastroesophageal junction, often caused by retching, is thought to create the tear. In up to 50% of patients with Mallory-Weiss syndrome, a hiatal hernia is present. However whether the presence of a hiatal hernia is etiologic to the tear or not is not clear. Retrograde intussusception of the stomach into the esophagus has been suggested as a mechanism for the pathogenesis of a Mallory-Weiss tear. The classic history of a Mallory-Weiss Syndrome is antecedent retching or emesis, initially presenting with clear vomitus, followed subsequently by hematemesis. Although antecedent retching was previously thought to be a prerequisite for the syndrome, it is actually reported in only 30–50% of patients. A significant proportion of these patients report alcohol binging. The Mallory-Weiss Syndrome may also associated with a variety of other antecedent events that give rise to an increase in intra-abdominal pressure, such as blunt abdominal trauma, hiccupping, retching during endoscopy, coughing, parturition, epileptic convulsions, straining, and even bowel preparation for colonoscopy. Predisposing conditions to the development of a Mallory-Weiss Syndrome include a hiatal hernia and, perhaps, advanced age (30).

Angiodysplasia

Angiodysplasiae are etctatic, dilated, thin-walled vessels in the gastrointestinal tract. They occur mostly in the stomach and less frequently in the small bowel and colon. They account for 5–7% of patients presenting with gastrointestinal bleeding. Often found in patients with advanced age, angiodysplasias are associated with chronic renal failure, hereditary hemorrhagic telangiectasia (Osler-Weber-Rendu Syndrome), chronic mucosal ischemia, and prior radiation therapy. The previous belief that angiodysplasia was related to aortic valve disease has been a subject of hot debate (31, 32). The diagnosis can be made by visualizing small, punctate, bright red, vascular mucosal lesions during endoscopy.

Platelet dysfunction associated with chronic renal failure has been postulated as a cause for recurrent bleeding. Endoscopic treatment using thermal coagulation can be successful but the multiplicity and involvement of sites not easily accessible, often in the small bowel, make its management difficult. Estrogen-progesterone treatment has been used to prevent recurrent bleeding from angiodysplasia but efficacy not proven by clinical studies.

Gastric antral vascular ectasia

Gastric antral vascular ectasia (GAVE), also known as "watermelon stomach," is an uncommon acquired vascular malformation distinct from portal hypertensive gastropathy (33). The diagnosis is made by a distinctive endoscopic appearance, characterized by longitudinal, vascular antral gastric folds converging like stripes of a watermelon onto the pylorus. Most patients present with chronic occult blood loss and transfusion-dependent anemia. Approximately 30% of patients with GAVE syndrome have cirrhosis but portal hypertension is not an absolute necessity for the development of this condition. Antral predilection for GAVE and the diffuse nature of portal hypertensive gastropathy distinguish the two entities. There is some evidence to suggest that GAVE may actually be associated with autoimmune diseases. As the lesion is superficial, often involving a large surface in the stomach, cautery with argon plasma coagulation often represents a particularly well adapted therapeutic option. The treatment might need to be repeated for several sessions before eradication can be achieved.

Dieulafoy's lesion

A Dieulafoy's lesion, also known as cirsoid aneurysm or submucosal arterial malformation, is a rare cause of upper GI bleeding. The lesion was named "exulceratio simplex" by the French surgeon Georges Dieulafoy in 1896. The condition can cause significant bleeding and is often difficult to diagnose. The true incidence is unknown, but in one series, it accounted for 1–5.8% of cases presenting with GI bleeding. A Dieulafoy's lesion consists of an abnormally large submucosal artery, a "caliber-persistent artery," protruding through a minute 2–5 mm mucosal defect. The diameter of the abnormal and often tortuous artery ranges from 1 to 3 mm, almost 10 times the diameter of normal arteries in the submucosa. Dieulafoy's lesions can be found along the entire GI tract, most commonly in the stomach (74%), duodenum (14%), colon (5%), gastric anastomosis (5%), small bowel (1%), and esophagus (1%). The proximal stomach is by far the most common site, classically described in the proximal lesser curvature within 6 cm of the gastroesophageal junction (34). For reasons which are still unclear, Dieulafoy's lesion is more commonly found in the older individuals.

Lower gastrointestinal bleeding

Lower GI bleeding arises from a source distal to the ligament of Treitz. It accounts for 10–20% of acute GI bleeding. It is usually suspected when

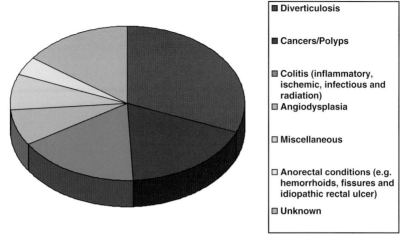

- ◼ Diverticulosis
- ◼ Cancers/Polyps
- ◻ Colitis (inflammatory, ischemic, infectious and radiation)
- ◻ Angiodysplasia
- ◻ Miscellaneous
- ◻ Anorectal conditions (e.g. hemorrhoids, fissures and idiopathic rectal ulcer)
- ◻ Unknown

Figure 1.4 Common causes of lower gastrointestinal bleeding (Modified from Zuckerman and Prakash (35) with permission from Elsevier.)

patients complain of hematochezia or passing blood clot instead of melena. Common causes of colonic bleeding include diverticular hemorrhage, angiodysplasia, radiation colo-proctitis, colonic polyps, carcinoma, and inflammatory bowel diseases (35) (Fig. 1.4). One emerging cause of lower GI bleeding relates to the increasing use of aspirin and NSAID in the elderly population. It is estimated that one-third of aspirin/non-aspirin NSAID induced ulcers or erosions occur beyond the level of the duodenum (36). The other important cause of lower GI bleeding would be related to bowel ischemia. This is usually found in the elderly patients as a result of heart failure, hypotension and cardiac arrhythmia. In a review of several large studies that include almost 1,600 patients with acute lower GI bleeding, the three most common causes of lower GI bleeding were diverticulosis, bowel ischemia, and anorectal conditions such as hemorrhoid, anal fissures and rectal ulcers (37).

Studies on lower gastrointestinal bleeding are much fewer than that of upper gastrointestinal bleeding. The severity of lower GIB is variable but past publications suggested the overall mortality to be low. A large-scale population-based study in Spain indicated that, while the incidence of upper gastrointestinal complication is declining, a rising trend of lower GI complications increased from 20/100,000 to 33/100,000 (38) (Fig. 1.5). This trend is attributed to the advancing age of patients, the higher number of comorbidities of the population and a decreased therapeutic effectiveness beyond the duodenum. With the development of balloon-assisted enteroscopy and wireless capsule endoscopy, there will be more cases of lower gastrointestinal bleeding confirmed with an identifiable cause.

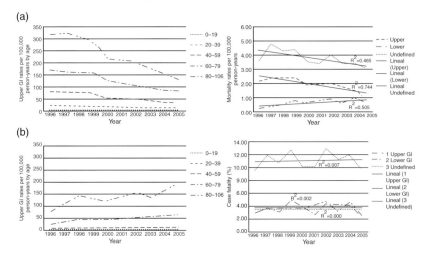

Figure 1.5 Time trend of upper and lower gastrointestinal bleeding and the associated mortality by year and by age groups (Modified from Lanas et al. (38) with permission from Wiley-Blackwell.)

Hospitalization due to the lower gastrointestinal bleeding was found mostly in patients older than 60 years of age. Mortality is relatively uncommon. Unlike the case of upper gastrointestinal bleeding which is found more commonly in males, in lower gastrointestinal bleeding, there is no gender difference between males and females. It will be a challenge to improve patient care in the future unless we develop new strategies to reduce the number of lower GI bleeding as well as reducing their associated mortality.

References

1. Longstreth GF. Epidemiology of hospitalization for acute upper gastrointestinal hemorrhage: A population-based study. Am J Gastroenterol 1995;90:206–10.
2. Van Leerdam M, Vreeburg E, Rauws E, Geraedts A, Tijssen J, Reitsma J. et al. Acute upper gastrointestinal bleeding: did anything change? Time trend analysis of incidence and outcome of acute upper GI bleeding between 1993 and 2000. Am J Gastroenterol 2003;98:1494–9.
3. Silverstein FE, Gilbert DA, Tedesco FJ. The national ASGE survey on upper gastrointestinal bleeding. Gastrointest Endosc 1981: 27:73–9.
4. Everhart JE. Recent developments in the epidemiology of *Helicobacter pylori*. Gastroenterol Clin North Am 2000;29:559–78.
5. Lassen A, Hallas J, Schaffalitzky, de Muckadell OB. Complicated and uncomplicated peptic ulcer in a Danish county 1993–2002. A population-based cohort study. Am J Gastro 2006;101:945–53.
6. Wilcox, CM, Alexander, LN, Cotsonis, G. A prospective characterization of upper gastrointestinal hemorrhage presenting with hematochezia. Am J Gastroenterol 1997;92:231.

7. Jutabha, R, Jensen, DM. Management of severe upper gastrointestinal bleeding in the patient with liver disease. Med Clin North Am 1996;80:1035.

8. Hung LC, Ching JY, Sung JJ, To KF, Hui AJ, Wong VW, et al. Long term outcome of Helicobacter pylori negative idiopathic bleeding ulcers: a prospective cohort study. Gastroenterol 2005;128:1845–50.

9. Sung JJY, Kuipers EJ, El-Serag HB. Systematic review: the global incidence and prevalence of peptic ulcer disease. Aliment Pharm Ther 2009;29:938–46.

10. Bardhan KD, Nayyar AK, Royston C. the outcome of bleeding duodenal ulcer in the era of H2 receptor antagonist therapy. QJM 1998;9:231–7.

11. Soplepmann J, Udd M, Peetsalu A, Palmu A. Acute upper gastrointestinal hemorrhage in Central Finland Province, Finland and in Tartu County, Estonia. Ann Chir Gynecol 1997;86:222–8.

12. Langman MJ. Ulcer complications associated with anti-inflammatory drug use. What is the extent of the disease burden? Pharmacoepidemiol Drug Saf 2001;10:13–19.

13. Blatchford O, Davidson LA, Murray WR, Blatchford M, Pell J. Acute upper gastro-intestinal bleeding in west of Scotland: case ascertainment study. BMJ 1997; 315:510.

14. Rockall TA, Logan, Devlin HB, Northfield TC. Variation in outcome after acute upper gastrointestinal hemorrhage, the National audit of acute upper gastrointestinal hem-orrhage. Lancet 1995;346:347–50.

15. Taha AS, Angerson WJ, Knill-Jones RP, Blatchford O. Upper gastrointestinal bleeding associated with low-dose aspirin and anti-thrombotic drugs a 6 year analysis and comparison with non-steroidal anti-inflammatory drugs. Aliment Pharma Ther 2005;22:285–9.

16. Chiu WY, Ng EKW, Cheung FKY, Chan FKL, Leung WK, Wu JCY, et al. Predicting mortality with bleeding peptic ulcers after therapeutic endoscopy. Clin Gastroenterol Hepatol 2009;7:311–16.

17. Ananthakrishnan AN, McGinley EL, Saeian K. Outcomes of weekend admissions for upper gastrointestinal hemorrhage: a nationwide analysis. Clin Gastroenterol Hepatol 2009;7:296–302.

18. Shaheen AAM, Kaplan GG, Myers RP. Weekend versus weekday admission and mortality from gastrointestinal bleeding caused by peptic ulcer disease. Clin Gastro-enterol Hepatol 2009;7:303–10.

19. Sung JJY, Tsoi KK, Ma TK, Yung MY, Lau JYW, Chiu PW. Causes of mortality in patients with peptic ulcer bleeding: a prospective cohort study of 10, 428 cases. Am J Gastroenterol 2010;105:84–9.

20. Sung JJY, Lau JYW, Ching JYL, et al. Continuation of low-dose aspirin therapy in peptic ulcer bleeding: a randomized trial. Ann Internal Med 2010;152:1–9.

21. Sonnenberg A. Time trends of ulcer mortality in non-European countries. Am J Gastroenterol 2007;102:1101–7.

22. Sonnenberg A. Time trends of ulcer mortality in Europe. Gastroenterol 2007;132:2320–7.

23. Moitinho E, Escorsell A, Bandi JC, et al. Prognostic value of early measurements of portal pressure in acute variceal bleeding. Gastroenterol 1999;117:626–31.

24. Prediction of the first variceal hemorrhage in patients with cirrhosis of the liver and esophageal varices. A prospective multicenter study. The North Italian Endoscopic Club for the Study and Treatment of Esophageal Varices. N Engl J Med 1988; 319: 983–9.

25. Beppu, K, Inokuchi, K, Koyanagi, N, et al. Prediction of variceal hemorrhage by esophageal endoscopy. Gastrointest Endosc 1981;27:213–18.

26. Goulis J, Patch D, Burroughs AK. Bacterial infection in the pathogenesis of variceal bleeding. Lancet 1999;352:139–42.

27. Hou MC, Lin HC, Liu TT, et al. Antibiotic prophylaxis after endoscopic therapy prevents rebleeding in acute variceal bleeding: a randomized trial. Hepatology 2004;29:746–53.

28. D'Amico G, de Francis R. Upper digestive bleeding in cirrhosis. Post-therapeutic outcome and prognostic indicators. Hepatology 2003;38:599.

29. Graham DY, Smith JL. The course of patients after variceal hemorrhage. Gastroenterology 1981;80:800–9.

30. Watts HD, Admirand WH. Mallory-Weiss syndrome: a reappraisal. JAMA 1974;230:1674–1675.

31. Shindler, DM. Aortic stenosis and gastrointestinal bleeding. Arch Intern Med 2004;164:103.

32. Imperiale, TF, Ransohoff, DF. Aortic stenosis, idiopathic gastrointestinal bleeding, and angiodysplasia: Is there an association? A methodologic critique of the literature. Gastroenterology 1988;95:1670–1676.

33. Payen, JL, Cales, P, Voigt, JJ, et al. Severe portal hypertensive gastropathy and antral vascular ectasia are distinct entities in patients with cirrhosis. Gastroenterology 1995;108:138–44.

34. Lee YT, Walmsley RS, Leong RWL, Sung JJY. Dielafoy's lesion. Gastrointest Endosc 2003;58:236–43.

35. Zuckerman, GR, Prakash, C. Acute lower intestinal bleeding. Part II: Etiology, therapy, and outcomes. Gastrointest Endosc 1999;49:228–38.

36. Lanas A, Sopena F. Nonsteroidal anti-inflammatory drugs and lower gastrointestainal complications. Gastroenterol Clin North Am 2009;38:333–52.

37. Strate, LL. Lower GI bleeding: epidemiology and diagnosis. Gastroenterol Clin North Am 2005;34:643–7.

38. Lanas A, Garcia-Rodriguez LA, Polo-Tomas M, et al. Time trends and impact of upper and lower gastrointestinal bleeding and perforation in clinical practice. Am J Gastro 2009;104:1633–41.

39. Canoy DS, Hart AR, Todd CJ. Epidemiology of duodenal ulcer perforation: a study on hospital admissions in Norfolk, United Kingdom. Dig Liver Dis 2002;34 (5): 322–7.

40. Higham J, Kang JY, Tinto A, Majeed A. Peptic ulceration in general practice in England and Wales 1994–98: period prevalence and drug management. Aliment Pharmacol Ther 2002;16 (6) 1067–1074.

41. Paimela H, Paimela L, Myllykangas-Luosujärvi R, Kivilaakso E. Current features of peptic ulcer disease in Finland: incidence of surgery, hospital admissions and mortality for the disease during the past twenty-five years. Scand J Gastroenterol 2002;37 (4): 399–403.

42. Bardhan KD, Williamson M, Royston C, Lyon C. Admission rates for peptic ulcer in the trent region, UK, 1972–2000. changing pattern, a changing disease? Dig Liver Dis 2004;36 (9): 577–88.

43. Ohmann C, Imhof M, Ruppert C, et al. Time-trends in the epidemiology of peptic ulcer bleeding. Scand J Gastroenterol 2005;40 (8): 914–20.

44. Ramsoekh D, van Leerdam ME, Rauws EA, Tytgat GN. Outcome of peptic ulcer bleeding, nonsteroidal anti-inflammatory drug use, and Helicobacter pylori infection. Clin Gastroenterol Hepatol 2005;3 (9): 859–64.

45. Kang JY, Elders A, Majeed A, Maxwell JD, Bardhan KD. Recent trends in hospital admissions and mortality rates for peptic ulcer in Scotland 1982–2002. Aliment Pharmacol Ther 2006;24 (1): 65–79.

CHAPTER 2

Gastrointestinal Bleeding: Resuscitation, ICU Care and Risk Stratification

Joseph Sung

Institute of Digestive Disease, The Chinese University of Hong Kong, Hong Kong, China

Initial management

The goals of managing a patient with acute GI bleeding are first to resuscitate; second, to control active bleeding; and third, to prevent recurrence of hemorrhage. The importance of resuscitation in the initial management of gastrointestinal bleeding cannot be over-emphasized.

Significant GI bleeding is indicated by syncope, continuous hematemesis and tachycardia, significant drop in systolic blood pressure, postural hypotension and requirement of blood or intravenous fluid to maintain blood pressure. Patients over age 60 and with multiple underlying diseases are at higher risk of negative outcomes. Those admitted for other medical problems (e.g. heart or respiratory failure, or cerebrovascular bleed) and who develop gastrointestinal bleeding during hospitalization also exhibit a higher risk of dying from the condition.

Vital signs should be closely monitored. In patients with hypovolaemic shock, central venous pressure and hourly urine output should be observed. Volume replacement, correction of bleeding diathesis, and emptying the stomach of gastric contents by nasogastric tube should be considered. Pre-endoscopic pharmacologic therapy using proton pump inhibitors or somatostatin should be considered on an individual basis. Following adequate resuscitation, management is directed to identify the lesion and identify the high-risk patient who is likely to require early endoscopic or surgical treatment.

Gastrointestinal Bleeding, Second Edition. Edited by Joseph J.Y. Sung, Ernst J. Kuipers and Alan N. Barkun. © 2012 Blackwell Publishing Ltd.
Published 2012 by Blackwell Publishing Ltd.

Fluid or blood replacement

The first priority is correcting fluid losses and restoring hemodynamic stability. Large bore intravenous access lines should be inserted to allow quick venous access. Volume resuscitation should be initiated with crystalloid intravenous fluid. Blood products including packed red cells, whole blood or plasma should be given as necessary. In order to maintain adequate oxygen-carrying capacity, the use of supplementary oxygen should be considered. Transfusions should be based on the patient's risk of developing complications from inadequate oxygenation rather than by a fixed hemoglobin, and are rarely indicated when Hb is >10 g/dL. Blood transfusion is indicated when Hb dropped to below 7 g/dL. International guidelines recommend that for critically ill patients in the absence of tissue hypoperfusion, coronary artery disease, or acute hemorrhage, red blood cell transfusions should be initiated when hemoglobin decreases to <7.0 g/dL (<70 g/L) and target a hemoglobin of 7.0–9.0 g/dL (70–90 g/L) (1). The Transfusion Requirements in Critical Care (TRICC) trial suggested that increased mortality was associated with a hemoglobin of 7–9 g/dL (70–90 g/L) compared with 10–12 g/dL (100–200 g/L) (2). In a prospective cohort study, a hemoglobin value <8.2 g/dL in patients with UGIB predicted myocardial injury (3). Overtransfusion, especially in elderly subjects with cardiopulmonary conditions, may lead to heart failure, adult respiratory distress syndrome and nosocomial infections. Close monitoring of central venous pressure is mandatory under such conditions.

Emptying gastric content

Nasogastric tube placement and aspiration can be considered in patients with hematemesis. Draining of blood and blood clots may facilitate the view of endoscopic examination This is, however, not routinely required and forceful suction on the nasogastric tube should be avoided as it may provoke bleeding from esophago-gastric varices.

The use of a promotility agent such as erythromycin or metoclopramide to hasten gastric emptying may be useful. A meta-analysis including a total of 371 patients showed that the use of a prokinetic agent significantly reduced the need for repeat endoscopy compared with placebo or no treatment (4). There were, however, no differences in length of stay, units of bloods transfused, or need for surgery as a result of this treatment. In addition, a cost-effectiveness analysis based on data from the three erythromycin trials found that the strategy of erythromycin prior to endoscopy is beneficial (5). Based on these data, promotility agents are recommended but should not be routinely used (1).

Correct bleeding diathesis

A bleeding diathesis can result from hepatic decompensation in patients with chronic liver disease, the use of anti-coagulants for the prevention of thrombosis, and the use of antiplatelet agents in patients with cardiac or cerebrovascular diseases. Correcting the coagulopathy is necessary in patients on anticoagulants, yet endoscopy should not be delayed (6).

Clinical evidence suggests that intensive interventions to aggressively correct coagulopathy can reduce mortality. Using a historical cohort comparison, Baradarian suggested that correcting an INR more aggressively to a value <1.8 led to lower mortality and fewer myocardial infarctions in the intervention group (7). There were no differences in length of stay, units of bloods transfused, or time to endoscopy. An exploratory analysis based on the RUGBE registry suggested that an INR of ≥1.5 was a significant predictor of mortality in patients with UGIB (RUBGE). Platelet count did not significantly predict mortality, and neither INR value nor platelet count predicted rebleeding. An INR of ≥1.5 may serve as target threshold for correction of a coagulopathy at initial resuscitation but, again, should not delay hemostatic therapy. Indeed, data suggest endoscopic treatment may be safely performed in patients with an INR of <2.5: An older cohort study comparing patients with or without using warfarin who underwent endoscopic treatment found no differences in rebleeding, surgery, mortality or complication rates between patients on warfarin who had INRs from 1.5 to 6.0 that were partially corrected using fresh frozen plasma to 1.5 to 2.5 (8).

Pharmacological treatment before endoscopy

Pre-Endoscopic proton pump inhibitors

Intravenous proton pump inhibitors can be used to provide a stop gap treatment while awaiting early endoscopy. In a study from Hong Kong in which over 380 patients were randomized to receive either intravenous high-dose omeprazole or placebo before endoscopy, proton pump inhibitor infusion was shown to reduce the frequency of active peptic ulcer bleeding and hence reduce the need for endoscopic therapy (9). There was, however, no significant difference in clinical outcomes such as rebleeding, surgery, or mortality. A subsequent cost-effectiveness analysis based on this study suggested that pre-endoscopic PPI therapy may be an economically dominant strategy compared to a no PPI approach (i.e. more effective and less costly) (10), while a North American analysis suggested conclusions were dependent on assumptions such as the presumed endoscopic findings and delay to surgery (11). Down-grading the lesion may be especially useful when endoscopy is being performed by inexperienced endoscopists.

A 2006 Cochrane meta-analysis that included five RCTs was recently updated with one additional trial (12). The updated meta-analysis of 2,233 patients, that included one study assessing oral and five assessing IV PPI strategies, showed no statistically significant differences in rates of mortality, rebleeding or surgery between PPI and control treatment. However, PPI treatment significantly reduced the proportion of patients with high-risk stigmata of recent hemorrhage (active bleeding, nonbleeding visible vessel, adherent clots) at index endoscopy, and the need for endoscopic therapy compared to control by about one-third.

Pre-Endoscopic vasoactive agents

Treatment of portal hypertension has been shown to effectively control bleeding from esophago-gastric varices and improve survival. The use of intravenous vasoactive agents such as somatostatin and octreotide (a long acting somatostatin analogue) is an effective method to control variceal hemorrhage before endoscopy. Randomized studies comparing endoscopic sclerotherapy and intravenous octreotide has shown that the pharmacologic agent can reduce portal pressure and offer temporally control of acute variceal bleeding (13). These findings were subsequently confirmed by pooled data from meta-analysis using various types of vasoactive agents (14). The benefit of vasoactive agents is found to be more evident when they are given as early as possible before endoscopic intervention can be offered (15–17). Rebleeding mortality was reduced and overall survival improved in patients received teripressin plus nitroglycerin, somatostatin or vapreotide (a long acting analogue of somatostatin). These agents are very safe with minimal adverse effects in short term usage. Because of their efficacy and safety profile, they should be started when there is any suspicion that the gastro-intestinal bleeding is related to portal hypertension.

Risk stratification

Patients with gastrointestinal bleeding should be stratified into low- and high-risk cases using validated prognostic scales. Early identification of high-risk patient is critical to allow appropriate intervention to minimize morbidity and mortality in patients with upper gastrointestinal bleeding. Furthermore, the identification of low-risk patients also allows triage for early discharge or obviation of hospitalization.

Peptic ulcer disease

There are various types of assessment instruments using either clinical and/or endoscopic findings in predicting the need for intervention, risk for recurrent bleeding or mortality of patients with UGIB (Box 2.1). One

Box 2.1 Commonly used risk scores for prediction of outcome of acute upper GI hemorrhage

Parameters	Score	Parameters	Score
Rockall Risk scoring system (19)		Baylor Bleeding score (24)	
A. Age (y)		A. Age (y)	
≥80	2	≥70	5
60-79	1	60-69	3
<60	0	50-59	2
		30-49	1
		<30	0
B. Shock		B. Number of illnesses (sum of diagnoses; irrespective of severity)	
Hypotension, SBP < 100 mm Hg	2	≥5	5
Tachycardia, SBP ≥ 100 mm Hg and pulse > 100 per min	1	3-4	4
		1-2	1
no shock, SBP ≥ 100 mm Hg and pulse <100 per min	0	None	0
C. Comorbidity		C. Severity of illnesses	
Renal failure, liver failure, disseminated malignancy	3	Acute (life-threatening illness *with* immediate threat to life)	5
Cardiac failure, ischemic heart disease any major comorbidity	2	Chronic (chronic, life-threatening illness *without* immediate threat to life)	4
		None	0
		D. Site of bleeding	

Continued p. 20

Box 2.1 (*continued*)

Parameters	Score	Parameters	Score
No major comorbidity	0	Posterior wall of duodenal bulb	4
D. Diagnosis at EGD		Other	0
Upper-GI cancer	2	E. SRH	
All other diagnosis	1	Active bleeding	5
No lesion, No SRH, MW tear	0	Visible vessel	3
E. Major SRH		Clot	1
Blood in Upper-GI tract, adherent clot, visibile or spurting vessel	2	None	0
None or dark spot only	0	Pre-endoscopy score: A + B + C. Postendoscopy score: A + B + C + D + E	
		Minimum score: 0 Maximum score: 24	
Pre-endoscopy score: A + B + C. Total score: A + B + C + D + E		Risk category: high (pre-endoscopy score >5 and/or postendoscopy score >10), and low (pre-endoscopy score ≤5 and/or postendoscopy score ≤10).	
Minimum score: 0 Maximum score: 11			
Risk category: high (≥5) intermediate (3-4), and low (0-2).			
Cedars-Sinai Medical Center Predictive Index (23)		Blatchford Risk score (20)	
A. EGD findings		A. Blood urea (mmol/L)*	
		≥25	6
Persistent hemorrhage, varices, upper-GI cancer	4	10-<25	4
		8-<10	3
Ulcer with non-bleeding visible vessel or SRH	2	6.5-<8	2
		<6.5	0
Ulcer with flat spot or	1	B. H (g/L)	

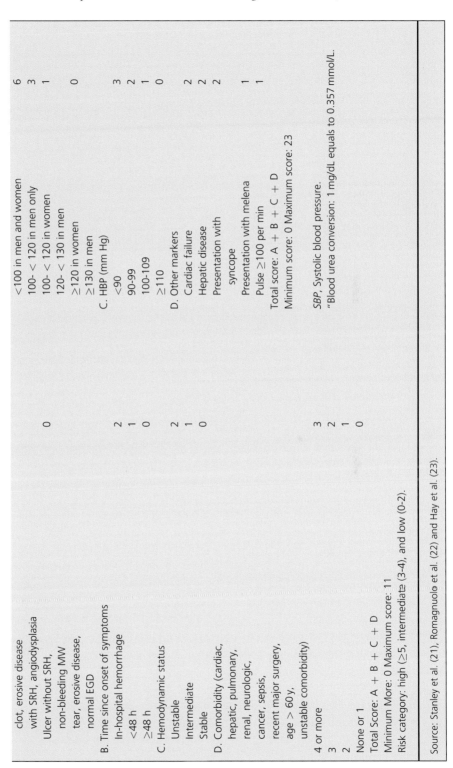

Scoring system (Total score: A + B + C + D; Minimum score: 0, Maximum score: 23)

A. Endoscopic diagnosis	Points
clot, erosive disease with SRH, angiodysplasia	6
Ulcer without SRH, non-bleeding MW tear, erosive disease, normal EGD	0

B. SBP (mm Hg)	Points
<100 in men and women	
100- < 120 in men only	
100- < 120 in women	
120- < 130 in men	
≥120 in women	
≥130 in men	

C. HBP (mm Hg)	Points
<90	3
90-99	2
100-109	1
≥110	0

D. Other markers	Points
Cardiac failure	2
Hepatic disease	2
Presentation with syncope	2
Presentation with melena	1
Pulse ≥100 per min	1

Total score: A + B + C + D

Minimum score: 0 Maximum score: 23

Scoring system (Total Score: A + B + C + D; Minimum score: 0, Maximum score: 11)

A. Endoscopic diagnosis	Points
clot, erosive disease with SRH, angiodysplasia	
Ulcer without SRH, non-bleeding MW tear, erosive disease, normal EGD	0

B. Time since onset of symptoms	Points
In-hospital hemorrhage	2
<48 h	1
≥48 h	0

C. Hemodynamic status	Points
Unstable	2
Intermediate	1
Stable	0

D. Comorbidity (cardiac, hepatic, pulmonary, renal, neurologic, cancer, sepsis, recent major surgery, age > 60 y, unstable comorbidity)	Points
4 or more	3
3	2
2	1
None or 1	0

Total Score: A + B + C + D

Minimum More: 0 Maximum score: 11

Risk category: high (≥5, intermediate (3-4), and low (0-2).

SBP, Systolic blood pressure.

"Blood urea conversion: 1 mg/dL equals to 0.357 mmol/L.

Source: Stanley et al. (21), Romagnuolo et al. (22) and Hay et al. (23).

Table 2.1 Comparison of the most commonly used scoring system for peptic ulcer bleeding.

Characteristics of Risk Scores	Baylor Score	Cedars-Sinai Score	Rockall Score	Blatchford Score
Primary outcome variable	Rebleeding	Rebleeding/ Mortality	Mortality	Clinical Intervention
Patient cohort	PUB	UGIB	UGIB	UGIB
Endoscopic findings	+	+	+	−
Patient's age	+	−	+	−
Comorbid conditions	+	+	+	+
Hemodynamic status	−	+	+	+
Time since onset of symptoms	−	+	−	−

must differentiate the objective of each score (for the prediction of rebleeding or mortality) and the specific target group they were developed for before using these scales (Table 2.1). A detail review on the topic was conducted by the ASGE in 2004 (18).

The Rockall score (19) is probably the best known of these scoring systems for prediction of mortality in upper gastrointestinal bleeding. It has two parts, the pre-endoscopic score which consists of three non-endoscopic variables (age, shock and comorbidity), and the complete score which uses both clinical and two endoscopic variables (endoscopic diagnosis and endoscopic stigmata of recent hemorrhage). The appearance of the ulcer, especially the presence of protuberant vessel at the ulcer base, is a strong indicator of recurrent bleeding risk (Fig. 2.1). This score was developed by determining independent risk factors of mortality and was prospectively validated in large scale studies in many countries.

The Blatchford score (20) is unique in two aspects. It uses only clinical and laboratory data before endoscopy, and it aims to identify patients presenting with upper gastrointestinal bleeding (non-variceal and variceal) who may require clinical intervention (blood transfusion, endoscopic or surgical treatment). It is a clinical (non endoscopic) risk score, which includes hemoglobin, blood urea, pulse, systolic blood pressure, the presence of syncope or melena, and evidence of hepatic disease or cardiac failure. It has been validated to identify low-risk patients. In addition, several studies have demonstrated that patients can be safely managed as outpatients without the need for early endoscopy using the Blatchford score (21, 22).

The Cedars-Sinai score was developed based on a retrospective cohort of UGIB targeting prediction of recurrent bleeding, requirement for and in-hospital death (23). It has taken into the formula time for onset of hemorrhage to arrival in hospital and in-hospital patients admitted for other medical illness.

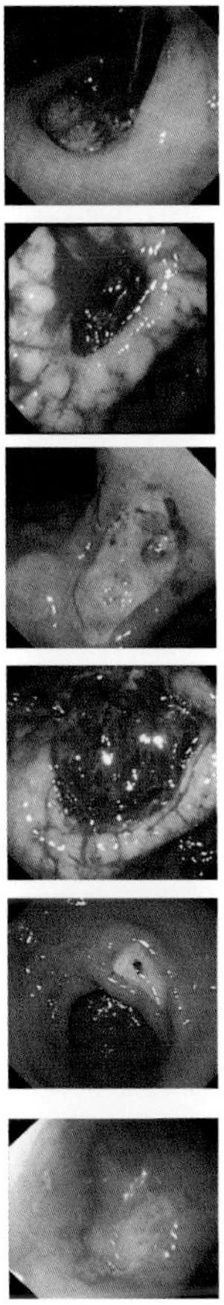

	Forrest class	Appearance	Risk of bleeding	Endoscopic Rx
	Ia	Arterial spurter	100%	Indicated
	Ib	Active oozing	55%	Indicated
	IIa	Protuberant vessels	43%	Indicated
	IIb	Adherent blood clot	22%	Indicated
	IIc	Pigmented spot	10%	Not indicated
	III	Clean ulcer base	5%	Not indicated

Figure 2.1 Stigmata of recent hemorrhage in bleeding peptic ulcers according to Forrest Classification and risk of recurrent bleeding

The Baylor score (24) was developed to predict recurrent bleeding primarily from peptic ulcer. The scoring system also has a pre-endoscopy score (age, number and severity of illness) and an endoscopic score (site and stigmata of hemorrhage).

Endoscopic predictors of increased risk include active bleeding and high-risk endoscopic stigmata, ulcer size (greater than 1 or 2 cm), and site of bleeding (i.e. the posterior lesser gastric curvature and posterior duodenal wall). A comparison of three prognostic scales (Baylor, Rockall, and Cedars-Sinai predictive indexes) found that Rockall best identified patients at low risk. Use of the Rockall risk score has also been shown to yield a more precise diagnosis and shorter duration of hospitalization, especially for patients at low-risk, compared to not using a prognostic scale. The Rockall scoring system has been validated in many different countries to date and shown to accurately predict mortality, but it performs poorly for rebleeding, particularly in patients at high risk.

Based on a large prospective cohort of over 3,300 patients with peptic ulcer bleeding, the Hong Kong group has recently reported a series of factors that predict recurrent bleeding after endoscopic therapy (25). These include hypotension, hemoglobin below 10 g/dL, finding fresh blood in stomach, ulcer with active bleeding and large ulcers. Using the same database, a scoring system to predict mortality in peptic ulcer bleeding was established (26). The scale included age over 70 years, presence of comorbidity, more than one listed comorbidity, hematemesis on presentation, systolic blood pressure below 100mmgHg, in-hospital bleeding, rebleeding and need for surgery.

Gastro-Esophageal varices

Several prognostic indices have been developed to predict which patients with esophageal varices are likely to bleed. Some of them are based on clinical parameters, others combined with endoscopic features, and the rest use a combination of endoscopic features, biochemical parameters and echo-Doppler ultrasound findings.

The most widely used index is still the North Italian Endoscopic Club Index (NIEC Index) (27) (Tables 2.2 and 2.3). This index is based on (1) severity of liver disease (Child-Pugh class), (2) size of varices and (3) presence of red markings on the varices (Table 2.2) (Fig. 2.2). Base on this index, cirrhotic patients has been classified into six risk classes, each with a prediction rate of bleeding (Table 2.3). The NIEC Index has been prospectively validated in independent patient populations. Yet, with the best prognostic index, one

Table 2.2 North Italian Endoscopy Club Index for Assessing the Risk of Variceal Bleeding (27).

Variable	Points to add
Child Class	
A	6.5
B	13.0
C	19.5
Size of varices	
Small	8.7
Medium	13.0
Large	17.4
Red wale marking	
Absent	3.2
Mild	6.4
Moderate	9.6
Severe	12.8

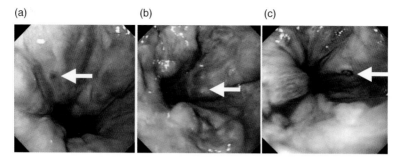

Figure 2.2 High risk varices with red dot sign (a), varices on varices appearance (b) and fibrin clot (c)

could only predict less than 40% of variceal bleeding. Obviously, many factors predisposing to variceal bleeding remain unknown.

Most variceal bleeding temporarily stops by the time the patient arrives in hospital. Without proper treatment, however, recurrent bleeding occurs in 30–40% within the next two to three days and up to 60% within one week. The risk of recurrent bleeding is presumably related to changes in hemodynamics of the portal system including an increase in portocollateral resistance after hypotension, increased splanchnic blood flow stimulated by blood in the gut and an increase in portal venous pressure as a result of overzealous volume expansion during resuscitation. After the index bleeding, mortality is highest in the first five days and returns to baseline levels by three to four months. This is the critical time window for optimal treatment to improve survival of variceal bleeders (28).

Lower gastrointestinal bleeding

There are less scoring systems available for the evaluation of lower gastrointestinal bleeding. A reliable predictive model that can accurately forecast

Table 2.3 Cumulative Percentages of Patients Bleeding among Patients with Cirrhosis and Varices Classified According to the NIEC Index (27).

Risk class	NIEC index	Rate of Bleeding (%)		
		6 months	1 year	2 year
1	<20.0	0.0	1.6	6.8
2	20.0–25.0	5.4	11.0	16.0
3	25.1–30.0	8.0	14.8	25.5
4	30.1–35.0	13.1	23.3	27.8
5	35.1–40.0	21.8	37.8	58.8
6	>40.0	58.5	68.9	68.9

the outcome of LGIB in terms of risk of recurrent bleeding, need for therapeutic intervention and mortality is needed. However, it is more difficult to develop a model for LGIB due to a plethora of disparate pathologies, with no single pathology having a predominant occurrence.

In a cohort of acute GIB patients admitted to a medical ICU, a group from St. Louis has identified a series of prognostic factors which predict poor clinical outcome in both upper and lower GIB (29). They found no significant difference in these factors comparing the group with UGIB versus the LGIB. To further develop an outcome prediction tool, the same group established the BLEED classification system (30) which included ongoing bleeding, low systolic blood pressure, elevated prothrombin time, erratic mental status, unstable comorbid illness. In a prospective study by Kollef, the BLEED classification system could predict outcome in patients hospitalized with acute LGIB when applied at the point of initial evaluation, the same classification instrument also was found to be useful for risk stratification for acute UGIB.

Management of patients with a serious and potentially life-threatening condition such as acute gastrointestinal bleeding requires rapid clinical decision, appropriate triage of high-risk patient to intensive care and low-risk patient to be discharged, and a multi-disciplinary management of complicated cases. An effective and reliable risk stratification system is very much in need. In order to establish these assessment instrument, large cohorts, prospective studies with proper randomization and preferably multi-center studies would be required.

References

1. Barkun A, Bardou M, Kuipers EJ, et al. International consensus recommendations on the management of patients with non-variceal upper gastrointestinal bleeding. Ann Intern Med 2010;152:101–13.
2. Hebert PC, Wells G, Blajchman MA, Marshall J, Martin C, Pagliarello G, et al. A multicenter, randomized, controlled clinical trial of transfusion requirements in critical care. Transfusion Requirements in Critical Care Investigators, Canadian Critical Care Trials Group. N Engl J Med 1999;340:409–17.
3. Bellotto F, Fagiuoli S, Pavei A, Gregory SA, Cati A, Silverj E, et al. Anemia and ischemia: myocardial injury in patients with gastrointestinal bleeding. Am J Med 2005;118:548–51.
4. Barkun A, Bardou M, Martel M, et al. Prokinetics in acute upper GI bleeding: a meta-analysis. GIE 2010;72:1138–45.
5. Winstead NS, Wilcox CM. Erythromycin prior to endoscopy for acute upper gastrointestinal haemorrhage: a cost-effectiveness analysis. Aliment Pharmacol Ther 2007;26:1371–7.
6. Barkun A, Bardou M, Gralnek I, Shingina A, Razzaghi A, Rostom A. Impact of elevated INR and of low platelet count on outcomes in acute upper GI bleeding (UGIB). Gastroenterology 2009; 134.

7. Baradarian R, Ramdhaney S, Chapalamadugu R, Skoczylas L, Wang K, Rivilis S, et al. Early intensive resuscitation of patients with upper gastrointestinal bleeding decreases mortality. Am J Gastroenterol 2004;99:619–22.

8. Choudari CP, Rajgopal C, Palmer KR. Acute gastrointestinal haemorrhage in anticoagulated patients: diagnoses and response to endoscopic treatment. Gut 1994;35:464–6.

9. Lau JWY, Lau JY, Leung WK, Wu JC, Chan FK, Wong VW, et al. Omeprazole before endoscopy in patients with gastrointestinal bleeding. N Engl J Med 2007. 19;356(16): 1631–40.

10. Tsoi KK, Lau JY, Sung JJ. Cost-effectiveness analysis of high-dose omeprazole infusion before endoscopy for patients with upper-GI bleeding. Gastrointest Endosc 2008;67:1056–63.

11. Al-Sabah S, Barkun AN, Herba K, Adam V, Fallone C, Mayrand S, et al. Cost-effectiveness of proton-pump inhibition before endoscopy in upper gastrointestinal bleeding. *Clin Gastroenterol Hepatol* 2008;6:418–25.

12. Naumovski-Mihalic S, Katicic M, Colic-Cvlje V, Bozek T, Prskalo M, Sabaric B, et al. Intravenous proton pump inhibitor in ulcer bleeding in patients admitted to an intensive care unit [Abstract W1578]. Gastroenterology 2005;128:A641.

13. Sung JJY, Chung SCS, Chan KL, Lai CW, Kassiandies C, Leung JWC, et al. Octreotide versus emergency sclerotherapy in the treatment of acute variceal haemorrhage. Lancet 1993;342:637–41.

14. Corley DA, Cello JP, Adkission W. et al. Octreotide for acute esophageal variceal bleeding: a meta-analysis. Gastroenterol 2001;120:946–54.

15. Waler S, Kreichgauer HP, Bode JC. Terlipressin vs somatostatin in bleeding esophageal varices: a controlled double-blind study. Hepatology 1992;15:1023–30.

16. Avgerinos A, Nevens F, Raptis S, Fevery J, and the ABOVE study group. Early administration of somatostatin and efficacy of sclerotherapy in acute oesophageal variceal bleeds: The European Acute Bleeding Oesophageal Variceal Episodes (ABOVE) randomized trial. Lancet 1997;350:1495.

17. Cales, P, Masliah, C, Bernard, B, et al. Early administration of vapreotide for variceal bleeding in patients with cirrhosis. French Club for the Study of Portal Hypertension. N Engl J Med 2001;344:23.

18. Das Ananya, Richard CK Wong. Prediction of outcome of acute GI hemorrhage: a review of risk scores and predictive models. GIE 2004;60:85–93.

19. Rockall TA, Logan RF, Devlin HB, Northfield TC. Risk assessment after acute upper gastrointestinal hemorrhage. Gut 1996;38:316–21.

20. Blatchford O, Murray WR, Blatchford MA. A risk score to predict need for treatment for upper gastrointestinal hemorrhage. Lancet 2000;356:1318–21.

21. Stanley AJ, Ashley D, Dalton HR, Mowat C, Gaya DR, Thompson E, et al. Outpatient management of patients with low-risk upper-gastrointestinal haemorrhage: multi-centre validation and prospective evaluation. Lancet 2009;373:42–7.

22. Romagnuolo J, Barkun AN, Enns R, Armstrong D, Gregor J. Simple clinical predictors may obviate urgent endoscopy in selected patients with nonvariceal upper gastrointestinal tract bleeding. Arch Intern Med 2007;167:265–70.

23. Hay JA, Lyubashevsky E, Elashoff J, Maldonado L, Weingarten SR, Ellrodt AG. Upper gastrointestinal hemorrhage clinical guideline: determining the optimal hospital length of stay. JAMA 1997;278 (24): 2151–2156.

24. Saeed ZA, Winchester CB, Michaletz PA, Woods KL, Graham DY. A scoring system to predict rebleeding after endoscopic therapy of non-variceal upper gastrointestinal hemorrhage with a comparison of heat probe and ethanol injection. Am J Gastroenterol 1993;88:1824–9.

25. Wong SKH, Yu LM, Lau JYW, Lam YH, Chan ACW, Ng EKW, et al. Prediction of therapeutic failure after adrenaline injection plus heater probe treatment in patients with bleeding peptic ulcers. Gut 2002;50:322–5.

26. Chiu PW, Ng EKW, Cheung FK, Chan FKL, Leung WK, Wu JC, et al. Predicting mortality in patients with bleeding peptic ulcers after therapeutic endoscopy. Clin Gastroenterol Hepol 2009;7:311–16.

27. North Italian Endoscopic Club for the Study and Treatment of Esophageal Varices prediction of the first variceal hemorrhage in patients with cirrhosis of the liver and esophageal varices. N Engl J Med 1988;319:983–9.

28. Graham DY, Smith JL. The course of patients after variceal hemorrhage. Gastroenterol 1981;80:800–9.

29. Kollef MH, O'Brien JD, Zuckerman GR, Shannon W. BLEED: a classification tool to predict outcomes in aptietns with acute upper and lower gastrointestinal hemorrhage. Crit Care Med 1997;25:1125–32.

30. Kollef MH, Canfield DA, Zuckerman GR. Triage considerations for patients with acute gastrointestinal hemorrhage admitted to a medical intensive care unit. Crit Care Med 1995;23:1048–54.

CHAPTER 3

Gastrointestinal Bleeding: Antiplatelets and Anticoagulants

Joseph Sung

Institute of Digestive Disease, The Chinese University of Hong Kong, Hong Kong, China

With the worldwide ageing population and an increasing usage of antiplatelets and anticoagulants for treatment and prevention of vascular diseases and malignancy, the proportion of patients with gastrointestinal bleeding are expanding. Antiplatelet agents can be the cause of upper and lower gastrointestinal bleeding by producing ulcers and erosions at different levels of the digestive tract. On the other hand, anticoagulants might precipitate bleeding from pre-existing lesions. Both classes of medication also make control of gastrointestinal bleeding more difficult.

Antiplatelet agents

Antiplatelet agents are increasingly used in the prevention and treatment of cardiovascular and cerebrovascular diseases. There are two main groups of antiplatelet agents. Aspirin produces its antiplatelet effect via irreversible acetylation of a serine moiety in the cyclooxygenase-1 enzyme of platelets. This irreversibly inhibits production of thromboxane A2 for the life of the platelet. On the other hand, thienopyridines such as clopidogrel, ticlopidine and prasugrel block the binding of ADP to a platelet receptor P2Y12, thereby inhibiting platelet aggregation. While the use of ticlopidine is limited by its hematological side effects (neutropenia), clopidogrel and prasugrel are widely used for varying durations of time in addition to aspirin for all patients having undergone coronary artery stenting to reduce the risk of stent thrombosis. All antiplatelet agents increase the risk of gastrointestinal bleeding by producing peptic ulcers or erosions. Administered together, they exhibit synergistic effect in increasing the risk of gastrointestinal bleeding.

Gastrointestinal Bleeding, Second Edition. Edited by Joseph J.Y. Sung, Ernst J. Kuipers and Alan N. Barkun. © 2012 Blackwell Publishing Ltd.
Published 2012 by Blackwell Publishing Ltd.

Aspirin

For many years, aspirin has been used to prevent cardiovascular thrombotic events. However, the strength of the data to support this practice varies depending on whether the use of aspirin is for primary or secondary prophylaxis. A meta-analysis of 287 randomized trials involving 135,000 patients comparing antiplatelet therapy versus control regimens and 77,000 comparing different antiplatelet regimens conducted by the Antithrombotic Trialists' Collaboration in 2002 showed that for every 1,000 such patients treated for a year, aspirin would be expected to prevent about 10–20 vascular events and cause 1–2 major gastrointestinal bleeding. In a wide range of high risk patients, antiplatelet therapy reduces the risk of combined outcome of any serious vascular event by approximately 25%. Therefore, aspirin or other antiplatelet drugs are clearly indicated in the context of secondary prevention, for patients with previous histories of vascular events (1).

The data are less compelling for the use of aspirin in primary prevention, that is, for patients without a prior history of cardiovascular events. A recommendation for the use of low-dose aspirin is based on an estimate of a patient's 10-year risk of suffering a cardiovascular event. The US Preventative Services Task Force states that any patient who has a 6% or greater 10-year risk of having a CV event should take low-dose aspirin (2); the American Heart Association recommends that patients with a 10% or greater 10-year risk receive low-dose aspirin (3). These recommendations are based on observations that aspirin treatment for primary prevention is safe at a coronary event risk of greater that 1.5% per year and unsafe at a coronary event risk of 0.5% per year (4). In another meta-analysis of studies assessing aspirin for the primary prevention of cardiovascular events, aspirin reduced the risk for the combined end point of non-fatal myocardial infarction and fatal coronary heart disease (OR = 0.72, 95% CI, 0.60 to 0.87) and increased the risk for hemorrhagic stroke (OR = 1.4, 95% CI 0.9 to 2.0) and major GI bleeding (OR = 1.7, 95% CI 1.4 to 2.1). All-cause mortality (OR = 0.93, 95% CI 0.84 to 1.02) was not significantly affected; the net benefit of aspirin increases with increasing cardiovascular risk (2).

A meta-analysis based on 14 trials approximated the pooled relative risk of major gastrointestinal bleeding in low-dose aspirin users at 2.07 (5). These results translate into an absolute rate increase with aspirin above placebo of 0.12% per year. In another meta-analysis by Derry et al. (6), 24 double-blinded placebo-controlled studies were pooled, for an odds ratio for bleeding with aspirin use of 1.68. The number of patients needed to be treated with low-dose aspirin to cause one additional gastrointestinal bleeding episode over one year (NNH) was 247. All in all, the relative risk of gastrointestinal bleeding with low-dose aspirin usage is around 2 to 2.5 with a range of approximately 1.5 to 3. The annualized incidence of major gastrointestinal bleeding attributable to aspirin use in placebo-controlled trials is 0.12%.

Risk factors for upper GI bleeding in aspirin users

Not all patients taking aspirin develop gastrointestinal injury leading to bleeding. A prior upper gastrointestinal event (i.e. peptic ulcer history or bleeding) has been identified to be an important risk factor for upper GI bleeding in low-dose aspirin user (7). Those with a history of gastrointestinal bleeding have a 6.5-fold increase in risk, while those with a prior history of ulcer exhibit a two-fold increased risk.

The gastrointestinal injury of aspirin appears to be related to dose and treatment duration. When used beyond the usual low-dose regimen, the risk of gastrointestinal bleeding and hospitalization is substantially increased (8). Increasing the dose of aspirin from 100 mg to 1,000 mg daily increases the risk of upper GI bleeding from 2.4 to almost 20 folds. On the other hand, treatment duration demonstrates an inverse relationship. Aspirin naïve subjects have the highest risk of developing complication in the first 30 days of treatment and those who have received aspirin for over one year show a substantially reduced bleeding risk (7). Furthermore, enteric-coated aspirin and buffered aspirin, both claimed to be safer than plain aspirin, have failed to demonstrate a better safety profile in clinical trials (9).

While advanced age is a well established factor for gastrointestinal complication in NSAID users, available data do not support such an association with low-dose aspirin use. Nevertheless, older patients taking low-dose aspirin do have a much greater absolute risk of gastrointestinal complications than younger patients because they have a much higher baseline risk of GI complications. Patrono et al. showed that the risk of ulcer complications in control subjects under 50 years old was below 0.5% while the risk of subjects aged 70–79 years was approximately 4%, and those over 80 was 6% (10) (Fig. 3.1).

Concomitant uses of other medications such as NSAIDs, warfarin and corticosteroid also increase the risk of aspirin-induced gastrointestinal bleeding. Three of four randomized controlled trials compared aspirin to aspirin combined with warfarin reported an increased risk of gastrointestinal bleeding. A cohort study from Denmark examining concomitant use of corticosteroid and low-dose aspirin found a relative risk of 5.3 compared to non-users (11) – about two-fold higher than using low-dose aspirin alone. Several studies have shown that the addition of non-aspirin NSAID to low-dose aspirin significantly increases the risk of developing upper GI bleeding by two- to four-folds. A five-year cohort study in Denmark showed that the annual incidence of hospital admissions for upper GI bleeding was more

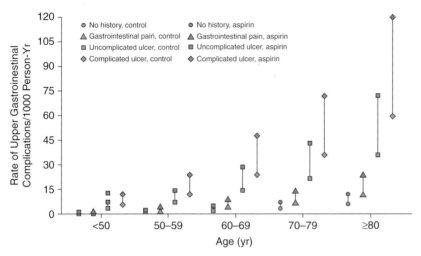

Figure 3.1 Estimated rate of upper gastrointestinal complications in men according to age and the presence or absence of a history of such complication and regular treatment with low-dose aspirin (Reproduced from Patrono et al. (10) with permission from Massachusetts Medical Society.)

than doubled when NSAIDs plus low-dose aspirin were used compared to low-dose aspirin alone (12).

As selective COX-2 inhibitor (Coxib) have been said to be safe for the digestive tract, an important question is whether combining aspirin with a Coxib would be less toxic to the gastrointestinal tract? In a 12-week double-blind endoscopic trial, the incidence of ulcers among users of concomitant Coxib and aspirin was two-fold greater than for aspirin users alone users (13), similar to a non-selective NSAID (Ibuprofen). In a large double-blind out-come trial (TARGET) comparing lumiracoxib to a non-selective NSAID, investigators stratified their population according low-dose aspirin use with 24% taking aspirin (14). The risk of complicated ulcer and symptomatic ulcer was not significantly different between the two groups. Aspirin, pre-sumably because of its effect as non-selective COX inhibitor, abolishes the gastro-protective effect of Coxibs.

H. pylori infection increases the risk of aspirin-induced peptic ulcer and ulcer bleeding. Randomized controlled trials have showed that among patients presented with peptic ulcer bleeding and confirmed to have *H. pylori* infection, treatment of the infection with triple antimicrobial therapy sig-nificantly reduces the risk of subsequent symptomatic ulcer and ulcer complications (15). The probability of recurrent ulcer bleeding during a 6-month follow-up of those who received anti-Helicobacter therapy was comparable to that of those who received maintenance proton pump inhibitors. Furthermore, the risk of recurrent UGIB after eradication of *H. pylori* continues to be reduced in long-term follow-up studies. In order to minimize the risk of recurrent ulcer and bleeding related to aspirin, *H. pylori* testing and treatment with confirmation of successful eradication is thus very important. Patients who develop recurrent ulcer bleeding on aspirin should be checked for successful eradication of *H. pylori* and absence of concomitant use of NSAID (16).

Clopidogrel

Unlike aspirin, clopidogrel is an inhibitor of ADP-induced platelet aggregation. Clopidogrel may be a more potent antiplatelet agent than aspirin and it is used for prevention of arterial thromboembolism in patients with atherosclerosis including those with peripheral vascular disease, myocardial infarction and acute coronary syndrome or thromboembolic stroke. It may be slightly more effective than aspirin alone and produces a synergistic effect when added to aspirin therapy. Clopidogrel has a specific and critical role in the prevention of occlusion of coronary artery stents. Although claimed to be safe among average-risk patients, clopidogrel used in patients with a history of peptic ulcer bleeding carries a substantially higher risk of inducing recurrent peptic ulcer bleeding. In a prospective randomized study comparing clopidogrel against aspirin combined with proton pump inhibitors, 8.6% of clopidogrel users developed recurrent GIB compared to 0.7% user of aspirin plus PPI (17). The superiority of proton pump inhibitor and aspirin combination over clopidogrel in preventing ulcer complication was confirmed in a separate clinical study (18) It is also worth noting that in this study, both treatments had resulted in lower GIB in 4.6%, indicating that the toxicity of aspirin and clopidogrel is not confined to the upper gastrointestinal tract.

Double antiplatelet agent therapy

The combination of two antiplatelet agents has been advocated for the prevention of drug-eluted and bare metal coronary stent from clogging Furthermore, antiplatelet agents are increasingly used in combination with anticoagulants in patients who have dual indications for treatment such as those with ischemic heart disease and atrial fibrillation. Case-control studies have shown that by combining aspirin with clopidogrel and dipyridamole, the risk of serious upper gastrointestinal bleeding is increased by two to seven folds (19). The number of treatment years needed to produce one excess case of upper GI bleeding is 124 for clopidogrel-aspirin combination. Therefore, as anti-thrombotic therapy is becoming more aggressive, bleeding upper GI complications are expected to rise. In view of the increasing

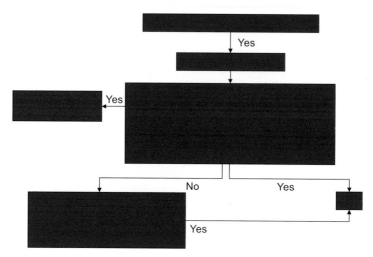

Figure 3.2 Algorithm to Assess GI risk with antiplatelet therapy (Reproduced form Bhatt et al. (20) with permission from *Nature.*)

trend of using antiplatelet agents in patients with a history of peptic ulcer disease or complications, the American Heart Association and the American College of Gastroenterology have proposed a management algorithm to assess GI risk before commencing antiplatelet therapy (20) (Fig. 3.2). The patient's age, history of ulcer and ulcer bleeding, concomitant use of corticosteroid or NSAID, and the presence of *H. pylori* infection are included in the assessment algorithm. Proton pump inhibitors are recommended in high risk patients that require antiplatelet agents. This consensus has recently been updated by the same expert group (21). In this update recommendation, the use of a PPI or H2 receptor antagonist in reducing the risk of upper GI bleeding in users of double antiplatelet is confirmed. PPI, however, are recommended only in patients with multiple risk factors and should not be given in low risk patients.

Discontinuation of aspirin during acute peptic ulcer bleeding

It is common practice that when patients taking aspirin for cardiovascular or cerebrovascular disease develop gastrointestinal bleeding, aspirin is stopped until the hemorrhagic complication stabilizes. Without clear agreement on when aspirin should be resumed, there is always a tension between gastroenterologists and cardiologists or neurologists about the safety/toxicity of antiplatelet agents. In a recent study which randomized patients with aspirin-induced ulcer bleeding to early (day 1) resumption of antiplatelet agents versus prolong discontinuation of antiplatelet agents (8 weeks) until ulcer was confirmed completely healed, recurrent bleeding and mortality was evaluated in these two strategies. The result shows that early resumption of aspirin, on day 1 after index bleeding, trends towards an increase in the risk of recurrent bleeding, yet on the other hand, when aspirin was discontinued for a prolonged period, the mortality related to cardiovascular and cerebrovascular causes were significantly increased (22). Therefore, in high risk patients, the most sensible strategy would be to discontinue aspirin or other antiplatelet medication for 3–5 days before resuming these drugs.

Interaction between antiplatelet agent and proton pump inhibitors

In 2009, the FDA issued a warning of possible interaction between clopidogrel and proton pump inhibitors. The FDA noted published reports that clopidogrel (Plavix) is less effective in some patients than it is in others. Differences in effectiveness may be due to genetic differences in the way the body metabolizes clopidogrel, or that using certain other drugs with clopidogrel can interfere with the body's metabolism of clopidogrel. As clopidogrel is a pro-drug that needs to be metabolized in the liver before becoming an active metabolite, a process that requires the enzyme P450 2C19[*], any drug that may interfere with this enzyme could theoretically interfere with the antiplatelet efficacy of clopidogrel. In a prospective study, patients requiring aspirin and clopidogrel after coronary artery stenting were randomized to receive omeprazole or placebo for one week (23). In the presence of omeprazole, the platelet reactivity index was found to be reduced to a lower degree. Other studies, however have not borne out such an association in *in vitro* measurements of platelet aggregation (24). Subsequently, two case-control studies have reported some disturbing data about the clinical outcomes of these patients.

In a population-based, nested case-control study, Juurlink et al. (25) showed that patients taking concomitant clopidogrel and proton pump inhibitors had a modest increase in the incidence of myocardial infarction (OR = 1.27, 95% CI 1.03–1.57). In a similar study by Ho et al. (26), concomitant use of clopidogrel and a proton pump inhibitor after hospital discharge for an acute coronary syndrome (ACS) was associated with an increased risk of adverse outcomes compared to exposure to clopidogrel without a PPI, suggesting that use of PPI may be associated with attenuation of benefits of clopidogrel after ACS. Death or repeated hospitalization for ACS occurred in 20.8% of patients prescribed clopidogrel without PPI and 29.8% of patients prescribed clopidogrel plus PPI. In multivariable analysis, use of clopidogrel plus a PPI at any point in time was associated with an increased risk of death or repeated hospitalization for ACS compared with the use of clopidogrel without a PPI (adjusted odds ratio = 1.25; 95% CI, 1.11–1.41). These data have raised a lot of concerns about the possible interaction between PPI and clopidogrel.

New light on this issue has recently been shed by the COGENT Trial (27). This is a multicenter, international, randomized, double-blind, double-dummy, placebo-controlled, parallel group, phase 3 efficacy and safety study of CGT-2168 (a fixed-dose combination of clopidogrel (75 mg) and omeprazole (20 mg)), compared with clopidogrel. The study aimed to evaluate the safety profile of clopidogrel and omeprazole combination versus clopidogrel alone in the digestive system as well as the efficacy of this regimen in the prevention of cardiovascular events. The initial planned sample size was 3200 patients, for an anticipated accrual over a period of one year, with a maximum follow up of two years. As a low rate of gastrointestinal events was observed as the trial was ongoing, the sample size target was increased to 4,200 and then approximately 5,000 (143 GI events). The study ended when the sponsor suddenly declared bankruptcy. However, the preliminary data based on 3,627 patients recruited from 393 sites and follow-up for a median of 133 days reported 136 cardiovascular events and 105 GI events. The results showed that combining clopidogrel with omeprazole significantly reduced the GI events (from 67 events in the placebo group to 38 events in the PPI group, HR = 0.55, 95% CI 0.36–0.85), with no associated demonstrable difference in the composite cardiovascular event and the rate of myocardial infarction between the two study groups (Fig. 3.3). The 95% confidence indicated that it does not rule out a small possible association with increase cardiovascular event but that the hazard ratio of the bleeding protection is much greater in magnitude than any small potential increase in cardiovascular event. The data of the COGENT study, albeit an unfinished study, provide strong reassurance that the benefits of proton pump inhibitor in protecting the gut outweigh the cardiovascular risk of using this drugs in patient requiring clopidogrel.

Anticoagulants

The most commonly used oral and intravenous anticoagulants are warfarin and heparin respectively. Warfarin is a coumarin derivative that inhibits vitamin K epoxide reductase which leads to intrahepatic depletion of the reduced form of vitamin K. Long term use of oral anticoagulant is particularly effective for the prevention and treatment of venous thromboembolism and prevention of embolization associated with atrial fibrillation or prosthetic heart valves. The major complication of treatment with warfarin is hemorrhage as well as a risk of excessive bleeding after trauma or surgery. The risk of bleeding is related to the INR, not the dose of warfarin. The higher

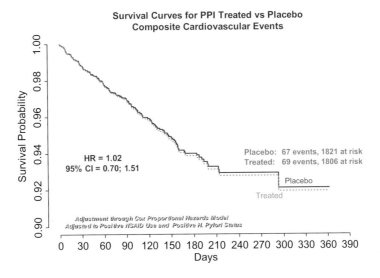

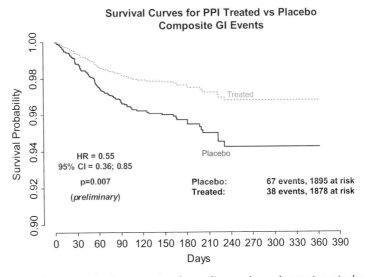

Figure 3.3 The Cogent Study comparing the cardiovascular and gastrointestinal event of patients using double antiplatelet agents with or without proton pump inhibitors (27)(Reproduced from Bhatt et al. (27) with permission from Massachusetts Medical Society.)

the INR, the greater will be the risk of bleeding. For elderly patients on warfarin, there is an annual risk of 1.5% of major hemorrhage including 0.3% of intracerebral hemorrhage (28).

Heparin is a naturally occurring glycosaminoglycan. The anticoagulant action of heparin is due to a combination of indirect antithrombin and anti-Xa activity. Heparin remains the most widely used parenteral antithrombotic agent. In recent years, unfractionated heparin (UFH) has gradually been replaced by low molecular weight heparin (LMWH) which is less protein bound than UF) and therefore has a more predictable dose-response profile. The anticoagulation effect of heparin is monitored by the APTT ratio. A typical regimen would be to prolong APTT to 2.0 times normal. The risk of gastrointestinal bleeding associated with heparin is not clear.

Patients with acute bleeding should be evaluated immediately on presentation. Resuscitation, including stabilization of blood pressure and restoration of intra-vascular volume should precede further diagnostic and therapeutic measures. Correcting coagulopathy is only necessary in patients on anticoagulants. There is some evidence from Baradarian et al. (29) that intensive resuscitation and interventions with aggressive correction of the coagulopathy to, on average, an INR of 1.8, can reduce myocardial infarctions and mortality. An INR of $\geq$1.5 may serve as target threshold for correction of a coagulopathy at initial resuscitation but should not delay hemostatic therapy. A recent consensus conference suggested that endoscopic therapy may safely be performed with an elevated INR as long as it is not supratherapeutic (i.e. up to an INR of 2.5) such as not to delay the benefits of early endoscopic intervention (30).

References

1. Antithrombotic Trialists' Collaboration. Collaborative meta-analysis of randomised trials of anti-platelet therapy for prevention of death, myocardial infarction, and stroke in high risk patients. BMJ 2002 12;324(7329):71–86.
2. Hayden M, Pignone M, Phillips C, Mulrow C. Aspirin for the primary prevention of cardiovascular events: a summary of the evidence for the U.S. Preventive Services Task Force. Ann Intern Med 2002;136(2):161–72.
3. Pearson TA, Blair SN, Daniels SR, et al. AHA Guidelines for Primary Prevention of Cardiovascular Disease and Stroke: 2002 Update: Consensus Panel Guide to Comprehensive Risk Reduction for Adult Patients Without Coronary or Other Atherosclerotic Vascular Diseases. American Heart Association Science Advisory and Coordinating Committee. *Circulation* 2002;106:388–91.
4. Sanmuganathan PS, Ghahramani P, Jackson PR, et al. Aspirin for primary prevention of coronary heart disease: safety and absolute benefit related to coronary risk derived from meta-analysis of randomised trials. Heart 2001;85(3):265–71.
5. McQuaid KR, Laine L. System review and meta-analysis of adverse events of low-dose aspirin and clopidogrel in randomized controlled trials. Am J Med 2006;119:624–38.
6. Derry S, Loke YK. Risk of gastrointestinal hemorrhage with long term use of aspirin: meta-analysis. BMJ 2000;32:1183–7.
7. Lanas A, Bajador E, Serrano P, et al. Nitrovasodilators, low-dose aspirin, other non-steroidal antiinflammatory drugs and the risk of upper gastrointestinal bleeding. N Engl J Med 2000;343:834–9.

8. Slattery J, Warlow CP, Shorrock CJ, Langman MJ. Risk of gastrointestinal bleeding during secondary prevention of vascular events with aspirin – analysis of gastrointestinal bleeding during the UK-TIA trial. Gut 1995;37:509–11.

9. Kelly JP, Kaufman DW, Jurgelon JM, Sheehan J, Koff RS, Shapiro S. Risk of aspirin-associated major upper gastrointestinal bleeding with enteric coated or buffered product. Lancet 1996;348:1413–16.

10. Patrono C, Garcia Rodriguez LA, Landolfi R, Baigent C. Low-dose aspirin for the prevention of atherothrombosis. N Engl J Med 2005;353:2373–83.

11. Nielsen GL, Sorensen HT, Mellemkjoer L, et al. Risk of hospitalization resulting from upper gastrointestinal bleeding among patients taking corticosteroids: a register-based cohort study. Am J Med 2001;111:541–5.

12. Sorensen HT, Mellemkjaer I, Blot WH, et al. Risk of upper gastrointestinal bleeding associated with use of low-dose aspirin. Am J Gastroenterol 2000;95:2218–24.

13. Laine L, Maller ES, Yu C, Quan H, Simon T. Ulcer formation with low-dose enteric-coated aspirin and the effect of COX-2 selective inhibition: a double-blind trial. Gastroenterology 2004;127:395–402.

14. Schnitzer TJ, Bumester GR, Mysler E, et al. Comparison of lumiracoxib with naproxen and ibuprofen in the Therapeutic Arthritis Research and Gastrointestinal Event Trial (TARGET): randomized controlled trial. Lancet 2004;364:665–74.

15. Chan FKL, Chung SCS, Suen BY, et al. Preventing recurrent upper gastrointestinal bleeding in patients with Helicobacter pylori infection who are taking low-dose aspirin or naproxen. NEJM 2001;344:967.

16. Lai KC, Lam SK, Chu KM, et al. Lansoprazole for the prevention of recurrence of ulcer complications from long-term low-dose aspirin use. N Engl J Med 2001;346:2033–8.

17. Chan FK, Ching JY, Hung LC, et al. Clopidogrel versus aspirin and esomeprazole to prevent recurrent ulcer bleeding. N Engl J Med 2005;352:238–44.

18. Lai KC, Chu KM, Hui WM, et al. Esomeprazole with aspirin versus clopidogrel for prevention of recurrent gastrointestinal ulcer complications. Clin Gastroenterol Hepatol 2006;4:860–5.

19. Hella J, Dall M, Andries A, Andersen BS, et al. Use of single and combined anti-thrombotic therapy and risk of serious upper gastrointestinal bleeding: population based case-control study. Br Med J 2006;333:726–30.

20. ACCF/ACG/AHA 2008 expert consensus document on reducing the gastrointestinal risks of antiplatelet therapy and NSAID use. Bhatt DL, Scheiman J, Abraham NS, et al. American College of Cardiology Foundation; American College of Gastroenterology; American Heart Association. Am J Gastroenterol 2008;103:2890–2907.

21. ACCR/ACG/AHA 2010 expert consensus document on the concomitant use of proton pump inhibitors and thienopyridines: a focused update of the ACCF/ACG/AHA 2008 expert consensus document on reducing the gastrointestinal risk of antiplatelet therapy and NSAID use. Abraham NS, Haltky MA, Antman EM, et al. Am J Gastroenterol 2010;105:2533–49.

22. Sung JJ, Lau JY, Ching JY, Wu JC, Lee YT, Chiu PW, et al. Continuation of low-dose aspirin therapy in peptic ulcer bleeding: a randomized trial. Ann Intern Med 2010;152:1–9.

23. Gilard M, Arnaud B, Cornily JC, Le Gal G, Lacut K, Le Calvez G, et al. Influence of omeprazole on the antiplatelet action of clopidogrel associated with aspirin: the randomized, double-blind OCLA (Omeprazole CLopidogrel Aspirin) study. Am Coll Cardiol 2008 22;51(3):256–60.

24. O'Donoghue ML, Braunwald E, Antman EM, et al. Pharmacodynamic effect and clinical efficacy of clopidogrel and prasugrel with or without a proton pump inhibitor: an analysis of two randomized trial. Lancet 2009;374:989–97.

25. Juurlink DN, Gomes T, Ko DT, Szmitko PE, Austin PC, Tu JV, et al. A population-based study of the drug interaction between proton pump inhibitors and clopidogrel. CMAJ 2009 31;180(7):713–18. Epub 2009 Jan 28.

26. Ho PM, Maddox TM, Wang L, Fihn SD, Jesse RL, Peterson ED, et al. Risk of adverse outcomes associated with concomitant use of clopidogrel and proton pump inhibitors following acute coronary syndrome. JAMA 2009 4;301(9):937–44.

27. Bhatt DL, Cryer BL, Contant CT, et al. Clopidogrel with or without omperazole in coronary artery disease. N Engl J Med 2010;363:1909–17.

28. Shireman TI, Howard PA, Kresowik TF, Ellerbeck EF. Combined anticoagulant-antiplatelet use and major bleeding events in elderly atrial fibrillation patients. Stroke 2004;35(10):2362–7.

29. Baradarian R, Ramdhaney S, Chapalamadugu R, Skoczylas L, Wang K, Rivilis S, et al. Early intensive resuscitation of patients with upper gastrointestinal bleeding decreases mortality. Am J Gastroenterol 2004;99:619–22.

30. Laine L. Gastrointestinal bleeding with low-dose aspirin: what is the risk? Aliment Pharma Ther 2006;24:897–908.

CHAPTER 4

Peptic Ulcer Bleeding: Endoscopic Diagnosis, Endoscopic Therapy and Pharmacotherapy

I. Lisanne Holster, Caroline M. den Hoed & Ernst J. Kuipers
Department of Gastroenterology and Hepatology, Erasmus MC University Medical Center, Rotterdam, The Netherlands

Introduction

Endoscopy is the mainstay for diagnosis and treatment of upper gastrointestinal bleeding, the most common gastrointestinal emergency. The importance of endoscopy is fourfold. It firstly allows identification of the bleeding focus. It secondly supports assessment of the underlying cause such as *Helicobacter pylori* infection or a malignancy. It then allows application of treatment, and finally determines the risk of recurrence and mortality, and thus allows dedicated use of resources. These aspects firstly require uniform nomenclature using a few definitions. A *peptic ulcer* is a mucosal defect in stomach or proximal duodenum with a minimal diameter of 0.5 cm and appreciable depth, mostly defined as penetrating the muscularis mucosae. Lesions of smaller size are defined as erosions. Ulcers are subclassified according to location and endoscopic appearance. *Gastric ulcers* are mainly located along the smaller curvature, including the angulus, and in the antrum. Ulcers above the transitional zone between corpus and antrum are called proximal ulcers, those at the angulus and below the transitional zone distal ulcers. *Duodenal ulcers* are mostly located in the bulbus either on the anterior or posterior wall, occasionally at both sites ("kissing" ulcers). As the transitional zone between antral and duodenal type mucosa often lies at the antral side of the pylorus, pyloric ulcers can be considered proximal duodenal ulcers. Postbulbar ulcers are located distal to the duodenal bulb. After a distal gastric resection (Billroth I or II procedure), ulceration may occur at the gastroduodenal anastomosis (*anastomotic ulcer*), or after a Billroth II reconstruction in the jejunal mucosa at the junction between the afferent and efferent loops (*ulcus jejuni pepticum*). Peptic ulcers may also

Gastrointestinal Bleeding, Second Edition. Edited by Joseph J.Y. Sung, Ernst J. Kuipers and Alan N. Barkun. © 2012 Blackwell Publishing Ltd.
Published 2012 by Blackwell Publishing Ltd.

develop in metaplastic or heterotopic gastric mucosa, such as in a Meckel's diverticulum, or the rectum. Gastric ulceration can also occur in a large hiatus hernia, usually at the level of the herniation. These ulcers are known as *Cameron's ulcers*. *Dieulafoy ulcers* are small mucosal defects over an intramural arteriole. Two thirds of these lesions are found in the stomach, but they can occur in the complete gastrointestinal tract.

Most peptic ulcers develop against a background of chronic mucosal inflammation. Depending on the location, this inflammation is termed *gastritis, duodenitis, or bulbitis.* With the current high resolution endoscopy equipment, this inflammation can often be recognized by signs of edema, reddening, and swelling of the mucosa. In patients with peptic ulcer disease, the inflammation should be confirmed histologically as this may provide further clues into the etiology of the ulcer, in particular by demonstration of *Helicobacter pylori.*

This chapter deals with endoscopic diagnosis, and endoscopic and pharmacotherapy of peptic ulcer disease.

Endoscopy timing and preparation

Timing of endoscopy

The position of endoscopy in the management of patients with gastrointestinal disorders has changed dramatically over the past 25 years. One of the first areas in which this change became apparent was upper gastrointestinal bleeding (UGIB). In the 1980s, it was still argued that there was no role for routine endoscopy in patients with upper GI bleeding (1–2). It took another ten years to establish that role by showing that endoscopic hemostasis was feasible and could reduce the risk of recurrent bleeding, shorten hospital stay, reduce the need for surgery, and reduce mortality (3). This was subsequently supported by a large amount of studies, in particular showing that endoscopic hemostasis improves outcome of high-risk cases (4). The overall magnitude of effect in terms of reduction of rebleeding can amount to above 75%.

These observations led to the search for the optimal timing for endoscopy in patients with UGIB. It was considered that early endoscopy allowed for early hemostasis, but also potentially could lead to complications such as oxygen desaturation and aspiration in insufficiently stabilized patients. Furthermore, the presence of large amounts of blood in stomach and duodenum can hamper adequate endoscopy and require the need for repeat endoscopy. These arguments fed the debate on optimal timing of endoscopy, against a further background that many endoscopy units could not provide 7×24 hour service and thus could not guarantee early endoscopy. In addition, introduction of continuous profound acid suppressive therapy made clinicians falsely confident to delay endoscopy. The need for initial resuscitation or other measures, such as correction of INR in patients using anticoagulants, was often presented as another reason to delay endoscopy. These issues have been adequately settled by further studies which showed that endoscopy within 24 hours of presentation can reduce the need for transfusion and surgery, as well as the length of hospital stay without any major increase in endoscopy-related complications (Table 4.1) (5–6). These effects were obtained in the era of profound acid suppressive therapy, and established the position of endoscopy as first-line modality not only for the diagnosis, but also for the treatment of acute upper GI bleeding. This led international guidelines to recommend endoscopy within 24 hours of first presentation in most patients with upper gastrointestinal bleeding, and that initial resuscitation and the need for INR correction should not lengthen this time window (7–10). The only exception pertains to the minority of patients with very low risk for rebleeding and need for intervention, such as for instance assessed by means of the Blatchford score (see Chapter 2). The 24-hour time frame as the most optimal window of opportunity was further supported by the observation that the risk of rebleeding is the highest in the initial period of admission. This is relevant as severe and persistent bleeding as well as rebleeding are all associated with poor outcome. The time-related incidence of rebleeding was illustrated by a large multicenter international trial in which 767 patients with high-risk peptic ulcer bleeding were followed for 30 days after endoscopic hemostasis. A rebleed occurred in 82 (11%) patients, 76% of these rebleeds occurred within the first 72 hours (11). For these reasons, the 24-hour time frame for endoscopy has been widely accepted and included in international guidelines endorsed by various gastroenterology associations worldwide (10). This implies that units which can not guarantee the 24-hour time frame for instance for patients presenting during weekends, should not take care of this patient population, and vice versa that all units which accept patients with upper gastrointestinal bleeding have to organize their endoscopy service to be able to meet these emergency demands and perform endoscopy by an experienced team at all times. Unfortunately, many units fail to meet these internationally accepted demands despite the available evidence for their relevance. In a recent survey within the UK in 208 endoscopy units providing emergency care for patients with upper GI bleeding, 6750 patients were included (12). Only 50% of medium and high-risk patients underwent endoscopy within 24 hours, and the presence of high-risk characteristics did not influence the timing of endoscopy. Units without formal out-of-office hour endoscopy rota more often provided delayed endoscopy services. As this was a survey and not an interventional study, it could not directly assess an effect of delayed endoscopy on outcome. The authors however concluded that their survey showed continuing delays in performance of endoscopy in patients with upper GI bleeding. In a Canadian multicenter observational study, 90% of 1675 patients with upper GI bleeding underwent endoscopy within 48 hours.

Table 4.1 Outcome of urgent endoscopy for non-variceal upper GI bleeding.

Timing of endoscopy (hrs after presentation)	Study (ref)	Design	Numbers of patients per study arm	Rebleeds (%)	Mortality (%)	Need for blood products (units)	Length of hospital stay (days)
2–3 hours	Lee (112)	RCT: EEE vs endoscopy <48 hrs	56 vs 54	3.6 vs 5.6	0 vs 3.7	1.2 vs 1.1	1 vs 2
	Schacher (15)	Retrospective: EEE vs endoscopy <24 hrs	43 vs 38	14 vs 15.8	0 vs 0	NR	5.9 vs 5.1
6–8 hours	Bjorkman (113)	RCT: endoscopy <6 hrs vs <48 hrs	47 vs 46	8.5 vs 2.2	0 vs 0	2.1 vs 1.5	4.0 vs 3.3
	Targownik (16)	Retrospective: endoscopy <6 hrs vs <24 hrs	77 vs 92	9 vs 8	8 vs 6	3.3 vs 2.9	4 vs 4
	Tai (114)	Retrospective: endoscopy <8 hrs vs <24 hrs	88 vs 101	3 vs 2	1 vs 6	3.5 vs 3.4	5.1 vs 6.0
<12 hours	Lin (115)	RCT: endoscopy <12 hrs vs >12 hrs	162 vs 163	3.7 vs 4.9	0.6 vs 0.6	450 ml vs 666 ml*	4 vs 14.5*
<24 hours	Cooper (116)	Observational cohort study: endoscopy <24 hrs vs >24 hrs	2240 vs 3247	NR	2.9 vs 2.8	NR	4 vs 6
	Cooper (117)	Retrospective: endoscopy < 24 hrs vs > 24 hrs	583 vs 326	14.2 vs 11.4**	NR	NR	5.0 vs 6.4

EEE: early endoscopy in emergency room, RCT: randomized controlled trial, NR: not reported, Underlined: significant difference (p < 0.05).
*no overall data available, significant benefit was found in a subgroup of patients with a bloody nasogastric aspirate.
**rebleeding and surgery.

The proportion undergoing endoscopy within 24 hours of presentation approximated 75% (13). Presence of an endoscopy-nurse on-call and admission to a hospital unit were predictors for earlier endoscopy, whereas the presence of chest pain, dyspneu, and inpatient status at the onset of bleeding were predictors for delayed endoscopy. The latter is remarkable as these patients almost invariably suffer from comorbidity as recommendation for early endoscopy. Finally, in an observational study from the US among 2592 elderly patients (>65 years) presenting with upper GI bleeding, 71% underwent endoscopy within 24 hours. Early endoscopy was associated with an on average 2-days shorter hospital stay, and a 63% reduction in the need for surgery, but no significant effect on mortality (14). All these observational data from various countries confirm the benefit of early endoscopy, and simultaneously show that major further improvements have to be made to ensure early intervention for all eligible patients as 10–50% still fail to be treated according to well-established guidelines.

There have been several studies to determine whether immediate endoscopy within the first 2 to 12 hours after presentation improves outcome in comparison with endoscopy within 24 hours. These studies have not shown that immediate endoscopy has a benefit with respect to the need for transfusion, repeat endoscopy, hospital stay, surgery, and mortality (Table 4.1). For example, one study assessed in 81 patients whether endoscopy within the first two hours had an effect of outcome. The mean hospital stay was 5.9 days in those who had undergone immediate endoscopy, versus 5.1 days in the controls undergoing regular endoscopy within 24 hours (15). The timing of endoscopy within the first 24-hour time frame did also not affect rebleeding and complication rates, nor the need for surgery. In a Canadian study in 169 patients, the rebleeding rate was 11.7% in those who had undergone endoscopy within 12 hours, versus 8.7% in those undergoing endoscopy within 24 hours (16). Similarly, very early endoscopy within 6 hours of presentation did not affect transfusion requirements, length of hospital stay, or any adverse bleeding outcome. Based on these findings, endoscopy is required within 24 hours, but does not routinely need to be performed within a shorter time interval. Nevertheless, immediate endoscopy should be considered for patients with signs of severe or persistent bleeding, even more so in the presence of comorbidity increasing the risk for poor outcome.

Medical therapy prior to endoscopy

While planning emergency endoscopy, most clinicians will administer high dose proton pump inhibitor (PPI) therapy intravenously. The potential benefit of such an approach firstly depends on the proportion of upper GI bleedings attributable to peptic ulcer disease as the condition which is most likely to benefit from profound acid suppression. In most cases, this proportion will vary between 40 to 60% (17). In a study from Hong Kong,

638 patients with upper GI bleeding were randomized to receive 80 mg omeprazole or placebo prior to endoscopy (18). During subsequent endoscopy, 19% of those having received omeprazole versus 28% of those receiving placebo needed a therapeutic intervention because of the presence of high-risk stigmata. This difference was significant, subgroup analysis showed that the difference in endoscopic intervention rate was also significant for patients with peptic ulcer disease, but not for patients with other bleeding causes. On endoscopy, fewer patients in the omeprazole arm had active bleeding ulcers. However, the benefit of iv proton pump inhibitor therapy did not translate in any difference with respect to other relevant parameters, such as need for transfusion, hospital stay, or rebleeding and mortality rates. The result of this study was later confirmed by others (19). A systematic review of 6 randomized trials including 2223 patients showed that PPI treatment prior to endoscopy reduced the prevalence of stigmata of recent hemorrhage during endoscopy from 46 to 37% (placebo vs PPI treatment, OR 0.67, 95% CI 0.54–0.87). This led to a reduction in the need for endoscopic treatment from 11.7% to 8.7% (placebo vs PPI treatment) (19). Based on these results, the international consensus recommends that pre-endoscopic proton pump inhibitor therapy may be considered to downstage the bleeding lesion and reduce the need for endoscopic therapy. However, because pre-endoscopic PPI therapy has no proven benefit on other clinically relevant outcome parameters such as the need for transfusion, hospital stay, further interventions and mortality, the same guidelines also stress that PPI therapy should not delay endoscopy (10).

Apart from profound acid suppression, another pharmacotherapeutic approach in UGIB patients is the use of promotility agents, in particular erythromycin and metoclopramide. These drugs have been tested under the assumption that they may clear the stomach and proximal duodenum of blood and thus improve the diagnostic yield of endoscopy and facilitate endoscopic therapy, while simultaneously perhaps decrease the risk of aspiration. This has been assessed in several randomized trials. A meta-analysis of five placebo-controlled trials on erythromycin and metoclopramide in patients who were suspected to have blood in the stomach found that the use of these agents was associated with an almost two-fold reduction in the need for repeat endoscopy (odds ratio 0.51, 95% CI 0.30–0.88), but prokinetic treatment had no effect on the need for transfusion or any other outcome parameter (10). Cost-efficacy analysis of the data from the three erythromycin trials showed a cost-effective outcome based on reduction in the need for repeat endoscopy from an average of 1.33 to 1.18 endoscopy per UGIB patient (20). Based on these data, the international guidelines concluded that promotility agents such as erythromycin or metoclopramide should not routinely be used prior to endoscopy in all patients presenting with UGIB. However, they should be considered in patients who have recently eaten and in those who are suspected to have considerable amounts of blood in the stomach as promotility agents improve visibility, and thus the diagnostic yield and the possibility to apply adequate endoscopic treatment. Both aspects explain the reduction in need for second-look endoscopy (10).

Gastric lavage prior to endoscopy

Gastric lavage has for long been widely used in patients with UGIB both for diagnostic and therapeutic purposes, the latter for instance under the assumption that cold-water lavage would reduce gastroduodenal blood flow and thus help to stop any ongoing bleeding. This practice dates from the era prior to endoscopy and profound acid suppressive therapy, there is very little place for gastric lavage in the current clinical setting (21). Lavage is first of all not of any major benefit to clear the stomach and thus improve the yield of endoscopy. In a small randomized trial involving 39 patients comparing pre-endoscopic gastric lavage with up to 15 litres of tap water versus no intervention prior to endoscopy, lavage somewhat improved visualization of the gastric fundus, but not of any other parts of the upper GI tract. It had no effect on identification and treatment of the bleeding source, nor on any other parameter (22). Secondly, nasogastric aspiration with or without lavage is also not very helpful in identification of the source of bleeding, being in the upper or lower GI tract. Clinical signs give in a large proportion of patients sufficient clues to direct the diagnostic approach without the need for further investigation prior to endoscopy. Furthermore, nasogastric aspiration has been shown to be a poor predictor of the source of bleeding. In a study from the US involving 220 patients presenting with signs of GI bleeding, 23% had positive nasogastric aspiration prior to gastroscopy (23). The sensitivity of aspiration to detect upper GI bleeding was 42%, the specificity 91%, with positive and negative predictive values of respectively 92% and 64%. The authors concluded that a positive nasogastric aspiration indicates probable upper GI bleeding, but a negative test, seen in almost three quarters of patients, provides little information (23). Likewise, aspiration is also inadequate to differentiate between persistent and stopped bleeding. In an older study, almost one-fifth of patients with active bleeding had negative aspiration, and almost half of patients without persistent bleeding had a positive aspiration of blood remnants in the stomach (24). Lavage and aspiration are to some extent helpful in identification of high-risk cases. In a retrospective, Canadian study of 520 patients who underwent nasogastric aspiration and subsequent endoscopy, a bloody aspirate had a specificity of 76% (95%CI 70–80%) for the presence of high-risk lesions. Patients with bloody aspirates were 2.8-fold (95% CI 1.8–4.3) more likely to have a high-risk lesion than patients with coffee-ground aspirates, and 4.8-fold (2.3–10.1) than those with clear/bile aspirates (25). With the retrospective design of the study, it remained unclear whether nasogastric aspiration can be used to plan patients for immediate endoscopy. Also, the results of lavage do not predict long-term outcome after endoscopy as shown in an Italian study of 1020 patients, in which patients with bloody or coffee-ground aspirates had a similar mortality as those without (26). Finally, nasogastric lavage is associated with patient burden, and also with a risk of further bleeds such as from nasal origin, and aspiration and pneumonia. For these reasons, there is nowadays very little place for nasogastric aspiration and lavage in the initial pre-endoscopic management of patients with UGIB (10, 21).

Other measures prior to endoscopy

Initial resuscitation is of major importance in patients with UGIB and is required prior to endoscopy, yet should not delay the procedure and thus the contact with the endoscopy team. The initial resuscitation includes the administration of intravenous fluids to restore blood pressure and tissue perfusion, transfusion of blood, and correction of marked coagulation disorders. Blood transfusion is generally recommended in patients with a hemoglobin level of 70 g/l or less, aiming for a level between 70 and 90 g/l. The decision for transfusion also depends on the rate of bleeding, medical condition, in particular vital signs, and the presence of comorbidity. INR correction is required but there are limited data as to the optimal level. Correction should also not delay endoscopy, unless the INR is supratherapeutic. For a more detailed description of these measures, see Chapters 2 and 3.

Endoscopy

Endoscopy team

Endoscopy for acute UGIB not only requires adequate preparation of the patient, but also of the team and equipment. An emergency physician first sees most patients, in-hospital bleeders are seen by a ward doctor. These physicians take care of the initial resuscitation and coordinate the first contacts to other physicians. A gastroenterologist should be available on call at all times, and be able to reach the hospital at short notice. Although there are no direct data that determine an exact time limit, a limit of one hour is generally assumed. The background of this time interval is that it allows ample time to prepare the patient for the procedure and at the same time not unnecessarily delay the procedure in patients with obvious signs of ongoing bleeding and difficult stabilization. Likewise, during office hours an endoscopy unit taking care of UGIB patients should be able to provide an experienced endoscopist for an emergency procedure when needed. The endoscopist should have ample experience with the treatment of acute upper GI bleeding, and be familiar with the equipment at the unit. The team should at all times also consist of an experienced endoscopy nurse who has full experience with the procedure, is aware of the place of storage and preparation of all equipment that is potentially needed, and experienced in assisting in all diagnostic and therapeutic aspects of the procedure. The team also requires a third person at short hand to monitor the patient, take care of transfusion and medication needs, and assist in any emergency. The endoscopy nurse assisting in the endoscopy procedure itself cannot safely do this. The procedure is for reasons of available equipment preferentially performed at the endoscopy suite if the patient can be transported and adequately monitored, otherwise it should be done at an emergency unit or intensive care. At any location, the endoscopy team should be fully prepared for the procedure. Depending on the severity of the bleed, early involvement of an intensivist is recommended with transfer to an ICU when needed. A full treatment team requires close collaboration with a gastrointestinal surgeon and intervention radiologist for further management in case of failure of endoscopic treatment, either at the first presentation, or during a recurrent bleeding episode. These physicians should have consensus and a local protocol for management of this most common emergency condition in gastroenterology practice. In many cases, the protocol requires early contact with surgeon and/or radiologist even before the endoscopy, in particular in high-risk and unstable patients.

The relevance of having an experienced endoscopy team available 7×24 hours was supported by studies reporting that UGIB patients who were admitted during weekends had worse outcomes than those admitted during weekdays. In an analysis of 237.412 patients admitted with upper GI bleeding in the period of 1993–2005 to 3.166 US hospitals, patients admitted on weekends had to wait longer for endoscopy (mean 2.21 vs 2.06 days, $p < 0.001$), and were less likely to undergo endoscopy on the day of admission (30 vs 34%, $p < 0.001$) (27). This was associated with prolonged hospital stay, in-hospital costs, need for surgery, and mortality (OR 1.12, 95% CI 1.05–1.20). The results of this large study were supported by other studies from the US (28–29). Together, these results were likely due to the combination of lack of on-call emergency endoscopy teams, lack of experience of on-call endoscopists, and the tendency to delay interventions in case of weekend admission. This explanation was supported by a large study from Hong Kong which showed that the presence of continuous 24-hour endoscopy service with an experienced team led to similar outcome for patients admitted during weekdays and weekends (30). These studies support guideline recommendations for 7×24 hour endoscopy rota and endoscopy within 24 hours in all patients except very low risk cases.

Endoscopy kit

The endoscopy unit requires a room with sufficient space for emergency handling by an endoscopy and emergency team if needed. The required equipment needs to be available within the room; this needs to be checked prior to the procedure. The room needs to be equipped with oxygen supply, and patient monitoring equipment, in particular automated registration of blood pressure, pulse, and peripheral oxygen saturation. It is important that the results of these measurements are stored in the patient charts for retrospective evaluation in case of events and overall safety measurement.

Endoscopy should be performed under continuous monitoring of vital functions, in particular blood pressure, pulse, and saturation. Endoscopy should preferentially be performed with an endoscope with a large diameter working channel, or if available two large working channels. A large diameter working channel improves the ability to remove blood and clots. Two large working channels enable combined removal of fluids and intervention procedures. A side viewing endoscope can be helpful for diagnosis and treatment of duodenal lesions. Equipment for treatment of the cause of the bleed should be directly available in the endoscopy room and the nursing staff should be acquainted with their use. A jet/pump system is helpful for cleansing of the stomach and duodenum in the presence of larger amounts of blood or active bleeding, as well as for removal of adherent clots. A separate suction device should be directly available for removal of blood from mouth and throat in particular in case patients are not intubated.

Endoscopy procedure

Intubation of the patient prior to the endoscopy can ease the procedure and prevent aspiration of blood, in particular in case of massive bleeding. If the patient is not intubated, some clinicians prefer to administer a benzodiazepine for conscious sedation. This may ease the procedure for the patient, but may also increase the risk of aspiration and potentially impair vital functions in patients at risk. Physicians should monitor vital signs of their patients. If complications occur, the endoscopist should try to determine whether or not these were related to the use or lack of conscious sedation. After introduction of the endoscope, adequate inspection of the full upper gastrointestinal tract is performed. This should not stop with identification of a bleeding source, as multiple bleeding sources may be present. For adequate inspection, the endoscopist will attempt to remove most of blood remnants if present. This may be more difficult in the presence of large clots, which may block the view and the suction channel of the endoscope, sometimes requiring removal of the endoscope for cleaning. In the presence of massive amounts of bloods and clots, an alternative approach is to try and locate the bleeding source by looking for the presence of fresh rood blood as a flagging sign amongst darker older blood and clots. This should be followed by endoscopic treatment of the bleeding source, after which full inspection can be performed.

Once a peptic ulcer is identified, the endoscopist should assess its appearance and thus determine the risk for persistent or recurrent bleeding, and the need for endoscopic therapy. This is done by determination of signs of

Table 4.2 Risk of recurrent bleeding in patients with bleeding peptic ulcer after medical therapy alone (31, 118–120).

Ulcer characteristics at endoscopy	Incidence (%)	Risk of recurrent bleeding (%)
Active bleeding		
Spurting bleeding	6–10	80–90
Oozing bleeding	4–10	10–30
Signs of recent hemorrhage		
Non-bleeding visible vessel	8–25	39–60
Adherent clot	8–17	22–35
Flat spot	10–23	0–13
Lesions without active bleeding		
Clean ulcer base	35–58	0–12

active bleeding, either spurting or oozing, and stigmata of recent hemorrhage, in particular a visible vessel or an adherent clot. International consensus guidelines do not indicate endoscopic hemostatic therapy for patients with low-risk stigmata (a clean-based ulcer or a flat pigmented spot in an ulcer bed), because of their low risk of rebleeding (Table 4.2) (10). In contrast, endoscopic therapy is mandatory in patients with high risk lesions, in particular those with signs of active bleeding or a visible vessel (Fig. 4.1) (4, 10). The role of endoscopic therapy for ulcers with adherent clots is controversial (10).

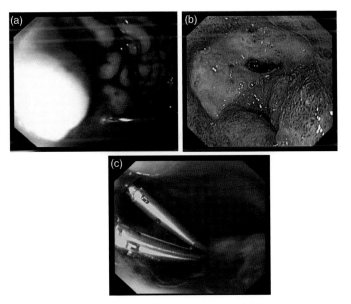

Figure 4.1 A: Active ulcer bleeding, with a spurting vessel (Forrest IA). **B**: Ulcer with visible vessel (Forrest IIA). **C**: Ulcer with visible vessel after hemoclip treatment.

Box 4.1 Endoscopic therapies used for the treatment of bleeding peptic ulcer

Injection therapy
- Epinephrine
- Normal saline
- Sclerosant (e.g. polidocanol, ethanolamine, and ethanol)
- Thrombin
- Fibrin sealant

Ablative therapy
- Thermocoagulation (e.g. heater probe)

- Electrocoagulation (e.g. Gold probe, BICAP probe, hemostatis forceps with soft coagulation)
- Argon plasma coagulation
- Laser photocoagulation

Mechanical therapy
- Hemoclip placement
- Band ligation

Combination therapy (injection therapy plus ablative therapy/ mechanical therapy)

Different endoscopic treatment options have been widely studied over the last 25 years (Box 4.1 and Table 4.3). These include (a) injection therapy with substances as ephinephrine, normal saline, ethanol, sclerosant, thrombin and fibrin sealant, (b) ablative treatment with techniques as thermocoagulation, electrocoagulation, argon plasma coagulation and laser therapy, and (c) mechanical therapy in particular hemoclips and band ligation. These methods have also been tested in a variety of combination therapies.

Injection therapy

Injection therapy with epinephrine is one of the most widely used methods for initial treatment of bleeding peptic ulcers, because it is effective, relatively inexpensive and easy to administer. It promotes hemostasis by a combination of local tamponade, vasospasm and induction of thrombosis and accordingly produces a cleaner field permitting further targeted treatment of the bleeding focus. Injection is performed with a standard sclerotherapy needle, introducing it tangentially into the submucosa. Injection is started in quadrants around the bleeding site, followed by central injection. When injecting in the right plane, local swelling occurs with whitening of the surrounding mucosa. Epinephrine typically reduces or stops bleeding initially, but rebleeding may recur from 20 minutes after injection when epinephrine is absorbed and a permanent clot has not yet been formed. Therefore epinephrine injection therapy should be combined with a more durable hemostatic technique (31). The optimal injection volume of epinephrine for endoscopic treatment of an actively bleeding ulcer is still a matter of debate. In a Chinese study of 228 patients with actively bleeding ulcers (spurting or oozing), injection with either 20, 30 or 40 mL diluted

Table 4.3 List of randomized controlled trials published over the last 10 years comparing different endoscopic treatments for peptic ulcer bleeding.

Author (ref)	Forrest classification of included patients	Treatment per study arm (n)	Primary hemostasis (%)	Rebleeding (%)	Surgery (%)	Bleeding related mortality (%)
Cipolletta (121)	Ia + Ib + IIa	hemoclips (56) / heater probe (57)	86 / 89	1.8 / 21	3.6 / 7	3.6 / 3.5
Lin (48)	Ia + Ib + IIa	hemoclips (40) / heater probe (40)	85 / 100	8.8 / 5	5 / 2.5	5 / 2.5
Lin (42)	Ia + Ib + IIa	epi (25) / fibrin sealant (26)	100 / 100	15 / 56	8 / 8	0 / 0
Laine (122)	Ia + Ib + IIa	bipolar (52) / saline injection (48)	71 / 88	NR	4.2 / 1.9	6 / 2
Pescatore	Ia + Ib + IIa + IIb	Epi (70) / epi + fibrin sealant (65)	100 / 100	24.3 / 21.5	10 / 6	3 / 3
Gevers (123)	Ia + Ib + IIa	epi + poli (34) / hemoclips (35) / hemoclips + epi + poli (32)	80 / 86 / 91	15 / 37 / 25	NR	0 / 0 / 9.3
Chau (124)	Ia + Ib + IIa + IIb	heater probe + epi (88) / argon plasma + epi (97)	95.9 / 97.7	21.6 / 17	9.3 / 4.5	6.2 / 5.7
Soon (125)	Ia + Ib + IIa + IIb	heater probe + epi (43) / monopolar (56)	96.4 / 76.7	0 / 14	0 / 0	0 / 0
Lin (126)	Ia + Ib + IIa	heater probe + epi (47) / hemoclips (46)	95.1 / 100	10.3 / 6.4	0 / 4.7	0 / 0
Chou (127)	Ia + Ib + IIa	distilled water (40) / hemoclips (39)	100 / 97.5	10.3 / 28.2	5.1 / 12.5	2.6 / 5.0
Church (41)	Ia + Ib + IIa	heater probe (120) / heater probe + thrombin (127)	97 / 97	15 / 15	13 / 11	6 / 12
Shimoda (37)	Ia + Ib + IIa	hemoclips (42) / etha (42) / hemoclips + etha (42)	85.7 / 90.5 / 92.9	14.3 / 9.5	7.1 / 0 / 0	0 / 2.4 / 7.1 / 2.4
Skok (56)	Ia + Ib + IIa + IIb	argon plasma (50) / epi + poli (50)	94 / 90	14 / 18	6 / 8	8 / 10
Ljubicic (128)	Ia + Ib	hemoclips + epi (31) / poli + epi (30)	96.8 / 96.7	6.5 / 13.3	3.2 / 3.3	3.2 / 0

Continued p.54

Table 4.3 (continued)

Author (ref)	Forrest classification of included patients	Treatment per study arm (n)	Primary hemostasis (%)	Rebleeding (%)	Surgery (%)	Bleeding related mortality (%)
Bianco (61)	Ia + Ib + IIa	bipolar + epi (58)	100	8.2	1.8	1.7
		bipolar (56)	68.4	14.3	7.1	5.3
Park (62)	Ia + Ib + IIa	hemoclips/band ligatie ± epi (45)	97.8	4.5	0	0
		epi (45)	97.8	20.5	2.2	2.2
Saltzman (129)	Ia + Ib + IIa + IIb	hemoclips (26)	100	15.4	11.5	0
		bipolar + epi (21)	95.2	23.8	4.8	9.5
Lo (130)	Ia + Ib + IIa + IIb	hemoclips + epi (52)	98	3.8	0	2
		epi (53)	92	21	9	0
Taghavi (52)	Ia + Ib + IIa + IIb	argon plasma + epi (89)	96.6	11.2	2.2	2.2
		hemoclips + epi (83)	98.8	4.8	0	1.2
Arima (49)	Ia + Ib + IIa	hemostatic forceps (48)	85	2	0	2
		hemoclips (48)	79	10	0	0

epi: epinephrine, etha: ethanol, poli: polidocanol, NR: Not reported, Underlined: significant difference ($p < 0.05$).

epinephrine (1:10.000) was equally effective for initial hemostasis, but 30 mL injection was more effective in preventing rebleeding than 20 mL, and gave rise to fewer perforations than 40 mL (32). In another study of 72 patients with actively bleeding ulcer or non-bleeding visible vessel, 35–45 mL diluted epinephrine (1:10.000) was more effective than injection of 15–25 mL of the same solution for prevention of recurrent bleeding (33). A similar observation was done in a trial in 156 patients randomized to 1:10.000 epinephrine injection in a volume of either 5–10 mL or 13–20 mL (34). The higher volume reduced rebleeding rates from 31 to 15%. Although these observations support the recommendation to use higher volume epinephrine injection, they are insufficient evidence for routine use of large volume injection, in particular because epinephrine injection should preferentially be combined with a second treatment modality for durable hemostasis. Furthermore, larger volumes of injected epinephrine may result in tachycardia, cardiac arrhythmias and hypertension and can potentially produce angina in patients at risk, in particular in the presence of anemia and hypotension. This risk may be reduced by further dilution of epinephrine to 1:20.000 in high risk cases. Normal saline is safer in use for patients with severe coronary artery disease, although it has been suggested that it is less effective in achieving initial hemostasis, because it only causes mechanical tamponade but no vasospasm or platelet aggregation (35). Sclerosants (e.g. polidocanol, ethanolamine, and ethanol) are used as addition or alternative to ephinephrine. They produce local tissue inflammation, acute chemical fixation and edema, resulting in tamponade of the bleeding and promotion of the thrombogenesis (31). However, the use of sclerosants for the treatment of peptic ulcer bleeding is nowadays limited, since local side effects are considerable and the benefit over epinephrine is marginal (36–39). Sclerosants may in particular induce enlargement of the ulcer, leading to impaired healing, recurrent bleeding, and in some eventually marked scarring or even perforation. An alternative is formed by thrombin injection, which has been experimentally used for the treatment of bleeding ulcers, both as monotherapy and as accessory agent, however without impressive results. An Italian study compared polidocanol versus thrombin injection in 82 consecutive patients with recent or ongoing ulcer hemorrhage. The rebleeding rate of patients treated with thrombin did not significantly differ from those treated with polidocanol (14.6% vs 9.1%) (40). In a randomized trial of 247 patients in the United Kingdom, the combination of thrombin and heater probe treatment did not confer an additional benefit over heater probe and placebo for the treatment of bleeding peptic ulcer (41). Fibrin sealant or glue is a two-component system which promotes thrombogenesis by mixing thrombin and fibrin locally at the site of bleeding after injection. In one randomized controlled trial of 51 patients with ulcer bleeding, fibrin sealant was equally effective as epinephrine in attaining primary hemostasis, but more effective in preventing rebleeding (15% vs. 56%) (42). Another randomized trial compared the use of fibrin sealant (single application and daily repeated doses) with the use of polidocanol 1% in 854 patients with actively bleeding ulcers or ulcers with a visible vessel. Repeated injection with fibrin sealant was significantly more effective in preventing rebleeding than injection with polidocanol (43). Nevertheless, repeated injections are uncomfortable for the patient, costly and increase workload. Therefore fibrin sealant is not generally used in clinical practice. Several recent meta-analyses compared the results of various endoscopic therapies. Although the use of epinephrine injection alone was more effective than medical therapy alone in patients with high risk lesions, monotherapy with epinephrine was significantly inferior in prevention of rebleeding compared with other monotherapies, as well as epinephrine followed by another modality. Therefore, epinephrine should be used in combination with another method (4, 44–47). According to a Cochrane review, additional endoscopic treatment after epinephrine injection significantly reduced rebleeding from 18.8% to 10.4% (OR, 0.51 [95% CI, 0.39–0.66]), need for emergency surgery (10.8% to 7.1%; OR, 0.63 [95% CI 0.45–0.89]), and mortality (5% to 2.5%; OR, 0.50 [95% CI 0.30–0.82]) in patients with bleeding peptic ulcer. This risk reduction was regardless of which second procedure was applied (47).

Ablative therapy

Ablative therapies can be divided into contact methods (e.g. thermocoagulation and electrocoagulation) and non-contact methods (e.g. argon plasma coagulation and laser photocoagulation). Hemostasis is promoted by the delivery of intense energy, which causes coagulation of tissue proteins, edema and vasoconstriction. It also activates thrombocoagulation and destroys tissue (31). Contact devices require placement of the probe directly to the bleeding focus for optimal effect and minimal scatter injury. Widely used devices for thermocoagulation are the heater probe and for electrocoagulation the Gold and BICAP probes. In a comparative study of 80 patients with bleeding peptic ulcer or non-bleeding visible vessel, heater probe treatment was significantly better in achieving ultimate hemostasis than endoscopic hemoclip placement (97.5% vs 77.5%). This result was especially seen in a subgroup of 21 patients with a difficult-to-approach bleeding focus such as in the posterior duodenal bulb. Nine patients (82%) in the heater probe group and three patients (30%) in the hemoclip group eventually achieved hemostasis (48). An alternative approach comes from the new developments in endoscopic mucosal resection and submucosal dissection, techniques which are associated with frequent bleeds. These are often treated by means of coagulation via grasping forceps. Recent studies show promising results for the use of this same forceps technique with soft coagulation in active gastrointestinal bleeding. Soft coagulation was as effective and safe as hemoclip placement, according one randomized trial and two retrospective studies (49–51).

Argon plasma coagulation offers fairly controlled, non-contact electro-coagulation. This technique uses monopolar electrocoagulation to ionize argon gas into a plasma that coagulates tissue nearest to the catheter tip. Argon plasma coagulation has some advantages; it is safe and has lower cost compared to laser, it can be learned easily, is repeatable and induces limited tissue destruction. Furthermore, it can be used for tangentially located or indirectly visualized bleeding sites (31). On the other hand, the depth of injury is unpredictable; it may be too shallow to produce sufficient hemostasis or too deep resulting in the risk of perforation (52). The risk of gastrointestinal perforation is about 0.5% or lower (53). In a series of 2,193 sessions in 1,062 patients with gastric vascular ectasia, the risk of perforation was 0.2% (54). Argon plasma coagulation was previously shown effective for the treatment of angiodysplasia, gastric antral vascular ectasia and radiation proctitis (54–55). A few published studies confirm this efficacy for bleeding peptic ulcers (52, 56–57). However, newer techniques which allow more targeted, dosed treatment such as heater prober and clips are more efficient and have replaced the use of argon plasma coagulation for bleeding peptic ulcer. Likewise, laser photocoagulation has also become obsolete, because the relatively high risk of gastrointestinal perforation (approximately 3%), the high kit cost, and the inferiority in achieving hemostasis compared to other therapies (31). In a meta-analysis, with a subgroup-analysis of four trials comparing hemoclips versus thermocoagulation with or without injec-tions, initial hemostasis was significantly different between hemoclips (88.7%) and thermocoagulation (94.5%). Definitive hemostasis, rebleeding rate, the need for surgery and all-cause mortality were similar (46). Accord-ing to another meta-analysis, a significant decrease in rebleeding attributable to clips compared with thermal therapy was noted (OR, 0.24 [95% CI, 0.06–0.95]). No differences were seen for surgery or mortality (4).

Mechanical therapy

Mechanical therapies compress the bleeding source by placement of a device (e.g. a clip or a rubber band). The device achieves hemostasis in a manner similar to surgical ligation. A study on 100 patients with peptic ulcer bleeding compared the effect of hemoclip placement with triclip (a novel clipping device with three prongs over the distal end) placement. Hemoclip placement was superior in obtaining primary hemostasis (94% vs 76%) and was easier to place in difficult-to-approach sites. Rebleeding rates, volume of blood transfusion and mortality rate did not significantly differ (58). Metallic hemoclips or endoclips are currently the most popular mechanical therapy. They immediately and securely occlude the bleeding vessel, arresting the bleeding. Side-effects are seldom reported. The clips may also seal small gastrointestinal tears or perforations caused by other endoscopic techniques.

Proper hemoclip placement, however, can be challenging and requires a highly skilled endoscopist. Furthermore, application of the clips can be difficult in tangentially located bleeding sites or when massive hemorrhage obscures the visual field (31). Hemoclips normally fall off 7–14 days after application, when the lesion has partly healed. Rebleeding at that time is unlikely. Sometimes clips dislodge prematurely, giving rise to a recurrent bleeding. An Iranian randomized trial compared the effect of argon plasma coagulation plus epinephrine injection with hemoclip placement plus epinephrine injection in 172 patients with major stigmata of peptic ulcer bleeding. The investigators found no significant difference in initial and definitive hemostasis and rebleeding rate between the two groups (52). Endoscopic band ligation is the most popular method for the treatment of esophageal varices, but it is incidentally used to treat bleeding peptic ulcers. In a study of patients with upper gastrointestinal hemorrhage from peptic ulcer in whom at least two attempts to control bleeding by injection therapy failed, definitive hemostasis could be performed in all eleven patients (59). A meta-analysis of nine studies including 699 patients, compared endoscopic clipping with heater probe alone, thermal therapy plus injection, and injection therapy alone for the treatment of peptic ulcer bleeding. The rate of initial hemostasis was not significantly different between the hemo-clip group and the controls (92% vs 96%, OR 0.58 [95% CI, 0.19–1.75], p = 0.33). The rebleeding rate was nonsignificantly decreased with hemo-clips compared to controls (8.5% vs 15.5%, OR 0.56 [95% CI, 0.30–1.05], p = 0.07). Emergency surgery and mortality rates showed no significant differences. A subgroup analysis comparing hemoclips with injection mono-therapy showed similar results (60). In a similar designed meta-analysis of 15 studies including 1156 patients, however, definitive hemostasis was higher with hemoclips (86.5%), than injection therapy alone (75.4%). In line with the previously mentioned meta-analysis, no significant differences between the hemoclip placement and thermocoagulation were found with respect to definitive hemostasis, rebleeding, need for surgery, and mortality (46).

Combination therapy

It is generally accepted that epinephrine injection alone is inferior to mechanical or ablative therapy for definitive hemostasis and prevention of rebleeding and should be used in combination with another endoscopic therapy, especially in high risk ulcers (10, 45, 61–62). The most suitable (combination of) therapies, however, has not yet been defined. In a meta-analysis of 20 randomized clinical trials encompassing 2,472 patients with recent bleeding from peptic ulcers with high-risk lesions, dual endoscopic therapy was significantly superior to epinephrine injection alone, but had no advantage over thermal or mechanical monotherapy (45). Another recent meta-analysis concluded that all endoscopic treatments were superior to pharmacotherapy alone. Thermal therapy or clips, either alone or in combination with other methods, showed similar effects with respect to rebleeding, surgery and mortality (4). Data fail to demonstrate any superiority of dual therapies over ablative therapy or hemoclip placement alone. It is hypothesized, that different subgroups of patients (e.g. large visible vessel, or tangentially located site) benefit from specific therapies. In a subgroup of patients with difficult-to-approach bleedings, heater probe was superior to hemoclip placement (48). Larger trials need to be done to confirm this hypothesis. Clinicians may choose the method based on their own experience, availability of equipment and ulcer and patient characteristics. In addition, new developments may add to the current mono and combination treatments. One potentially very important new development is the introduction of nanopowder spray to seal the bleeding lesion and induce hemostasis. This technique was highly effective in a first proof-of-principle study (63).

Treatment of adherent clots

The risk of rebleeding of ulcers with adherent clots depends on finding a vessel underlying the clot (64) and treatment of that vessel can reduce the risk of rebleeding. For that reasons, there is international consensus that clot removal should be attempted by vigorous irrigation (10). This leads to removal of the adherent clot in some 26 to 43% of cases (65–66). In a study of 46 patients with peptic ulcer bleeding and an adherent clot, vigorous irrigation for 5 minutes led to removal of the clot in 43%, revealing in almost equal frequency oozing bleeding, a visible vessel, or flat pigmented spots, and only in rare cases either a spurting bleed or a clean ulcer (65). If vigorous irrigation does not lead to removal of the clot, further endoscopic management can be considered. This is generally done by epinephrine injection at the base of the clot, followed by cold snaring, leaving the clot pedicle intact. This approach leads to higher clot removal rates. In an international study on 764 patients with peptic ulcer bleeding and stigmata of active or recent hemorrhage, 22% of patients had adherent clots (11). More than half of these clots were successfully removed by a combination of irrigation and snaring if needed, again in particular revealing oozing bleeds and visible vessels. These data together, show that some 70% of cases with adherent clots have high-risk lesions underneath. The rebleeding risk of irremovable clots varied in different studies between 0 to 35% (66–69). A systematic review on endoscopic therapy for adherent clots reported that endoscopic management is not associated with increased risk (45). Several systematic reviews suggested that endoscopic therapy for adherent clots reduced the risk of rebleeding (relative risks for rebleeding ranging from 0.30 – 0.45), although most of these results did not reach statistical significance given the limited patient numbers included in the analysis (45, 64, 70). Independent risk factors for a higher chance of rebleeding are comorbid illness, shock, and initial hemoglobin level of $\leq 10\,\text{gm/dL}$ (66).

Pharmacotherapy

Introduction

Pharmacotherapy plays a second, major role after endoscopic therapy, together they form the mainstay of treatment for patients with peptic ulcer bleeding. While endoscopic therapy is only applied in patients with high-risk stigmata, pharmacotherapy is relevant for both patients with and without these stigmata. In the absence of high-risk stigmata (active bleeding, visible vessel, or adherent clot), endoscopic therapy is not required and pharmacotherapy can be the sole treatment option. In the presence of high risk stigmata, the current standard of care is endoscopic treatment followed by profound acid suppressive therapy. Already since 1953 it is known that a strongly acidic environment may lead to clot lysis (71). Further studies demonstrated that lowering of environmental pH below 6.0 leads to inhibition of platelet aggregation (72), and lowering the pH below 5.0 inhibits plasma coagulation (73–74). These data led to the hypothesis that acid inhibition and the consequent increase of intragastric pH could contribute to the treatment of patients with peptic ulcer bleeding. Therefore, histamine H2 receptor antagonists (H2RA), somatostatin and octreotide were used and studied as treatment options for peptic ulcer bleeding. Although all these agents inhibit acid secretion by receptor blockage, no studies provided convincing evidence for the beneficial effect of any of these drugs (75). The introduction of proton pump inhibitors (PPIs) allowed more effective suppression of acid secretion. PPIs directly and irreversibly block the acid pump instead of the receptor and have a higher anti-secretory potential than the previously mentioned agents (67, 76–83).

Protonpump inhibitors

PPIs inhibit gastric hydrochloric secretion by irreversible binding to the H^+, K^+-ATPase proton pump, which blocks the final step in acid production (84–86). This block is maintained during the lifetime of the proton pump, which lies around three days (87). As binding of the PPI to the acid pump requires activation of the drug by protonation, a single dose of PPIs only leads to blocking of active pumps, and thus not to a total blocking of acid secretion (77).

Omeprazole was the first PPI to be developed and since then several other PPIs have emerged on the market, in particular pantoprazole, lansoprazole, rabeprazole and esomeprazole. Omeprazole is the most widely studied PPI (80, 88–90). Several studies demonstrated that omeprazole is more effective than placebo in the treatment of peptic ulcer bleeding in high risk patients in terms of bleeding recurrence, hospital days, and the need for transfusion (11, 78, 82, 91–94). Other studies demonstrated a positive effect of omeprazole on rebleeding, surgery, hospital stay and death in patients with low risk peptic ulcer bleeding (89, 95). Differences between the different PPIs lie in pharmacokinetic characteristics and metabolization, and, in the case of esomeprazole, in consisting only of the active isomer. Several meta-analyses concluded that high dose PPIs were effective in consistently increasing intragastric pH to 6.0 and above and decreasing the rebleeding rates (76, 96). This conclusion was based on studies giving the PPI as a bolus followed by continuous infusion for 72 hours, after which the drug was continued as once daily oral dose. However, these conclusions were in particular based on the results of studies in Asian populations, with fewer, non-conclusive data from Western populations. This difference is relevant as Asian subjects often have lower acid output than Caucasians and African-Americans. Furthermore, they usually have higher *H. pylori* prevalence rates, in particular of *cagA*-positive strains, which is associated with active gastritis which further impairs acid production. Finally, Asian populations have a higher prevalence of low-metabolizing CYP2C19 polymorphisms, which is associated with a smaller first-pass effect of most PPIs, and thus a higher efficacy of a given dose of PPIs. Taking all these effects together explains why high dose PPI therapy has more pronounced acid suppressive effect in Asians than in European and US populations (78–79, 93, 97). Based on these discrepancies and the lack of a convincing effect in non-Asian populations of high-dose i.v. treatment with the first generation PPIs on outcome of peptic ulcer bleeding, no PPI was until recently registered for this indication. However, this changed recently when the results of a large multicenter, international trial became available. This trial was conducted in a multiethnic population with high risk peptic ulcer bleeding. Study subjects were randomized to either intravenous esomeprazole given as 80 mg bolus followed by continuous infusion of 8 mg/h or placebo for 72 hours after adequate haemostatic endoscopic therapy. In this study, a significant difference was found between both treatments with respect to the rates of recurrent bleeding, being 5.9 vs 10.3% (p = 0.026) and the need for endoscopic retreatment (6.4 vs 11.63%; p 0.01) (11). A further cost-effectiveness study showed that high dose intravenous administration of esomeprazole after successful endoscopic therapy improves patient outcomes at a modest increase of costs (Table 4.4) (98).

Administration method

PPIs can be administered orally as well as intravenously. Most indications for PPI therapy, e.g. GERD, can be treated with oral administration of a low daily dose of PPI. In the case of peptic ulcer bleeding the preferred administration method differs between high risk and low risk bleeders. In case of low risk peptic ulcer bleeding, the highest concern is to induce

Table 4.4 Literature PPI in peptic ulcer bleeding (131).

Study, year (ref.)	Area	Study design	Patients	(n)	Treatment	Results	Study period
Jensen et al. 2006 (132)	US	RCT	Peptic ulcer bleeding (high risk)	153	Endoscopic treatment and PPI i.v. 80 + 8 mg/h (72 h) or H_2RA 50 mg + 6.25 mg/h (72 h) After 72 h p.o. PPI 20 mg for 30 days.	Stopped early because slow enrolment Rebleeding 6.9% vs. 14.3%, mortality 4% vs. 4%. No significant differences.	30 days
Sung et al. 2003 (67)	Asia	RCT	Peptic ulcer bleeding (high risk)	156	Endoscopic therapy + PPI i.v. 80 mg + 8 mg/h (72 h) or only PPI i.v. 80 + 8 mg/h (72 h) After 72 h both groups PPI 20 mg p.o.	Rebleeding 1.1% vs. 11.6% (p 0.009) Mortality 2.6% vs. 5.1%. Endoscopic therapy important	30 days
Zargar et al. 2006 (133)	Asia	RCT	Peptic ulcer bleeding (high risk)	203	Endoscopic therapy + PPI iv 80 mg + 8 mg/h (72 h) or placebo (72 h) After 72 h all pts PPI 40 mg p.o. 6 weeks	Rebleeding 7.8% vs. 19.8% (p 0.01), fewer transfusions (p 0.003), fewer days in hospital (p 0.0003)	30 days
Lau et al. 2000 (134)	Asia	RCT	Peptic ulcer bleeding (high risk)	240	Endoscopic therapy + PPI 80 mg + 8 mg/h or placebo for 72 h. After 72 h all pts PPI 20 mg p.o. 2 months	Rebleeding 6.7% vs. 22.5% (HR 3.9), mortality 4.2% vs. 10%	30 days

Kaviani et al. 2003 (91)	Middle East	RCT	Peptic ulcer bleeding (high risk)	160	Endoscopic therapy + p.o. PPI 20 mg/6 h or placebo	Mean hospital stay 62.8 ± 28.6 vs. 75 ± 35 h (p 0.032), mean transfusion 1.13 ± 1.36 vs. 1.68 ± 1.68 bags (p 0.029) rebleeding 12 vs. 26 pts (p 0.022)	3 weeks
Schaffalitzky de Muckadell et al. 1997 (94)	Eur	RCT	Peptic ulcer bleeding (high risk)	274	Endoscopic therapy + PPI 80 mg + 8 mg/h i.v. or placebo After 72 h both PPI 20 mg p.o. till day 21	Overall outcome score difference in favor of omeprazole (p 0.004), less blood transfusions (p 0.01), shorter degree and duration of bleeding (p 0.02) and less surgery (p 0.003) or additional endoscopic therapy (p 0.04)	21 days
Khuroo et al. 1997 (92)	Asia	RCT	Peptic ulcer bleeding (high risk)	220	PPI 40 mg BID for 5 days or placebo	Further bleeding/rebleeding 10.9% vs. 36.45 (p <0.001) surgery 8 vs. 26 pt (p < 0.001) Mortality 2 vs. 6 pts. Transfusions 29.1% vs. 70.9% (p < 0.001) Significant reduction in pt with NBVB and adherent clots, no significant reduction in pts with oozing or arterial spurting	30 days

Continued p.64

Table 4.4 (continued)

Study, year (ref.)	Area	Study design	Patients	(n)	Treatment	Results	Study period
Lin et al. 2006 (82)	Asia	RCT	Peptic ulcer bleeding (high risk)	200	Endoscopic therapy + PPI i.v. 40 mg/6 h or PPI i.v. 40 mg/12 h or H₂RA 400 mg/12 h. After 72 h both PPI 20 mg p.o. 2 months	Rebleeding omeprazole 40 mg/6 h 9% vs. 32.8% in cimetidine ($p < 0.01$). Volume of transfusion less in OME mg/6 h than OME 40 mg/12 h and CIM ($p < 0.001$) No statistical difference: hospital stay, surgery and mortality	14 days
Lin et al. 1998 (83)	Asia	RCT	Peptic ulcer bleeding (high risk)	100	Endoscopic therapy + PPI i.v. 40 mg + 160 mg/24 h or H₂RACimetidine i.v. 300 mg + 1200 mg/24 h If necessary second look and therapy and after 72 h all pts PPI 20 mg p.o. 2 weeks	Intragastric pH > 6 84.4% ± 22.9% vs. 53.5% ± 32.3% ($p < 0.001$) Rebleeding 4% vs. 24% ($p = 0.004$), less transfusion median 0 (0–2500 ml) vs. median 0 (0–5000 ml) ($p = 0.08$). No difference in mortality, hospital stay or surgery rate	14 days
Hasselgren et al. 1997 (89)	Eur	RCT	Peptic ulcer bleeding	333	Endoscopic therapy + PPI i.v. 80 mg + 8 mg/h or placebo. After 72 h groups PPI 20 mg p.o. 2 weeks	Overall outcome (scale) omeprazole better (p 0.017) Need for surgery omeprazole vs. placebo (p 0.003), degree of bleeding (p 0.003) and treatment failure (p 0.0009). Mortality identical. Subgroup oozing: outcome omeprazole better (p 0.01)	21 days

Study	Region	Type	Condition	N	Intervention	Results	Follow-up
Sung et al. 2009 (11)	Worldwide	RCT	Peptic ulcer bleeding (high risk)	767	Endoscopic therapy + PPI i.v. 80 mg + 8 mg/h or placebo for 72 h. After 72 h all pt PPI p.o. 40 mg for 27 days	Recurrent bleeding 5.9% vs. 10.3% (p 0.026), retreatment 6.4% vs. 11.6% (p 0.012), surgery 2.7% vs. 5.4% and all cause mortality 0.8% vs. 2.1% (last 2 not significant)	30 days
Li et al. 2000 (88)	Asia	Retrospective	Peptic ulcer bleeding (excl arterial spurt)	607	Endoscopic therapy in oozing bleeding H_2RA 400 mg bolus BID for 5 days or PPI iv. 40 mg for 5 days	Surgery 3.8% vs. 9.28% (p < 0.05) mortality rate 1.49% vs. 2.66% not significant. Transfusion not significantly different in number and volume.	30 days

re-epithelialization of the ulcer and treatment of the underlying cause. The risk of rebleeding is however low and therapy therefore aims at maintaining a pH above 4. Oral and intravenous administration of PPI are both effective in reaching this goal, and thus low-risk patients can be adequately managed by oral PPI therapy with early discharge (10).

In high risk peptic ulcer bleeding the first concern is the prevention of rebleeding and thus rapid increase of intragastric pH. Several administration methods and schemes have been studied and current guidelines recommend treatment with an intravenous bolus followed by continuous infusion of PPI in patients with high risk stigmata who have undergone successful endoscopic therapy (10). Because the proton pumps are continuously being regenerated and the bio-availability of a PPI in the circulation is short, the rationale for this regimen is to first inactivate all actively secreting proton pumps with a bolus injection, then prevent further activation of remaining proton pumps with the continuous infusion (99).

Dosage

In patients without high-risk stigmata, treating in particular aims at re-epithelialization of the ulcer. For this purpose, a daily PPI dosage to 20–40 mg omeprazole is sufficient. In patients with high-risk stigmata, treatment also aims at maintaining hemostasis. For this purpose, continuous high-dose intravenous PPI therapy is needed. A double blind cross-over study in *H. pylori*-positive healthy volunteers measured the intragastric pH during intravenous treatment with 80 mg omeprazole given as a bolus followed by continuous infusion with either 2, 4, or 8 mg/h. The 8 mg/h infusion led to higher mean pH levels than the other treatment regimens (103). Another study evaluated the intragastric pH in bleeding peptic ulcer patients during intravenous treatment with pantoprazole 80 mg bolus followed by either 6 or 8 mg/h intravenously. Again, the 8 mg/h regimen showed a lower intra-individual variability of the intragastric pH and a greater proportion of time with an intragastric pH above 6 (104).

Current practice

The current standard of care for patients with low-risk ulcers consists of standard dose oral PPI treatment for a period determined by the underlying cause of peptic ulcer disease. No head to head studies have been conducted comparing the different PPI agents in the treatment of high risk peptic ulcer bleeding. In patients with a high risk for rebleeding, the first 3 days after endoscopic therapy are crucial since most recurrent bleeding occurs within 72 hours. It is generally accepted based on the literature mentioned earlier that the aim for these patients is to maintain the intragastric pH > 6 during those initial 3 days. This goal can be approached by continuous high dose i.v. esomeprazole treatment, starting with a bolus of 80 mg followed by 8 mg/hr continuously, as was decided in the latest guidelines (10–11). Esomeprazole i.v. has recently been the first PPI to be approved in the EU and other markets for the short-term maintenance of haemostasis and prevention of rebleeding in patients following therapeutic endoscopy for acute bleeding gastric or duodenal ulcers. Earlier, no such approval existed for any PPI anywhere in the world.

Follow-Up

Management of peptic ulcer bleeding consists not only of acute therapy, but should also include diagnosis and treatment of the underlying cause. The most common causes of peptic ulcers are *H. pylori* infection and use of NSAIDs (non steroidal anti-inflammatory drugs) and low dose acetylsa-licylic acid (ASA) use (10, 105–106). In the case of underlying *H. pylori* infection, eradication of *H. pylori* is mandatory. *H. pylori* eradication does not affect the early rebleeding rates, eradication therapy can thus be scheduled after discharge (107–108). In fact, some studies have demonstrated a faster and higher increase of intragastric pH in *H. pylori*-positive patients during PPI treatment, related to the fact that *H. pylori* gastritis augments the acid-suppressive effect of the PPI. Once the acute episode has passed, *H. pylori* eradication should be prescribed as it is the most efficient strategy, also better than maintenance acid suppressive treatment, to prevent renewed bleeding from recurrent ulcers. In determining whether a bleeding ulcer is related to *H. pylori*, it is of importance to note that active bleeding as well as PPI therapy can cause false negative outcomes in *H. pylori* testing (109). For this reason, guidelines recommend to retest patients with a negative *H. pylori* test-result obtained in the acute setting (10). Eradication therapy can consist of several medication combinations from the standard triple therapy (PPI and 2 different kinds of antibiotics), quadruple therapy (containing a PPI, bis-muth, and two antibiotics or a PPI and three antibiotics), to sequential therapy or the more recent hybrid sequential therapy, with treatments schedules varying from 7 to 14 days (Table 4.5). The more extensive therapies such as quadruple therapy are more effective, in particular in patients with strains carrying antimicrobial resistance. The effect of erad-ication therapy should be assessed at least 4 weeks after the end of therapy, as patients in whom eradication treatment failed have a significant risk for recurrent ulcer bleeding.

In the case of NSAIDs or low dose ASA use the important question is whether or not the medication can be permanently withdrawn. This is not possible in the majority of patients receiving low dose ASA, as they use this medication for secondary cardiovascular prophylaxis. In fact, a study from Hong Kong showed that low dose aspirin should be restarted as soon as possible in these patients despite their bleeding ulcer, to prevent early occurrence of cardiovascular events. For secondary prophylaxis of bleeding during ongoing low dose aspirin treatment, *H. pylori*-negative patients

Table 4.5 Overview of antibiotics used for *H. pylori* eradication (135–136).

Drug class	Drug	Triple therapy[a]	Quadruple therapy[b,c]	Quadruple therapy[b]	Sequential therapy[d]	Sequential-hybrid[e]
		Dose	Dose	Dose	Dose	Dose
Acid suppression	proton pump inhibitor	20–40 mg bid[f]	20–40 mg bid[f]	20–40 mg bid[f]	20–40 mg bid[f]	20–40 mg bid[f]
Standard antimicrobials	bismuth compound[g]	2 tablets bid	2 tablets bid			
	Amoxicillin	1 g bid		1 g bid	1 g bid	1 g bid
	Metronidazole[h]	500 mg bid	500 mg tid	500 mg tid	500 mg bid	500 mg bid
	Clarithromycin	500 mg bid		500 mg bid	500 mg bid	500 mg bid
	Tetracycline		500 mg qid			
Salvage antimicrobials	Levofloxacin	300 mg bid				
	Rifabutin	150 mg bid				
	Furazolidone	100 mg bid				

[a] Triple therapy consists of a PPI or bismuth compound, together with two of the listed antibiotics, usually given for 7–14 days.

[b] Quadruple therapy consists of a PPI plus bismuth compound with two antibiotics as listed given for 4 – 10 days or PPI plus three antibiotics as listed given for 4–10 days.

[c] Bismuth, metronidazole and tetracycline can be administered in a single capsule 1 times daily (Pylera ®).

[d] Sequential therapy consists of 10 days of treatment with a PPI, plus amoxicillin for the first five days and a combination of clarithromycin and metronidazole for the second five days (9).

[e] Sequential Hybrid consists of 14 days of PPI and amoxicillin during the last seven days combined with clarithromycin and metronidazole (98).

[f] PPI dose equivalent to omeprazole 20 mg bid.

[g] Bismuth subsalicylate or subcitrate.

[h] Alternative = tinidazole 500 mg bid.

required PPI maintenance treatment in a dose equivalent to 20 mg omeprazole once daily. In *H. pylori*–positive patients, PPI maintenance treatment and *H. pylori* eradication are equally effective to prevent rebleeding. Replacing aspirin by clopidogrel is an inferior strategy to prevent rebleeding. A considerable proportion of patients who present with peptic ulcer bleeding during NSAID therapy, this medication can be stopped. This is sufficient prophylaxis for rebleeding, unless subjects are also infected with *H. pylori*. In that case, additional *H. pylori* eradication is recommended. Patients who need to continue NSAIDs, should be preferentially treated with a combination of a COX-2 inhibitor and a PPI in a dose equivalent to omeprazole 20 mg once daily, as alternative strategies of a COX-2 inhibitor alone or a PPI with a conventional NSAID are still associated with a significant risk of rebleeding.

Patients with non-NSAID non-*H. pylori* idiopathic ulcer disease require maintenance treatment with a PPI in a dose equivalent to 20 mg omeprazole once daily. They further need to be assessed for the underlying cause of the ulcer. Once identified, the underlying cause should be treated if possible. Finally, patients with gastric ulcer disease need to adequately assessed for the possibility that the ulcer is due to underlying gastric malignancy (110–111).

Conclusions

The management of peptic ulcer bleeding has changed dramatically over the past 20 years. Early endoscopy is crucial for initial diagnosis and risk assessment. For cases with high risk stigmata, in particular active bleeding or visible vessel or adherent clot, endoscopic treatment is the mainstay in management. Endoscopic treatment primarily consists of clips placement or thermal coagulation, alone or in combination with epinephrine injection. After adequate hemostasis, high risk cases should receive profound acid suppressive therapy, for the first 72 hours given as continous infusion. Recurrent bleedings can usually firstly be managed again by endoscopic treatment. Failures should either undergo surgery or trans-arterial embolization. During follow-up, adequate attention should be given to identify and manage the underlying cause of the bleeding ulcer. With this multistep approach, the outcome of bleeding has strongly improved over the years.

References

1. Graham DY. Limited value of early endoscopy in the management of acute upper gastrointestinal bleeding. Prospective controlled trial. Am J Surg. 1980 Aug;140 (2):284–90.
2. Peterson WL, Barnett CC, Smith HJ, Allen MH, Corbett DB. Routine early endoscopy in upper-gastrointestinal-tract bleeding: a randomized, controlled trial. N Engl J Med. 1981 Apr 16;304(16):925–9.

3. Cook DJ, Guyatt GH, Salena BJ, Laine LA. Endoscopic therapy for acute nonvariceal upper gastrointestinal hemorrhage: a meta-analysis. Gastroenterology. 1992 Jan;102 (1):139–48.

4. Barkun AN, Martel M, Toubouti Y, Rahme E, Bardou M. Endoscopic hemostasis in peptic ulcer bleeding for patients with high-risk lesions: a series of meta-analyses. Gastrointest Endosc. 2009 May;69(4):786–99.

5. Spiegel BM, Vakil NB, Ofman JJ. Endoscopy for acute nonvariceal upper gastrointestinal tract hemorrhage: is sooner better? A systematic review. Arch Intern Med. 2001 Jun11;161(11):1393–404.

6. Spiegel BM. Endoscopy for acute upper GI tract hemorrhage: sooner is better. Gastrointest Endosc. 2009 Aug;70(2):236–9.

7. Barkun A, Bardou M, Marshall JK. Nonvariceal Upper GIBCCG. Consensus recommendations for managing patients with nonvariceal upper gastrointestinal bleeding. Ann Intern Med. 2003 Nov 18;139(10):843–57.

8. British Society of Gastroenterology,Non-variceal upper gastrointestinal haemorrhage: guidelines. Gut. 2002 Oct;51Suppl 4:iv1–6.

9. Adler DG, Leighton JA, Davila RE, Hirota WK, Jacobson BC, Qureshi WA, et al. ASGE guideline: The role of endoscopy in acute non-variceal upper-GI hemorrhage. Gastrointest Endosc. 2004 Oct;60(4):497–504.

10. Barkun AN, Bardou M, Kuipers EJ, Sung J, Hunt RH, Martel M, et al. International consensus recommendations on the management of patients with nonvariceal upper gastrointestinal bleeding. Ann Intern Med. 2010 Jan 19;152(2):101–13.

11. Sung JJ, Barkun A, Kuipers EJ, Mossner J, Jensen DM, Stuart R, et al. Intravenous esomeprazole for prevention of recurrent peptic ulcer bleeding: a randomized trial. Ann Intern Med. 2009 Apr 7;150(7):455–64.

12. Hearnshaw SA, Logan RF, Lowe D, Travis SP, Murphy MF, Palmer KR. Use of endoscopy for management of acute upper gastrointestinal bleeding in the UK: results of a nationwide audit. Gut. 2010 Aug;59(8):1022–9.

13. da Silveira EB, Lam E, Martel M, Bensoussan K, Barkun AN. The importance of process issues as predictors of time to endoscopy in patients with acute upper-GI bleeding using the RUGBE data. Gastrointest Endosc. 2006 Sep;64(3):299–309.

14. Cooper GS, Kou TD, Wong RC. Use and impact of early endoscopy in elderly patients with peptic ulcer hemorrhage: a population-based analysis. Gastrointest Endosc. 2009 Aug;70(2):229–35.

15. Schacher GM, Lesbros-Pantoflickova D, Ortner MA, Wasserfallen JB, Blum AL, Dorta G. Is early endoscopy in the emergency room beneficial in patients with bleeding peptic ulcer? A "fortuitously controlled" study. Endoscopy. 2005 May;37(4):324–8.

16. Targownik LE, Murthy S, Keyvani L, Leeson S. The role of rapid endoscopy for high-risk patients with acute nonvariceal upper gastrointestinal bleeding. Can J Gastroenterol. 2007 Jul;21(7):425–9.

17. van Leerdam ME. Epidemiology of acute upper gastrointestinal bleeding. Best Pract Res Clin Gastroenterol. 2008;22(2):209–24.

18. Lau JY, Leung WK, Wu JC, Chan FK, Wong VW, Chiu PW, et al. Omeprazole before endoscopy in patients with gastrointestinal bleeding. N Engl J Med. 2007 Apr 19;356 (16):1631–40.

19. Sreedharan A, Martin J, Leontiadis GI, Dorward S, Howden CW, Forman D, et al. Proton pump inhibitor treatment initiated prior to endoscopic diagnosis in upper gastrointestinal bleeding. Cochrane Database Syst Rev. 2010;7:CD005415.

20. Winstead NS, Wilcox CM. Erythromycin prior to endoscopy for acute upper gastrointestinal haemorrhage: a cost-effectiveness analysis. Aliment Pharmacol Ther. 2007 Nov 15;26(10):1371–7.

21. Pitera A, Sarko J. Just say no: gastric aspiration and lavage rarely provide benefit. Ann Emerg Med. 2010 May;55(4):365–6.

22. Lee SD, Kearney DJ. A randomized controlled trial of gastric lavage prior to endoscopy for acute upper gastrointestinal bleeding. J Clin Gastroenterol. 2004 Nov–Dec;38(10):861–5.

23. Witting MD, Magder L, Heins AE, Mattu A, Granja CA, Baumgarten M. Usefulness and validity of diagnostic nasogastric aspiration in patients without hematemesis. Ann Emerg Med. 2004 May;43(4):525–32.

24. Cuellar RE, Gavaler JS, Alexander JA, Brouillette DE, Chien MC, Yoo YK, et al. Gastrointestinal tract hemorrhage. The value of a nasogastric aspirate. Arch Intern Med. 1990 Jul;150(7):1381–4.

25. Aljebreen AM, Fallone CA, Barkun AN. Nasogastric aspirate predicts high-risk endoscopic lesions in patients with acute upper-GI bleeding. Gastrointest Endosc. 2004 Feb;59(2):172–8.

26. Marmo R, Koch M, Cipolletta L, Capurso L, Pera A, Bianco MA, et al. Predictive factors of mortality from nonvariceal upper gastrointestinal hemorrhage: a multicenter study. Am J Gastroenterol. 2008 Jul;103(7):1639–47; quiz 48.

27. Shaheen AA, Kaplan GG, Myers RP. Weekend versus weekday admission and mortality from gastrointestinal hemorrhage caused by peptic ulcer disease. Clin Gastroenterol Hepatol. 2009 Mar;7(3):303–10.

28. Dorn SD, Shah ND, Berg BP, Naessens JM. Effect of weekend hospital admission on gastrointestinal hemorrhage outcomes. Dig Dis Sci. Jun;55(6):1658–66.

29. Ananthakrishnan AN, McGinley EL, Saeian K. Outcomes of weekend admissions for upper gastrointestinal hemorrhage: a nationwide analysis. Clin Gastroenterol Hepatol. 2009 Mar;7(3):296–302e1.

30. Tsoi K, Pang S, Chiu P, Yung M, Lau J, Sung J. The risk of ulcer-related death in relation to hospital admission on public holidays: a cohort study on 10.428 cases of upper gastrointestinal bleeding. Presentation #891p. Digestive Disease Week New Orleans, 2010.

31. Cappell MS. Medscape. Therapeutic endoscopy for acute upper gastrointestinal bleeding. Nat Rev Gastroenterol Hepatol. 2010 May;7(4):214–29.

32. Liou TC, Lin SC, Wang HY, Chang WH. Optimal injection volume of epinephrine for endoscopic treatment of peptic ulcer bleeding. World J Gastroenterol. 2006 May 21;12(19):3108–13.

33. Park CH, Lee SJ, Park JH, Lee WS, Joo YE, Kim HS, et al. Optimal injection volume of epinephrine for endoscopic prevention of recurrent peptic ulcer bleeding. Gastrointest Endosc. 2004 Dec;60(6):875–80.

34. Lin HJ, Hsieh YH, Tseng GY, Perng CL, Chang FY, Lee SD. A prospective, randomized trial of large- versus small-volume endoscopic injection of epinephrine for peptic ulcer bleeding. Gastrointest Endosc. 2002 May;55(6):615–9.

35. Liou TC, Chang WH, Wang HY, Lin SC, Shih SC. Large-volume endoscopic injection of epinephrine plus normal saline for peptic ulcer bleeding. J Gastroenterol Hepatol. 2007 Jul;22(7):996–1002.

36. Koyama T, Fujimoto K, Iwakiri R, Sakata H, Sakata Y, Yamaoka K, et al. Prevention of recurrent bleeding from gastric ulcer with a nonbleeding visible vessel by endoscopic injection of absolute ethanol: a prospective, controlled trial. Gastrointest Endosc. 1995 Aug;42(2):128–31.

37. Shimoda R, Iwakiri R, Sakata H, Ogata S, Kikkawa A, Ootani H, et al. Evaluation of endoscopic hemostasis with metallic hemoclips for bleeding gastric ulcer: comparison with endoscopic injection of absolute ethanol in a prospective, randomized study. Am J Gastroenterol. 2003 Oct;98(10):2198–202.

38. Chung SC, Leong HT, Chan AC, Lau JY, Yung MY, Leung JW, et al. Epinephrine or epinephrine plus alcohol for injection of bleeding ulcers: a prospective randomized trial. Gastrointest Endosc. 1996 Jun;43(6):591–5.

39. Choudari CP, Palmer KR. Endoscopic injection therapy for bleeding peptic ulcer; a comparison of adrenaline alone with adrenaline plus ethanolamine oleate. Gut. 1994 May;35(5):608–10.

40. Benedetti G, Sablich R, Lacchin T. Endoscopic injection sclerotherapy in non-variceal upper gastrointestinal bleeding. A comparative study of polidocanol and thrombin. Surg Endosc. 1991;5(1):28–30.

41. Church NI, Dallal HJ, Masson J, Mowat NA, Johnston DA, Radin E, et al. A randomized trial comparing heater probe plus thrombin with heater probe plus placebo for bleeding peptic ulcer. Gastroenterology. 2003 Aug;125(2):396–403.

42. Lin HJ, Hsieh YH, Tseng GY, Perng CL, Chang FY, Lee SD. Endoscopic injection with fibrin sealant versus epinephrine for arrest of peptic ulcer bleeding: a randomized, comparative trial. J Clin Gastroenterol. 2002 Sep;35(3):218–21.

43. Rutgeerts P, Rauws E, Wara P, Swain P, Hoos A, Solleder E, et al. Randomised trial of single and repeated fibrin glue compared with injection of polidocanol in treatment of bleeding peptic ulcer. Lancet. 1997 Sep 6;350(9079):692–6.

44. Laine L, McQuaid KR. Endoscopic therapy for bleeding ulcers: an evidence-based approach based on meta-analyses of randomized controlled trials. Clin Gastroenterol Hepatol. 2009 Jan;7(1):33–47; quiz 1–2.

45. Marmo R, Rotondano G, Piscopo R, Bianco MA, D'Angella R, Cipolletta L. Dual therapy versus monotherapy in the endoscopic treatment of high-risk bleeding ulcers: a meta-analysis of controlled trials. Am J Gastroenterol. 2007 Feb;102(2):279–89; quiz 469.

46. Sung JJ, Tsoi KK, Lai LH, Wu JC, Lau JY. Endoscopic clipping versus injection and thermo-coagulation in the treatment of non-variceal upper gastrointestinal bleeding: a meta-analysis. Gut. 2007 Oct;56(10):1364–73.

47. Vergara M, Calvet X, Gisbert JP. Epinephrine injection versus epinephrine injection and a second endoscopic method in high risk bleeding ulcers. Cochrane Database Syst Rev. 2007(2):CD005584.

48. Lin HJ, Hsieh YH, Tseng GY, Perng CL, Chang FY, Lee SD. A prospective, randomized trial of endoscopic hemoclip versus heater probe thermocoagulation for peptic ulcer bleeding. Am J Gastroenterol. 2002 Sep;97(9):2250–4.

49. Arima S, Sakata Y, Ogata S, Tominaga N, Tsuruoka N, Mannen K, et al. Evaluation of hemostasis with soft coagulation using endoscopic hemostatic forceps in comparison with metallic hemoclips for bleeding gastric ulcers: a prospective, randomized trial. J Gastroenterol. 2010 May;45(5):501–5.

50. Fujishiro M, Abe N, Endo M, Kawahara Y, Shimoda R, Nagata S, et al. Retrospective multicenter study concerning electrocautery forceps with soft coagulation for nonmalignant gastroduodenal ulcer bleeding in Japan. Dig Endosc. 2010 Jul;22 Suppl 1:S15–8.

51. Nagata S, Kimura S, Ogoshi H, Hidaka T. Endoscopic hemostasis of gastric ulcer bleeding by hemostatic forceps coagulation. Dig Endosc. 2010 Jul;22 Suppl 1:S22–5.

52. Taghavi SA, Soleimani SM, Hosseini-Asl SM, Eshraghian A, Eghbali H, Dehghani SM, et al. Adrenaline injection plus argon plasma coagulation versus adrenaline injection plus hemoclips for treating high-risk bleeding peptic ulcers: a prospective, randomized trial. Can J Gastroenterol. 2009 Oct;23(10):699–704.

53. Havanond C, Havanond P. Argon plasma coagulation therapy for acute non-variceal upper gastrointestinal bleeding. Cochrane Database Syst Rev. 2005(2):CD003791.

54. Herrera S, Bordas JM, Llach J, Gines A, Pellise M, Fernandez-Esparrach G, et al. The beneficial effects of argon plasma coagulation in the management of different types of

gastric vascular ectasia lesions in patients admitted for GI hemorrhage. Gastrointest Endosc. 2008 Sep;68(3):440–6.

55. Karamanolis G, Triantafyllou K, Tsiamoulos Z, Polymeros D, Kalli T, Misailidis N, et al. Argon plasma coagulation has a long-lasting therapeutic effect in patients with chronic radiation proctitis. Endoscopy. 2009 Jun;41(6):529–31.

56. Skok P, Krizman I, Skok M. Argon plasma coagulation versus injection sclerotherapy in peptic ulcer hemorrhage–a prospective, controlled study. Hepatogastroenterology. 2004 Jan–Feb;51(55):165–70.

57. Yap LM, Hagan S, Craig A, Hebbard GG, Young GP, Bampton PA. An audit of argon plasma coagulation, epinephrine injection, and proton-pump infusion therapy in the management of bleeding peptic ulcer disease. Endoscopy. 2004 May;36(4):371–2; author reply 2–3.

58. Lin HJ, Lo WC, Cheng YC, Perng CL. Endoscopic hemoclip versus triclip placement in patients with high-risk peptic ulcer bleeding. Am J Gastroenterol. 2007 Mar;102 (3):539–43.

59. Misra SP, Dwivedi M, Misra V, Kunwar B, Arora JS, Dharmani S. Endoscopic band ligation as salvage therapy in patients with bleeding peptic ulcers not responding to injection therapy. Endoscopy. 2005 Jul;37(7):626–9.

60. Yuan Y, Wang C, Hunt RH. Endoscopic clipping for acute nonvariceal upper-GI bleeding: a meta-analysis and critical appraisal of randomized controlled trials. Gastrointest Endosc. 2008 Aug;68(2):339–51.

61. Bianco MA, Rotondano G, Marmo R, Piscopo R, Orsini L, Cipolletta L. Combined epinephrine and bipolar probe coagulation vs. bipolar probe coagulation alone for bleeding peptic ulcer: a randomized, controlled trial. Gastrointest Endosc. 2004 Dec;60(6):910–5.

62. Park CH, Joo YE, Kim HS, Choi SK, Rew JS, Kim SJ. A prospective, randomized trial comparing mechanical methods of hemostasis plus epinephrine injection to epinephrine injection alone for bleeding peptic ulcer. Gastrointest Endosc. 2004 Aug;60 (2):173–9.

63. Sung J, Luo D, Wu J, Chan F, Lau J, Mack S, et al. Nanopowders are highly effective in achieving hemostasis in severe peptic ulcer bleeding: an interim report of a prospective human trial. Presentation S1575. Digestive Disease Week New Orleans, 2010.

64. Kahi CJ, Jensen DM, Sung JJ, Bleau BL, Jung HK, Eckert G, et al. Endoscopic therapy versus medical therapy for bleeding peptic ulcer with adherent clot: a meta-analysis. Gastroenterology. 2005 Sep;129(3):855–62.

65. Laine L, Stein C, Sharma V. A prospective outcome study of patients with clot in an ulcer and the effect of irrigation. Gastrointest Endosc. 1996 Feb;43 (2 Pt 1):107–10.

66. Lin HJ, Wang K, Perng CL, Lee FY, Lee CH, Lee SD. Natural history of bleeding peptic ulcers with a tightly adherent blood clot: a prospective observation. Gastrointest Endosc. 1996 May;43(5):470–3.

67. Sung JJ, Chan FK, Lau JY, Yung MY, Leung WK, Wu JC, et al. The effect of endoscopic therapy in patients receiving omeprazole for bleeding ulcers with nonbleeding visible vessels or adherent clots: a randomized comparison. Ann Intern Med. 2003 Aug 19;139(4):237–43.

68. Bleau BL, Gostout CJ, Sherman KE, Shaw MJ, Harford WV, Keate RF, et al. Recurrent bleeding from peptic ulcer associated with adherent clot: a randomized study comparing endoscopic treatment with medical therapy. Gastrointest Endosc. 2002 Jul;56(1):1–6.

69. Jensen DM, Kovacs TO, Jutabha R, Machicado GA, Gralnek IM, Savides TJ, et al. Randomized trial of medical or endoscopic therapy to prevent recurrent ulcer hemorrhage in patients with adherent clots. Gastroenterology. 2002 Aug;123 (2):407–13.

70. Laine L. Systematic review of endoscopic therapy for ulcers with clots: Can a meta-analysis be misleading? Gastroenterology. 2005 Dec;129(6):2127; author reply -8.

71. Barkham P, Tocantins LM. Action of human gastric juice on human blood clots. J Appl Physiol. 1953 Jul;6(1):1–7.

72. Green FW, Jr., Kaplan MM, Curtis LE, Levine PH. Effect of acid and pepsin on blood coagulation and platelet aggregation. A possible contributor prolonged gastroduodenal mucosal hemorrhage. Gastroenterology. 1978 Jan;74(1):38–43.

73. Chaimoff C, Creter D, Djaldetti M. The effect of pH on platelet and coagulation factor activities. Am J Surg. 1978 Aug;136(2):257–9.

74. Patchett SE, Enright H, Afdhal N, O'Connell W, O'Donoghue DP. Clot lysis by gastric juice: an in vitro study. Gut. 1989 Dec;30(12):1704–7.

75. Leontiadis GI, Howden CW. Pharmacologic Treatment of Peptic Ulcer Bleeding. Curr Treat Options Gastroenterol. 2007 Mar;10(2):134–42.

76. Andriulli A, Annese V, Caruso N, Pilotto A, Accadia L, Niro AG, et al. Proton-pump inhibitors and outcome of endoscopic hemostasis in bleeding peptic ulcers: a series of meta-analyses. Am J Gastroenterol. 2005 Jan;100(1):207–19.

77. Hirschowitz BI, Keeling D, Lewin M, Okabe S, Parsons M, Sewing K, et al. Pharmacological aspects of acid secretion. Dig Dis Sci. 1995 Feb;40 (2 Suppl):3S–23S.

78. Khuroo MS, Farahat KL, Kagevi IE. Treatment with proton pump inhibitors in acute non-variceal upper gastrointestinal bleeding: a meta-analysis. J Gastroenterol Hepatol. 2005 Jan;20(1):11–25.

79. Kovacs TO, Jensen DM. The short-term medical management of non-variceal upper gastrointestinal bleeding. Drugs. 2008;68(15):2105–11.

80. Labenz J, Peitz U, Leusing C, Tillenburg B, Blum AL, Borsch G. Efficacy of primed infusions with high dose ranitidine and omeprazole to maintain high intragastric pH in patients with peptic ulcer bleeding: a prospective randomised controlled study. Gut. 1997 Jan;40(1):36–41.

81. Leontiadis GI, Sharma VK, Howden CW. Proton pump inhibitor therapy for peptic ulcer bleeding: Cochrane collaboration meta-analysis of randomized controlled trials. Mayo Clin Proc. 2007 Mar;82(3):286–96.

82. Lin HJ, Lo WC, Cheng YC, Perng CL. Role of intravenous omeprazole in patients with high-risk peptic ulcer bleeding after successful endoscopic epinephrine injection: a prospective randomized comparative trial. Am J Gastroenterol. 2006 Mar;101(3):500–5.

83. Lin HJ, Lo WC, Lee FY, Perng CL, Tseng GY. A prospective randomized comparative trial showing that omeprazole prevents rebleeding in patients with bleeding peptic ulcer after successful endoscopic therapy. Arch Intern Med. 1998 Jan 12;158(1):54–8.

84. Johnson TJ, Hedge DD. Esomeprazole: a clinical review. Am J Health Syst Pharm. 2002 Jul 15;59(14):1333–9.

85. McKeage K, Blick SK, Croxtall JD, Lyseng-Williamson KA, Keating GM. Esomeprazole: a review of its use in the management of gastric acid-related diseases in adults. Drugs. 2008;68(11):1571–607.

86. Spencer CM, Faulds D. Esomeprazole. Drugs. 2000 Aug;60(2):321–9; discussion 30–1.

87. Junghard O, Hassan-Alin M, Hasselgren G. The effect of the area under the plasma concentration vs time curve and the maximum plasma concentration of esomeprazole on intragastric pH. Eur J Clin Pharmacol. 2002 Oct;58(7):453–8.

88. Li Y, Sha W, Nie Y, Wu H, She Q, Dai S, et al. Effect of intragastric pH on control of peptic ulcer bleeding. J Gastroenterol Hepatol. 2000 Feb;15(2):148–54.

89. Hasselgren G, Lind T, Lundell L, Aadland E, Efskind P, Falk A, et al. Continuous intravenous infusion of omeprazole in elderly patients with peptic ulcer bleeding. Results of a placebo-controlled multicenter study. Scand J Gastroenterol. 1997 May;32(4):328–33.

90. Netzer P, Gaia C, Sandoz M, Huluk T, Gut A, Halter F, et al. Effect of repeated injection and continuous infusion of omeprazole and ranitidine on intragastric pH over 72 hours. Am J Gastroenterol. 1999 Feb;94(2):351–7.

91. Kaviani MJ, Hashemi MR, Kazemifar AR, Roozitalab S, Mostaghni AA, Merat S, et al. Effect of oral omeprazole in reducing re-bleeding in bleeding peptic ulcers: a prospective, double-blind, randomized, clinical trial. Aliment Pharmacol Ther. 2003 Jan;17(2):211–6.

92. Khuroo MS, Yattoo GN, Javid G, Khan BA, Shah AA, Gulzar GM, et al. A comparison of omeprazole and placebo for bleeding peptic ulcer. N Engl J Med. 1997 Apr 10;336 (15):1054–8.

93. Lanas A, Artal A, Blas JM, Arroyo MT, Lopez-Zaborras J, Sainz R. Effect of parenteral omeprazole and ranitidine on gastric pH and the outcome of bleeding peptic ulcer. J Clin Gastroenterol. 1995 Sep;21(2):103–6.

94. Schaffalitzky de Muckadell OB, Havelund T, Harling H, Boesby S, Snel P, Vreeburg EM, et al. Effect of omeprazole on the outcome of endoscopically treated bleeding peptic ulcers. Randomized double-blind placebo-controlled multicentre study. Scand J Gastroenterol. 1997 May;32(4):320–7.

95. Yilmaz S, Bayan K, Tuzun Y, Dursun M, Canoruc F. A head to head comparison of oral vs intravenous omeprazole for patients with bleeding peptic ulcers with a clean base, flat spots and adherent clots. World J Gastroenterol. 2006 Dec 28;12(48):7837–43.

96. Stedman CA, Barclay ML. Review article: comparison of the pharmacokinetics, acid suppression and efficacy of proton pump inhibitors. Aliment Pharmacol Ther. 2000 Aug;14(8):963–78.

97. Gisbert JP, Gonzalez L, Calvet X, Roque M, Gabriel R, Pajares JM. Proton pump inhibitors versus H2-antagonists: a meta-analysis of their efficacy in treating bleeding peptic ulcer. Aliment Pharmacol Ther. 2001 Jul;15(7):917–26.

98. Barkun AN, Adam V, Sung JJ, Kuipers EJ, Mossner J, Jensen D, et al. Cost effectiveness of high-dose intravenous esomeprazole for peptic ulcer bleeding. Pharmacoeconomics. 2010 Mar 1;28(3):217–30.

99. Barkun AN, Cockeram AW, Plourde V, Fedorak RN. Review article: acid suppression in non-variceal acute upper gastrointestinal bleeding. Aliment Pharmacol Ther. 1999 Dec;13(12):1565–84.

100. Wang CH, Ma MH, Chou HC, Yen ZS, Yang CW, Fang CC, et al. High-dose vs non-high-dose proton pump inhibitors after endoscopic treatment in patients with bleeding peptic ulcer: a systematic review and meta-analysis of randomized controlled trials. Arch Intern Med. 2010 May 10;170(9):751–8.

101. Barkun A, Sabbah S, Enns R, Armstrong D, Gregor J, Fedorak RN, et al. The Canadian Registry on Nonvariceal Upper Gastrointestinal Bleeding and Endoscopy (RUGBE): Endoscopic hemostasis and proton pump inhibition are associated with improved outcomes in a real-life setting. Am J Gastroenterol. 2004 Jul;99(7):1238–46.

102. Simon-Rudler M, Massard J, Bernard-Chabert B, V DIM, Ratziu V, Poynard T, et al. Continuous infusion of high-dose omeprazole is more effective than standard-dose omeprazole in patients with high-risk peptic ulcer bleeding: a retrospective study. Aliment Pharmacol Ther. 2007 Apr 15;25(8):949–54.

103. Hasselgren G, Keelan M, Kirdeikis P, Lee J, Rohss K, Sinclair P, et al. Optimization of acid suppression for patients with peptic ulcer bleeding: an intragastric pH-metry study with omeprazole. Eur J Gastroenterol Hepatol. 1998 Jul;10(7):601–6.

104. van Rensburg CJ, Hartmann M, Thorpe A, Venter L, Theron I, Luhmann R, et al. Intragastric pH during continuous infusion with pantoprazole in patients with bleeding peptic ulcer. Am J Gastroenterol. 2003 Dec;98(12):2635–41.

105. Bardou M, Toubouti Y, Benhaberou-Brun D, Rahme E, Barkun AN. Meta-analysis: proton-pump inhibition in high-risk patients with acute peptic ulcer bleeding. Aliment Pharmacol Ther. 2005 Mar 15;21(6):677–86.

106. Thomopoulos KC, Vagenas KA, Vagianos CE, Margaritis VG, Blikas AP, Katsakoulis EC, et al. Changes in aetiology and clinical outcome of acute upper gastrointestinal bleeding during the last 15 years. Eur J Gastroenterol Hepatol. 2004 Feb;16 (2):177–82.

107. Lin HJ, Tseng GY, Hsieh YH, Perng CL, Lee FY, Chang FY, et al. Will Helicobacter pylori affect short-term rebleeding rate in peptic ulcer bleeding patients after successful endoscopic therapy? Am J Gastroenterol. 1999 Nov;94(11):3184–8.

108. Schilling D, Demel A, Nusse T, Weidmann E, Riemann JF. Helicobacter pylori infection does not affect the early rebleeding rate in patients with peptic ulcer bleeding after successful endoscopic hemostasis: a prospective single-center trial. Endoscopy. 2003 May;35(5):393–6.

109. Gisbert JP, Abraira V. Accuracy of Helicobacter pylori diagnostic tests in patients with bleeding peptic ulcer: a systematic review and meta-analysis. Am J Gastroenterol. 2006 May;101(4):848–63.

110. Tulassay Z, Stolte M, Engstrand L, Butruk E, Malfertheiner P, Dite P, et al. Twelve-month endoscopic and histological analysis following proton-pump inhibitor-based triple therapy in Helicobacter pylori-positive patients with gastric ulcers. Scand J Gastroenterol. 2010 Sep;45(9):1048–58.

111. Pruitt RE, Truss CD. Endoscopy, gastric ulcer, and gastric cancer. Follow-up endoscopy for all gastric ulcers?Dig Dis Sci. 1993 Feb;38(2):284–8.

112. Lee JG, Turnipseed S, Romano PS, Vigil H, Azari R, Melnikoff N, et al. Endoscopy-based triage significantly reduces hospitalization rates and costs of treating upper GI bleeding: a randomized controlled trial. Gastrointest Endosc. 1999 Dec;50(6):755–61.

113. Bjorkman DJ, Zaman A, Fennerty MB, Lieberman D, Disario JA, Guest-Warnick G. Urgent vs. elective endoscopy for acute non-variceal upper-GI bleeding: an effectiveness study. Gastrointest Endosc. 2004 Jul;60(1):1–8.

114. Tai CM, Huang SP, Wang HP, Lee TC, Chang CY, Tu CH, et al. High-risk ED patients with nonvariceal upper gastrointestinal hemorrhage undergoing emergency or urgent endoscopy: a retrospective analysis. Am J Emerg Med. 2007 Mar;25(3):273–8.

115. Lin HJ, Wang K, Perng CL, Chua RT, Lee FY, Lee CH, et al. Early or delayed endoscopy for patients with peptic ulcer bleeding. A prospective randomized study. J Clin Gastroenterol. 1996 Jun;22(4):267–71.

116. Cooper GS, Chak A, Connors AF, Jr., Harper DL, Rosenthal GE. The effectiveness of early endoscopy for upper gastrointestinal hemorrhage: a community-based analysis. Med Care. 1998 May;36(4):462–74.

117. Cooper GS, Chak A, Way LE, Hammar PJ, Harper DL, Rosenthal GE. Early endoscopy in upper gastrointestinal hemorrhage: associations with recurrent bleeding, surgery, and length of hospital stay. Gastrointest Endosc. 1999 Feb;49(2):145–52.

118. Lau JY, Chung SC, Leung JW, Lo KK, Yung MY, Li AK. The evolution of stigmata of hemorrhage in bleeding peptic ulcers: a sequential endoscopic study. Endoscopy. 1998 Aug;30(6):513–8.

119. Katschinski B, Logan R, Davies J, Faulkner G, Pearson J, Langman M. Prognostic factors in upper gastrointestinal bleeding. Dig Dis Sci. 1994 May;39(4):706–12.

120. Laine L, Peterson WL. Bleeding peptic ulcer. N Engl J Med. 1994 Sep 15;331 (11):717–27.

121. Cipolletta L, Bianco MA, Marmo R, Rotondano G, Piscopo R, Vingiani AM, et al. Endoclips versus heater probe in preventing early recurrent bleeding from peptic

ulcer: a prospective and randomized trial. Gastrointest Endosc. 2001 Feb;53 (2):147–51.

122. Laine L, Estrada R. Randomized trial of normal saline solution injection versus bipolar electrocoagulation for treatment of patients with high-risk bleeding ulcers: is local tamponade enough?Gastrointest Endosc. 2002 Jan;55(1):6–10.

123. Gevers AM, De Goede E, Simoens M, Hiele M, Rutgeerts P. A randomized trial comparing injection therapy with hemoclip and with injection combined with hemoclip for bleeding ulcers. Gastrointest Endosc. 2002 May;55(4):466–9.

124. Chau CH, Siu WT, Law BK, Tang CN, Kwok SY, Luk YW, et al. Randomized controlled trial comparing epinephrine injection plus heat probe coagulation versus epineph-rine injection plus argon plasma coagulation for bleeding peptic ulcers. Gastrointest Endosc. 2003 May;57(4):455–61.

125. Soon MS, Wu SS, Chen YY, Fan CS, Lin OS. Monopolar coagulation versus conventional endoscopic treatment for high-risk peptic ulcer bleeding: a prospective, randomized study. Gastrointest Endosc. 2003 Sep;58(3):323–9.

126. Lin HJ, Perng CL, Sun IC, Tseng GY. Endoscopic haemoclip versus heater probe thermocoagulation plus hypertonic saline-epinephrine injection for peptic ulcer bleeding. Dig Liver Dis. 2003 Dec;35(12):898–902.

127. Chou YC, Hsu PI, Lai KH, Lo CC, Chan HH, Lin CP, et al. A prospective, randomized trial of endoscopic hemoclip placement and distilled water injection for treatment of high-risk bleeding ulcers. Gastrointest Endosc. 2003 Mar;57(3):324–8.

128. LJubicic N, Supanc V, Vrsalovic M. Efficacy of endoscopic clipping for actively bleeding peptic ulcer: comparison with polidocanol injection therapy. Hepatogas-troenterology. 2004 Mar-Apr;51(56):408–12.

129. Saltzman JR, Strate LL, Di Sena V, Huang C, Merrifield B, Ookubo R, et al. Prospective trial of endoscopic clips versus combination therapy in upper GI bleeding (PROTECCT–UGI bleeding). Am J Gastroenterol. 2005 Jul;100(7):1503–8.

130. Lo CC, Hsu PI, Lo GH, Lin CK, Chan HH, Tsai WL, et al. Comparison of hemostatic efficacy for epinephrine injection alone and injection combined with hemoclip therapy in treating high-risk bleeding ulcers. Gastrointest Endosc. 2006 May;63 (6):767–73.

131. den Hoed CM, Kuipers EJ. Esomeprazole for the treatment of peptic ulcer bleeding. Expert Rev Gastroenterol Hepatol. 2010 Dec;4(6):679–95.

132. Jensen DM, Pace SC, Soffer E, Comer GM. Continuous infusion of pantoprazole versus ranitidine for prevention of ulcer rebleeding: a U.S. multicenter randomized, double-blind study. Am J Gastroenterol. 2006 Sep;101(9):1991–9; quiz 2170.

133. Zargar SA, Javid G, Khan BA, Yattoo GN, Shah AH, Gulzar GM, et al. Pantoprazole infusion as adjuvant therapy to endoscopic treatment in patients with peptic ulcer bleeding: prospective randomized controlled trial. J Gastroenterol Hepatol. 2006 May;21(4):716–21.

134. Lau JY, Sung JJ, Lee KK, Yung MY, Wong SK, Wu JC, et al. Effect of intravenous omeprazole on recurrent bleeding after endoscopic treatment of bleeding peptic ulcers. N Engl J Med. 2000 Aug 3;343(5):310–6.

135. Malfertheiner P, Megraud F, O'Morain C, Bazzoli F, El-Omar E, Graham D, et al. Current concepts in the management of Helicobacter pylori infection: the Maastricht III Consensus Report. Gut. 2007 Jun;56(6):772–81.

136. Graham DY, Fischbach L. Helicobacter pylori treatment in the era of increasing antibiotic resistance. Gut. 2010 Aug;59(8):1143–53.

CHAPTER 5

Peptic Ulcer Bleeding: Surgery and Radiology

Irene M. Mulder[1], Ernst J. Kuipers[2] & Johan F. Lange[1]

[1]Department of Surgery, Erasmus MC University Medical Centre, Rotterdam, the Netherlands
[2]Department of Gastroenterology and Hepatology, Erasmus MC University Medical Centre, Rotterdam, the Netherlands

Introduction

The role of surgical therapy in peptic ulcer disease (PUD) has changed dramatically during the last two decades. Conservative treatment has improved with the development of anti-secretory agents and the discovery of the strong association of *Helicobacter pylori* with PUD. As a result of these improvements, surgery for peptic ulcer disease has become almost obsolete. The two main exceptions are surgery for ulcer bleeding refractory to endoscopic treatment, and for ulcer perforation. Other rare indications for surgical treatment for peptic ulcer disease include patients with refractory ulcers in the presence of severe fibrosis or local ischemia, and patients with gastric outlet stenosis due to stricturing as a result of recurrent pyloric or duodenal ulceration.

Before the development of therapeutic endoscopy, 35–55% of patients with significant upper gastrointestinal hemorrhage required emergency surgery. This was associated with a mortality rate of 10–30% (1–4). The need for surgery changed dramatically with the gradual introduction of endoscopic therapy, and the demonstration that such therapy was associated with a favorable outcome. This development was further enhanced by the demonstration that recurrent bleeding could also first be treated by endoscopy. In a randomized controlled trial comparing endoscopic retreatment and surgery in 92 patients with recurrent peptic ulcer bleeding (PUB) after initial endoscopic control, endoscopic retreatment reduced the need for surgery without increasing the risk of death (5). Rebleeding did not occur in 72% of patients undergoing repeat endoscopy. The 30-day mortality did not significantly differ for patients undergoing repeat endoscopy and those undergoing surgery (10% vs. 18%) (5).

Based on these results, surgery is nowadays restricted to cases with primary or secondary bleeding refractory to endoscopic treatment. For these cases, transcatheter arterial embolization (TAE) has evolved as alternative, less invasive treatment. With this new treatment modality, the need for surgery decreased to only 1.9–5.4% of patients presenting with PUB (5–8). This chapter deals with TAE and surgery for refractory and recurrent peptic ulcer bleeding.

Indications for transcatheter arterial embolization and surgical treatment

Severe bleeding despite conservative medical treatment and endoscopic intervention occurs in 5–14% of patients (7, 9–11). In these patients more invasive treatment is warranted. Indications for TAE or surgery are:

1 Significant PUB (transfusion requirement of at least 4 U blood/24 h) or hemodynamic instability (hypotension with systolic pressure <100 mmHg and heart rate of 100/min or clinical shock secondary to blood loss)
2 PUB that has failed to respond to conservative medical therapy, including volume replacement, antacids, H2-receptor blocking agents, or proton pump inhibitors
3 Bleeding that has failed to respond to at least one, and sometimes two, attempts at endoscopic control (12)
4 Confirmed presence (or very strong clinical suspicion) of malignancy, usually in a gastric ulcer.

Risk factors for recurrent bleeding are (13):
• age over 60
• high comorbidity, especially cardiopulmonary disease
• initial severe hemorrhage
• active bleeding grade Ia, according to the Forrest classification (endoscopy)
• clot or visible vessel classified IIa, according to Forrest classification
• large ulcers > 2 cm (5), especially when localized at the posterior wall of the duodenal bulb or minor curvature (14).

Transcatheter arterial embolization

TAE is based on arterial catheterization under fluoroscopic guidance. Feeding arteries in the bleeding area are selectively catheterized followed by contrast injection. Once a bleeding focus has been visualized by extravasation of contrast (Fig. 5.1), thrombogenic material can be injected selectively through the same catheter, leading to local thrombus formation

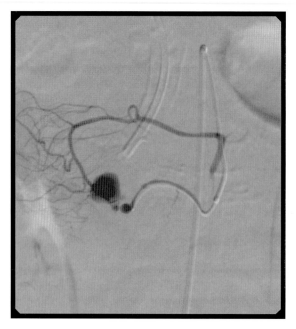

Figure 5.1 Contrast extravasation during angiography, showing an active bleeding focus

and arterial occlusion, thus stopping the bleed (Fig. 5.2). It is desirable to correct any coagulopathy before or directly following embolization because termination of bleeding and prevention of bleeding recurrence depend on technically successful embolization as well as effective coagulation.

This therapeutic embolization has been successfully applied in virtually every vascular territory to arrest hemorrhage, occlude congenital and acquired vascular abnormalities, palliate neoplasms, and ablate tissue (15). In 1972 TAE was first described for the treatment of acute gastrointestinal bleeding (16) and in 1974 for bleeding duodenal ulcer (17). The increased utilization of TAE in particular in the past 15 years reflects the general shift to minimally invasive treatment. This development was accelerated by major improvements in endovascular technology and embolization materials, enabling safe, selective catheterization of small vessels. Such superselective catheterization leads to more durable hemostasis and reduces ischemic complications.

Angiography

In most patients presenting with PUB, the cause and location of hemorrhage have been identified by previous endoscopy and angiography is only performed as a precursor to endovascular therapeutic intervention. Vascular access is usually obtained by inserting a sheath in the common femoral artery. In case of severe vascular stenosis the brachial artery can be used. Once vascular access has been obtained, arteriography is performed to

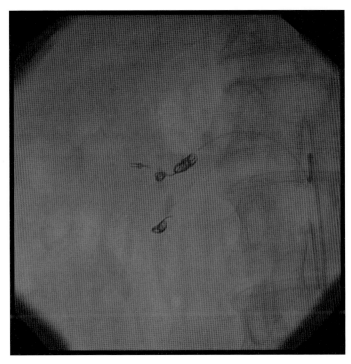

Figure 5.2 Coiling of the gastroduodenal artery in a patient with recurrent peptic ulcer bleeding. After coiling, there is no further extravasation of contrast

visualize the arterial anatomy of the mesenteric vessels and to identify contrast extravasation. For diagnostic angiography in PUB, knowledge on the anatomy of the celiac artery is indispensable.

Because significant hemorrhage mostly originates from the duodenum, our anatomical description starts here (Fig. 5.3). The duodenum is supplied

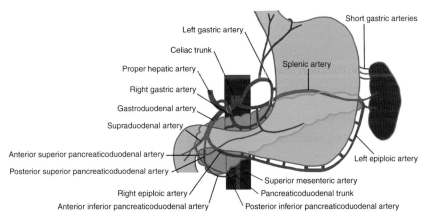

Figure 5.3 Anatomy of the arterial vascularization of the stomach and proximal small bowel

with arterial blood by the gastroduodenal artery (GDA), the superior mesenteric artery (SMA), and, rarely, the supraduodenal artery which originates from the proper hepatic artery. GDA originates from the common hepatic artery or celiac axis in the majority of patients, but may also originate from the right hepatic artery.

A rich arterial communication exists between GDA and SMA via the pancreatic arteries and inferior pancreatico-duodenal artery. Retrograde hemorrhage after embolization of the GDA may therefore be caused by the blood supply from this arcade.

Different parts of the stomach are supplied with blood by different arteries (Fig. 5.3). The lesser curvature of the stomach and the distal oesophagus are supplied by branches of the left gastric artery, which originates from the celiac artery. These branches are related to distal branches of the short gastric arteries from the splenic artery (*vasa brevia*) and branches of the right gastric artery.

The gastro-epiploic arcade supplies the greater curvature of the stomach and originates from the right gastro-epipolic artery, which originates from the gastroduodenal branch of the common hepatic artery, and the left gastro-epiploic artery, a branch of the distal splenic artery. The arcade is complete in about 65% of patients.

Extravasation of contrast into the lumen of the intestine or a false aneurysm-like lesion demonstrates the origin of the bleeding ulcer. Extravasation of contrast is observed in 54% to 63% of patients with bleeding PUB undergoing angiography (Fig. 5.1) (18, 19). Because of the intermittent nature of gastrointestinal bleeding, the site of bleeding can be missed by highly selective angiography. The likelihood of identifying the bleeding source is higher when the arteriogram is performed promptly after the start of or during active bleeding. Furthermore, a positive angiography requires more than oozing bleeding in order to obtain sufficient extravasation into the bowel and thus radiographically visualize the bleeding (20).

Clips placed during endoscopy at the junction of the ulcer mostly remain in position for several days and may help to localize the branches feeding the bleeding ulcer (21). Superselective angiography guided by clip position is more likely to visualize the extravasation, thus making blind coil placement unnecessary (Fig. 5.4). This increases the efficacy of the procedure, and decreases the risk of coil misplacement and inadvertent hepatic embolization (21, 22). It thus also reduces the need for repeat angiography after a negative procedure or misplaced coils. Clip placement is also helpful when the bleeding artery arises separately from the proper hepatic artery or the gastroduodenal artery. In rare cases, the size of the bleeding vessel may be thus large that the catheter can be forwarded directly into the gastric or duodenal lumen, with contrast filling of the lumen (Fig. 5.5).

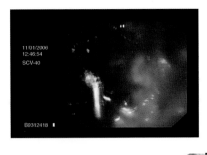

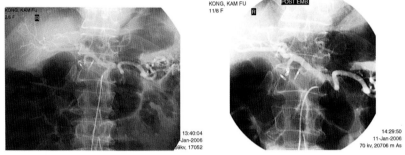

Figure 5.4 Endoscopically placed hemoclip marking the bleeding focus enabling highly selective angiography

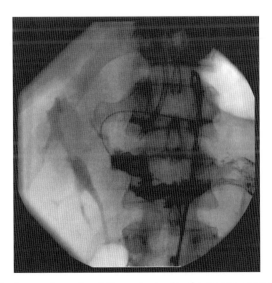

Figure 5.5 Selective angiography of the gastroduodenal artery in a patient with a large bleeding ulcer. The size of the vascular lesion allows passage of the cathether into the duodenum, with contrast filling of the lumen

Infusion of pharmacologic agents, such as t-PA, intra-arterial antic-oagulants or vasodilators, has been tried to temporarily increase the rate of hemorrhage during angiography to facilitate angiographic iden-tification and localization of the gastro-intestinal bleeding lesion (23, 24). There has been a large variation in rates of identification of the bleed-ing site in studies using this technique of provocative angiography. The reported rate of identification varies from 29% to 80%, probably reflecting differences in patient selection, drug regime used, routes of delivery (systemic vs. local), duration of time from bleeding, and operator experience (24–26).

Embolization

Once the bleeding vessel has been identified by extravasation of contrast, the vessel needs to be embolized as distal as possible. This leads to control of the bleed in 72 to 100% of patients (22, 27, 28). Recurrent bleeding occurs in 9–66% of patients, in particular in case of multiple or large duodenal ulcers, persistent coagulopathy, or multi-organ failure (29, 30).

Various embolic materials have been used including coils, polyvinyl alcohol (PVA) particles, blood clot, gelfoam, alcohol, and cyano-acrylate glue. Large embolic agents such as coils and gelfoam may be used for embolization of large vessels at sites with abundant collateral supply. These embolic agents cause, like surgical ligation, a decrease in arterial pressure at the site of hemorrhage. This can result in more effective clotting and a reduction in bleeding. Collateral supply will usually maintain ade-quate perfusion of the vascular bed to prevent ischemic complications. Liquid agents such as alcohol and glue will embolize up to the most distal vascular supply and cause infarction by occluding the smallest arterioles supplying the lesion. This results in necrosis. For bleeding peptic ulcer, however, the most optimal choice of embolic agent remains controversial. In most series the choice for an embolic agent was at the discretion of the interventional radiologist. Although many series were relatively small and non-comparative, some conclusions can be drawn. Firstly, mono-therapy with gelatin sponges was associated with low success rates. For instance, in a series of 29 patients treated with gelatin sponge TAE, the bleeding was stopped in only 62% (31). Monotherapy with PVA particles or gelfoam may lead to higher success rates, but has been reported to be associated with rates of recurrent bleeding up to 40% (32). The same group reported that the use of tissue adhesive for occlusion of the distal vasculature of GDA was effective but associated with later development of duodenal strictures in 40% of patients, which was likely related to embolization of terminal muscular branches. This is a serious contraindication for the use of tissue adhesives for this indication. The use of coils has been proven to be a successful approach for patients with PUB, if adequate care is taken to perform sandwich

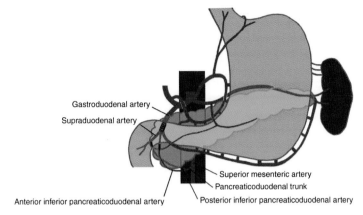

Gastroduodenal artery

Supraduodenal artery

Superior mesenteric artery

Pancreaticoduodenal trunk

Anterior inferior pancreaticoduodenal artery

Posterior inferior pancreaticoduodenal artery

Figure 5.6 Sandwich embolization of the gastroduodenal artery with use of proximal and distal coils

embolization with coiling of the arterial trunk of GDA (Fig. 5.6). In addition, it is well known that successful embolization with coils depends on the number of coils used. The use of n-butyl cyanoacrylate in combination with gelatine sponges or coils may significantly decrease the length of the TAE procedure. This is especially important in case of massive bleeding that requires urgent hemostasis, in particular in patients with coagulopathy. Early clinical success was reported in 22 (65%) of 34 patients treated by sandwich embolization of GDA using coils released distally and proximally in combination with gelatine sponge placed in the arterial trunk (28). Together, these results support the tendency for the use of coils as first approach in TAE for PUB.

Various series reported technical success rates of endovascular treatment ranging from 91 to 100% (27, 28, 33). Technical success was in most series defined as complete proximal and distal occlusion of the gastroduodenal artery with no residual extravasation of contrast at the end of the procedure (29). Reasons for failure of endovascular embolization are difficult vascular anatomy, presence of arterial dissection, vasospasm, false-negatively read angiogram, multiple bleeding sites, and tumorous bleeding (18).

After technically successful embolization, 72 to 100% of patients have a good clinical response with cessation of bleeding (22, 27, 28). When endoscopy is performed at this stage, a coil may occasionally be seen in the ulcer bed (Fig. 5.7). A small group has signs of ongoing bleeding despite lack of persistent extravasation of contrast during TAE. This is usually due to temporary stop of the bleed, multiple bleeding sites, or collateral feeding of the lesion. Rebleeding occurs in 35% (22). Possible predictors of rebleeding are presence of multiple or large duodenal ulcers, coagulopathy, longer time

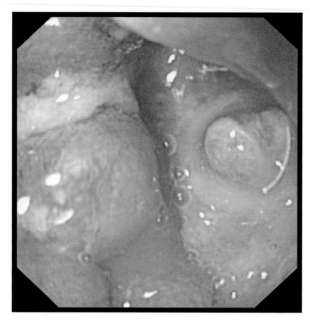

Figure 5.7 Visible coil in a duodenal ulcer several days after angiography of the gastroduodenal artery for recurrent bleeding refractory to endoscopic treatment

from shock onset to angiography, a larger number of RBC units transfused before angiography, having ≥ 2 comorbid conditions, previous surgery for bleeding, shock or multi-organ failure (22,27,34–37). More than half of patients who continue to bleed respond to repeat embolization (5).

In patients without contrast extravasation, blind embolization can be performed but the reported results of such an approach are disappointing. Patients without active bleeding on the angiogram have a lower likelihood of lasting hemostasis. In one study comparing 12 patients with extravasation versus 9 patients without extravasation during TAE, recurrent bleeding after targeted respectively blind embolization occurred in 25 versus 33% (38). In another study on 64 patients with upper gastrointestinal bleeding without angiographic evidence of contrast extravasation, the proportion of patients who required surgery for bleeding control was similar in the patients who did not undergo embolization as in the patients who underwent blind embolization (39). However, others reported similar clinical outcomes between patients who underwent blind embolization and those who underwent embolization after angiographic proof of bleeding (22, 30, 36).

During blind embolization a "sandwich technique" is used, in which both ends of the artery thought to be responsible for the bleeding are filled with embolic material to avoid retrograde bleeding from the collateral circulation (Fig. 5.6). This means that in many cases, approached from the celiac artery as well as from the superior mesenteric artery, both the gastroduodenal and pancreaticoduodenal vessels have to be catheterized and embolized (40).

Complications

Complications related to endovascular treatment occur in 5–26% of cases (18). Complications can be due to the angiographic procedure or the actual embolization. Complications associated with the angiography are access site thrombosis or hemorrhage, contrast reactions, and injury to the target vessels, specifically the superior mesenteric artery, inferior mesenteric artery and celiac artery including dissection and distal embolization (20). In a review on 819 patients embolization-related complications were reported in 9% of cases, including liver and spleen infarction, gastro-intestinal ischemia and duodenal stenosis. Ischemia is rare because of the rich collateral supply of the stomach and duodenum. However, the risk of ischemia is increased in patients with a history of previous upper abdominal surgery, as well as in patients in whom embolic agents that can advance far into the vascular bed such as liquid agents and very small particles are being used (34, 41–43). Duodenal stenosis was reported mostly after use of tissue adhesive (32) and is thought to be caused by severe hypoxia and resulting avascular necrosis. But stenosis has also been described after chronic peptic ulcer disease without bleeding. Endoscopic balloon dilatation can be attempted as a first step, but surgical correction is required in patients with persistent symptoms of duodenal obstruction.

Mortality

Mortality rates after TAE ranged in various series between 4 % and 46 % (32, 44). This wide range is similar to the rate described in some surgical series for emergent open repair of PUB (45, 46). However, in a large proportion of these patients, mortality is not directly related to persistent bleeding, but caused by concomitant disease and complications of the bleed, such as aspiration pneumonia and cerebrovascular events. Mortality and complication rates vary between series, and this is possibly related to case selection and TAE experience. Recent studies, however, showed that low mortality rates can be achieved in high volume centres with considerable expertise (47).

When interpreting mortality rates in various series, one should be aware that some accept TAE as immediate treatment after failed endoscopic treatment, whereas others only refer patients for TAE if open surgical repair is not feasible, in particular because of comorbidity and advanced age. In one series, mortality was significantly lower in patients with angiographic extravasation and successful embolization compared to patients requiring surgery after failed embolization (38 vs. 83% mortality rate) (39). Only 20% of the patients who initially underwent embolization finally needed surgical intervention to control recurrent bleeding. This indicates that TAE can decrease the need for surgery in patients with acute PUB.

Patients with recurrent bleeding not fit for surgery can be treated with embolization repeatedly. A previously performed embolization is not a contraindication for recurrent angiographic intervention in case of a rebleeding (44, 48).

Surgery

Introduction
Surgery is the salvage treatment of choice for patients in whom bleeding cannot be controlled by endoscopy or interventional radiology. With the increased efficacy of the former two methods, the definite indications and timing of surgery are a matter of debate (49).

Whether to consider repeated therapeutic endoscopy or surgical intervention as a first choice for patients with recurrent bleeding after primary endoscopic treatment has been investigated in a randomized controlled trial from Hong Kong (5). In this trial, 100 patients with rebleeding after previous successful endoscopic treatment for peptic ulcer bleeding were randomized to either undergo endoscopic retreatment or surgery. Permanent hemostasis was achieved in 73% of patients treated by endoscopy, versus 93% of those treated with surgery. Complications occurred in respectively 14 and 36% while mortality was equal in both groups. Predictors for failure of endoscopic treatment were hypotension prior to the second endoscopy and an ulcer diameter larger than 2 cm. The authors concluded that in patients with recurrent peptic ulcer bleeding, repeat endoscopic treatment is the approach of first choice, because it reduces the need for surgery without increasing the risk of death and with fewer complications than surgery.

Surgical techniques and outcome
The most important determinant of a successful surgical procedure to control hemorrhage from peptic ulcer disease is the ability to accurately locate the site or sites of hemorrhage (50). This is generally much easier to do endoscopically rather than by direct intra-operative inspection. Therefore presence of the surgeon during or performing preoperative endoscopy is advisable to optimize understanding of the anatomic location of the source of hemorrhage. The choice of operation is mainly determined by anatomical and pathological considerations, and the experience and judgement of the surgeon. Expertise in the surgical management of bleeding ulcers remains an important integral part of a dedicated upper gastrointestinal bleeding team (14). The choice for the most optimal surgical treatment strategy is

primarily based on trials using mortality as endpoint. In the presence of profound acid suppressive therapy and other measures to prevent ulcer recurrence, such as *Helicobacter pylori* eradication, the aim of emergency surgery is to control the hemorrhage, and no longer to cure ulcer diathesis. However, most of controlled clinical trials comparing various surgical techniques were done before the routine use of proton pump inhibitors and promoted more invasive surgery with addition of acid reduction procedures. Under these circumstances various procedures have been suggested to reduce acid secretion such as partial gastrectomy or vagotomy. Acid secretion by the parietal cells is normally stimulated by acetylcholine from the vagus nerve and gastrin release from the antrum. Thus, surgical approaches attempted to reduce this secretion by sectioning the vagal nerves (vagotomy), eliminating hormonal stimulation from the antrum (antrectomy), or by also decreasing the acid secretory capacity by means of a (sub-) total gastric resection). These definite approaches are nowadays reserved for the rare patients with PUD in whom all medical treatment fails. Complications that can arise after these procedures are continuing ulcer disease caused by incomplete vagotomy, postvagotomy diarrhea, dumping syndrome and reflux gastritis. Also complications of gastric resection such as anastomotic leakage, dumping syndrome, gastric stump carcinoma, and ulcer formation of the ascending jejunal limb are well known.

In the last two decades, most surgeons routinely perform "conservative" surgery for bleeding duodenal and pyloric ulcers. This firstly implies opening of the duodenal bulb and/or pylorus along its length at the anterior side (Fig. 5.8). Sometimes a wide pyloro-duodenotomy may be necessary to inspect the duodenal bulb and gastric antrum if endoscopy has failed to precisely identify the source of hemorrhage. Control of the hemorrhage is obtained by oversewing the (most frequently) bleeding gastroduodenal artery with non-absorbable suture material. Care must be taken not to include the distal retroduodenal common bile duct in the suture. In rare cases additional ligation of the gastroduodenal artery above and below the duodenum may be undertaken, and if necessary combined with ligation of the right gastro-epiploic and anterior superior pancreaticoduodenal arteries, but this is not the standard operation technique. The efficacy of this procedure has not been established and it may be difficult and dangerous when edema is present, because of risk of inducing pancreatitis. Subsequently the duodenum is closed transversely to prevent stenosis.

This limited approach was applied in 22 consecutive patients undergoing emergency surgery for PUB in one series (46). Only two patients had a rebleeding (9%) and five patients (22%) died of non-bleeding related causes (multivisceral failures). In the conservative treatment group with double GDA ligation, no patients experienced rebleeding. With these success of "conservative" surgical management, vagotomy alone or with antrectomy

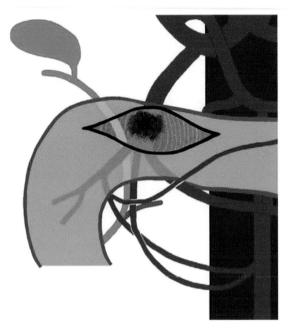

Figure 5.8 Duodenum opened by transverse incision for treatment of a bleeding peptic ulcer

has become outdated for most patients. Bleeding recurrence rate was reduced by conservative surgical treatment but mortality remained stable due to non-bleeding related causes. Oversewing of the ulcer appears the safest and easiest approach, but does not offer certainty about the histological character of the ulcer. The main indication for limited resection of the gastric ulcer or antrectomy is to rule out malignancy if suspected. When the ulcer is located high at the small curvature excision is most safely performed with a large nasogastric tube in the stomach to prevent stenosis. Subcardial ulcers, located within 2–5 cm of the esophageogastric junction, can sometimes not safely be excised without jeopardizing gastrointestinal continuity. For these ulcers sometimes partial gastrectomy with gastrojejunostomy has to be performed. Very rare cases with a stenotic pylorobulbic region sometimes also require gastric resection or gastrojejunostomy. These cases are often characterized by the presence of larger chronic ulcers (over 2 cm) at the posterior duodenal bulb. These chronic "giant" ulcers can also be found high at the lesser curve and then sometimes require partial gastrectomy.

Timing of surgery, complications and post-operative management

The optimal timing of surgical intervention remains a difficult clinical decision particularly for patients with a high risk of rebleeding. Various concepts of early elective surgery have been tested, mainly based on the bleeding activity at emergency endoscopy described according to the Forrest classification. From older studies it has become clear that if endoscopic treatment fails in patients with active bleeding or a visible vessel, surgery should be performed within 24 hours. In patients with a high risk of rebleeding a defensive strategy with early surgery is thought to neutralize the risk of recurrent bleeding and death. For such an approach with early elective surgery gastroenterologists should select patients with a high risk of rebleeding based on the view during endoscopy (14). Possible short-term complications of surgery are in particular recurrent bleeding, leakage of the pyloro-duodenal incision, and short term functional disorders (46). Further management is performed as after endoscopy, in particular with profound acid suppressive therapy, identification and treatment of the underlying cause of the bleeding ulcer, and early restitution of oral feeding.

TAE versus surgery

No randomized controlled trial has been conducted to compare TAE with surgery in PUB after failed endoscopic treatment. However, three retrospective studies reported similar results with both techniques in terms of recurrent bleeding, morbity, and mortality. Firstly, Ripoll et al. assessed 70 patients with refractory PUB who underwent TAE (31 patients) or surgery (39 patients) (51). The allocation to treatment was decided on an individual basis by attending physicians. Patients treated with TAE were older (mean age about 10 years higher) and had higher rates of cardiovascular disease and anticoagulation treatment. In the embolization group, the technical failure rate was 6.5% (n = 2) and the rebleeding rate was 29% (n = 9). Four of the patients with persistent bleeding underwent surgical exploration. In the surgery group, the rebleeding rate was 23% (n = 9); five of these patients underwent a repeat surgical procedure for bleeding control. In addition, seven other patients required repeat surgery for complications from the initial operation. Overall, the embolization and surgery groups were not significantly different regarding the need for additional surgery (16% vs. 31%, respectively) or survival (26% vs. 20%, respectively). However, the re-intervention rate was considerably higher in the surgery group.

Secondly, Eriksson et al. compared 91 patients with upper GI bleeding after failed endoscopic therapy. Forty patients were treated with angiographic embolization and 51 with surgery. The angiographic embolization group was older and had a higher comorbidity rate. Mortality after 30 days was lower in the patients undergoing angiographic embolization (3% vs. 14%) (52).

Finally, Venclauskas et al compared the efficacy of TAE and surgery after failed endoscopic therapy for acute duodenal ulcer bleeding in 74 patients (53). Treatment allocation was decided by the treating surgeon. Fifty patients underwent surgery and 24 patients were treated with embolization. The TAE group was older, had more concomitant disease, higher APACHE-scores, lower rates of active bleeding, and had undergone more endoscopies before the attempted definite treatment. However, there was no difference in rebleeding rate and mortality rate between the groups. Of note, in patients with an APACHE score > 16.5, the mortality rate was twice as high in the surgery group compared with the TAE group.

These findings raise the question whether TAE should be considered the first alternative treatment of choice in recurrent hemorrhage after endoscopic therapy. In many patients with concomitant disease, surgical treatment has a high incidence of morbidity and mortality. Negative or impractical endoscopy because of severe bleeding in hemodynamically unstable patients should prompt urgent angiography, whereas re-endoscopy should be first considered in stable patients (47). TAE is a promising treatment for these high-risk patients. But the higher rate of rebleeding after TAE with mortality rates similar to surgical therapy gives rise to the question if TAE should only be offered to patients with high APACHE-score (48, 53). Unfortunately TAE is not available in every hospital, and successful outcome of TAE, like other procedures such as endoscopy and surgery, requires a well trained team and a dedicated physician. Recently TAE performed by surgical staff has been proposed with advantages as continuous in-house availability of surgical staff and continuity-of-care (54). Irrespective of the background of the performing physician, the issue of TAE versus surgery therefore has to be addressed in a randomized controlled trial with stratification by APACHE-score.

Conclusions

A variety of alternatives for the treatment of PUB after endoscopic failure has emerged during the last two decades. The safety and efficacy of transcatheter embolization for the treatment of life-threatening bleeding peptic ulcer is now widely accepted and should, together with surgery, be considered the gold standard for endoscopy-refractory patients. The exact position of both treatments has to be further determined. The existing evidence suggests that there is no difference between conservative and radical surgery concerning mortality but this has to be proven by further data. Most clinical evidence with regard to the extent of the surgical approach is limited by the old date of the related research under totally different circumstances with regard to pharmacologic and endoscopic potencies. Conservative procedures seem to have benefited from early effective medical treatment and technical improvements thus outweighing the results of invasive surgery, which is associated with substantial morbidity. As a rule vagotomy is no longer performed due to a high recurrence rate and more effective prevention of ulcer recurrence by *Helicobacter pylori* eradication and PPI administration. As most surgical centers in Western countries nowadays perform fewer surgical interventions for bleeding peptic ulcer, procedures should be done by selected GI surgeons with sufficient experience with these procedures (55).

With the adequate further treatment options, surgical procedures in emergency situations should be limited to safe hemostasis. For bleeding gastric ulcer, ulcer excision is the operative procedure of choice, except for large, chronic, penetrating ulcers, in which a more radical procedure like gastric resection is still sometimes mandatory. Subsequently for bleeding duodenal ulcers ligation of GDA is preferable. The addition of acid reduction surgery must now be considered obsolete as a result of the availability of PPI (49). Only in very rare cases must gastric resection be considered.

References

1. Cook DJ, Guyatt GH, Salena BJ, Laine LA. Endoscopic therapy for acute nonvariceal upper gastrointestinal hemorrhage: a meta-analysis. Gastroenterology 1992;102(1): 139–48.
2. Goldman ML, Land WC, Bradley EL, Anderson RT. Transcatheter therapeutic embolization in the management of massive upper gastrointestinal bleeding. Radiology 1976;120(3):513–21.
3. Sacks HS, Chalmers TC, Blum AL, Berrier J, Pagano D. Endoscopic hemostasis. An effective therapy for bleeding peptic ulcers. JAMA 1990;264(4):494–9.
4. Vellacott KD, Dronfield MW, Atkinson M, Langman MJ. Comparison of surgical and medical management of bleeding peptic ulcers. Br Med J (Clin Res Ed) 1982; 284(6315):548–50.
5. Lau JY, Sung JJ, Lam YH, Chan AC, Ng EK, Lee DW, et al. Endoscopic retreatment compared with surgery in patients with recurrent bleeding after initial endoscopic control of bleeding ulcers. N Engl J Med 1999;340(10):751–6.
6. Hearnshaw SA, Logan RF, Lowe D, Travis SP, Murphy MF, Palmer KR. Use of endoscopy for management of acute upper gastrointestinal bleeding in the UK: Results of a nationwide audit. Gut 2010;59(8):1022–9.
7. Sung JJ, Barkun A, Kuipers EJ, Mossner J, Jensen DM, Stuart R, et al. Intravenous esomeprazole for prevention of recurrent peptic ulcer bleeding: a randomized trial. Ann Intern Med 2009;150(7):455–64.
8. Zargar SA, Javid G, Khan BA, Yattoo GN, Shah AH, Gulzar GM, et al. Pantoprazole infusion as adjuvant therapy to endoscopic treatment in patients with peptic ulcer bleeding: prospective randomized controlled trial. J Gastroenterol Hepatol 2006; 21(4):716–21.

9. Qvist P, Arnesen KE, Jacobsen CD, Rosseland AR. Endoscopic treatment and restrictive surgical policy in the management of peptic ulcer bleeding. Five years' experience in a central hospital. Scand J Gastroenterol. 1994;29(6):569–76.

10. Chiu PW, Lam CY, Lee SW, Kwong KH, Lam SH, Lee DT, et al. Effect of scheduled second therapeutic endoscopy on peptic ulcer rebleeding: a prospective randomised trial. Gut 2003;52(10):1403–7.

11. de Manzoni G, Catalano F, Festini M, Guglielmi A, Lombardo F, Kind R, et al. [Acute hemorrhage caused by duodenal ulcer. Results of endoscopic treatment of the first bleeding episode and of recurrences] Emorragia acuta da ulcera duodenale. Risultati del trattamento endoscopico del primo sanguinamento e delle recidive. Ann Ital Chir 2002;73(4):387–94; discussion 394–6.

12. Parente F, Anderloni A, Bargiggia S, Imbesi V, Trabucchi E, Baratti C, et al. Outcome of non-variceal acute upper gastrointestinal bleeding in relation to the time of endoscopy and the experience of the endoscopist: a two-year survey. World J Gastroenterol 2005;11(45):7122–30.

13. Schoenberg MH. Surgical therapy for peptic ulcer and nonvariceal bleeding. Langenbecks Arch Surg 2001;386(2):98–103.

14. Lau JY, Chung SC. Surgery in the acute management of bleeding peptic ulcer. Baillieres Best Pract Res Clin Gastroenterol 2000;14(3):505–18.

15. Drooz AT, Lewis CA, Allen TE, Citron SJ, Cole PE, Freeman NJ, et al Quality improvement guidelines for percutaneous transcatheter embolization. J Vasc Interv Radiol 2003;14(9 Pt 2):S237–42.

16. Rösch J, Dotter CT, Brown MJ. Selective arterial embolization. A new method for control of acute gastrointestinal bleeding. Radiology 1972;102(2):303–6.

17. White RI, Jr., Giargiana FA, Jr., Bell W. Bleeding duodenal ulcer control. Selective arterial embolization with autologous blood clot. JAMA 1974;229(5):546–8.

18. Loffroy R, Rao P, Ota S, De Lin M, Kwak BK, Geschwind JF. Embolization of acute nonvariceal upper gastrointestinal hemorrhage resistant to endoscopic treatment: results and predictors of recurrent bleeding. Cardiovasc Intervent Radiol 2010; 33(6):1088–1100.

19. Loffroy R, Guiu B, Mezzetta L, Minello A, Michiels C, Jouve JL, et al. Short- and long-term results of transcatheter embolization for massive arterial hemorrhage from gastroduodenal ulcers not controlled by endoscopic hemostasis. Can J Gastroenterol 2009;23(2):115–20.

20. Miller M, Jr., Smith TP. Angiographic diagnosis and endovascular management of nonvariceal gastrointestinal hemorrhage. Gastroenterol Clin North Am 2005; 34(4):735–52.

21. Eriksson LG, Sundbom M, Gustavsson S, Nyman R. Endoscopic marking with a metallic clip facilitates transcatheter arterial embolization in upper peptic ulcer bleeding. J Vasc Interv Radiol 2006;17(6):959–64.

22. Loffroy R, Guiu B, D'Athis P, Mezzetta L, Gagnaire A, Jouve JL, et al. Arterial Embolotherapy for Endoscopically Unmanageable Acute Gastroduodenal Hemorrhage: Predictors of Early Rebleeding. Clin Gastroenterol Hepatol 2009; 7(5):515–23.

23. Sandstede J, Wittenberg G, Schmitt S, Scheppach W, Hahn D. [The diagnostic localization of acute gastrointestinal bleeding in a primarily negative angiographic finding] Lokalisationsdiagnostik einer akuten gastrointestinalen Blutung bei primar negativem angiographischem Befund. Rofo 1997;166(3):258–9.

24. Johnston C, Tuite D, Pritchard R, Reynolds J, McEniff N, Ryan JM. Use of provocative angiography to localize site in recurrent gastrointestinal bleeding. Cardiovasc Intervent Radiol 2007;30(5):1042–6.

25. Bloomfeld RS, Smith TP, Schneider AM, Rockey DC. Provocative angiography in patients with gastrointestinal hemorrhage of obscure origin. Am J Gastroenterol 2000;95(10):2807–12.

26. Koval G, Benner KG, Rösch J, Kozak BE. Aggressive angiographic diagnosis in acute lower gastrointestinal hemorrhage. Dig Dis Sci 1987;32(3):248–53.

27. Defreyne L, Vanlangenhove P, De Vos M, Pattyn P, Van Maele G, Decruyenaere J, et al. Embolization as a first approach with endoscopically unmanageable acute nonvariceal gastrointestinal hemorrhage. Radiology 2001;218(3):739–48.

28. Loffroy R, Guiu B, Cercueil JP, Lepage C, Latournerie M, Hillon P, et al. Refractory bleeding from gastroduodenal ulcers: arterial embolization in high-operative-risk patients. J Clin Gastroenterol 2008;42(4):361–7.

29. Larssen L, Moger T, Bjørnbeth BA, Lygren I, Kløw NE. Transcatheter arterial embolization in the management of bleeding duodenal ulcers: a 5.5-year retrospective study of treatment and outcome. Scand J Gastroenterol 2008;43(2):217–22.

30. Padia SA, Geisinger MA, Newman JS, Pierce G, Obuchowski NA, Sands MJ. Effectiveness of coil embolization in angiographically detectable versus non-detectable sources of upper gastrointestinal hemorrhage. J Vasc Interv Radiol 2009;20(4): 461–6.

31. Encarnacion CE, Kadir S, Beam CA, Payne CS. Gastrointestinal bleeding: treatment with gastrointestinal arterial embolization. Radiology 1992;183(2):505–8.

32. Lang EK. Transcatheter embolization in management of hemorrhage from duodenal ulcer: long-term results and complications. Radiology 1992;182(3):703–7.

33. Ljungdahl M, Eriksson LG, Nyman R, Gustavsson S. Arterial embolisation in management of massive bleeding from gastric and duodenal ulcers. Eur J Surg 2002;168 (7):384–90.

34. Walsh RM, Anain P, Geisinger M, Vogt D, Mayes J, Grundfest-Broniatowski S, et al. Role of angiography and embolization for massive gastroduodenal hemorrhage. J Gastrointest Surg 1999;3(1):61–5; discussion 66.

35. Poultsides GA, Kim CJ, Orlando R, 3rd, Peros G, HalliseyMJ, Vignati PV. Angiographic embolization for gastroduodenal hemorrhage: safety, efficacy, and predictors of outcome. Arch Surg 2008;143(5):457–61.

36. Aina R, Oliva VL, Therasse E, Perreault P, Bui BT, Dufresne MP, et al. Arterial embolotherapy for upper gastrointestinal hemorrhage: outcome assessment. J Vasc Interv Radiol 2001;12(2):195–200.

37. Schenker MP, Duszak R, Jr., Soulen MC, Smith KP, Baum RA, Cope C, et al. Upper gastrointestinal hemorrhage and transcatheter embolotherapy: clinical and technical factors impacting success and survival. J Vasc Interv Radiol 2001;12 (11):1263–71.

38. Holme JB, Nielsen DT, Funch-Jensen P, Mortensen FV. Transcatheter arterial embolization in patients with bleeding duodenal ulcer: an alternative to surgery. Acta Radiol 2006;47(3):244–7.

39. Dempsey DT, Burke DR, Reilly RS, McLean GK, Rosato EF. Angiography in poor-risk patients with massive nonvariceal upper gastrointestinal bleeding. Am J Surg 1990;159(3):282–6.

40. van Lanschot JJ, van Leerdam M, van Delden OM, Fockens P. Management of bleeding gastroduodenal ulcers. Dig Surg 2002;19(2):99–104.

41. Shapiro N, Brandt L, Sprayregan S, Mitsudo S, Glotzer P. Duodenal infarction after therapeutic Gelfoam embolization of a bleeding duodenal ulcer. Gastroenterology 1981;80(1):176–80.

42. Rösch J, Keller FS, Kozak B, Niles N, Dotter CT. Gelfoam powder embolization of the left gastric artery in treatment of massive small-vessel gastric bleeding. Radiology 1984;151(2):365–70.

43. Loffroy R, Guiu B, Cercueil JP, Krause D. Endovascular therapeutic embolisation: an overview of occluding agents and their effects on embolised tissues. Curr Vasc Pharmacol 2009;7(2):250–63.

44. Loffroy R, Guiu B. Arterial embolization is the best treatment for pancreaticojejunal anastomotic bleeding after pancreatoduodenectomy. World J Gastroenterol 2009; 15(32):4090–1.

45. Imhof M, Schröders C, Ohmann C, Röher H. Impact of early operation on the mortality from bleeding peptic ulcer – ten years' experience. Dig Surg 1998;15(4):308–14.

46. Brehant O, Duval H, Dumont F, Fuks D, Deshpande S, Verhaeghe P, et al. Surgical conservative treatment of recurrent bleeding duodenal ulcer. Hepatogastroenterology 2008;55(85):1327–31.

47. Loffroy R. Bleeding peptic ulcers resistant to endoscopic treatment: Calling for a surgeon or an interventional radiologist? Presse Med 2011;40(2):123–5.

48. van Vugt R, Bosscha K, van Munster IP, de Jager CP, Rutten MJ. Embolization as treatment of choice for bleeding peptic ulcers in high-risk patients. Dig Surg 2009; 26(1):37–42.

49. Abe N, Takeuchi H, Yanagida O, Sugiyama M, Atomi Y. Surgical indications and procedures for bleeding peptic ulcer. Dig Endosc 2010;22 Suppl 1: S35–7.

50. Martin RF. Surgical management of ulcer disease. Surg Clin North Am 2005;85 (5):907–29, vi.

51. Ripoll C, Bañares R, Beceiro I, Menchén P, Catalina MV, Echenagusia A, et al. Comparison of transcatheter arterial embolization and surgery for treatment of bleeding peptic ulcer after endoscopic treatment failure. J Vasc Interv Radiol 2004;15(5):447–50.

52. Eriksson LG, Ljungdahl M, Sundbom M, Nyman R. Transcatheter arterial emboliza-tion versus surgery in the treatment of upper gastrointestinal bleeding after thera-peutic endoscopy failure. J Vasc Interv Radiol 2008;19(10):1413–18.

53. Venclauskas L, Bratlie SO, Zachrisson K, Maleckas A, Pundzius J, Jönson C. Is transcatheter arterial embolization a safer alternative than surgery when endoscopic therapy fails in bleeding duodenal ulcer? Scand J Gastroenterol 2010;45(3):299–304.

54. Burris JM, Lin PH, Johnston WF, Huynh TT, Kougias P. Emergent embolization of the gastroduodenal artery in the treatment of upper gastrointestinal bleeding. The experience from a surgeon-initiated interventional program. Am J Surg 2009; 198(1):59–63.

55. Johnson AG. Proximal gastric vagotomy: does it have a place in the future manage-ment of peptic ulcer? World J Surg 2000;24(3):259–63.

CHAPTER 6

Variceal Bleeding: Endoscopic Diagnosis, Endoscopic Therapy and Pharmacotherapy

Dennis M. Jensen, Thomas O.G. Kovacs & Disaya Chavalitdhamrong

CURE Digestive Diseases Research Center, David Geffen School of Medicine at UCLA and Divisions of Digestive Diseases, UCLA Medical Center and West Los Angeles VA Medical Center, Los Angeles, CA, USA

Introduction

A major cause of cirrhosis-related morbidity and mortality is the development of variceal bleeding (1). Esophageal varices are found in approximately 50% of patients with cirrhosis (40% and 60% of compensated and decompensated cirrhotic patients, respectively) (2, 3). Each episode of active variceal bleeding is associated with a 30% mortality and survivors of an episode of active bleeding have a 70% risk of recurrent bleeding within one year (4, 5). Varices are the source of bleeding in 50–90% of cirrhotic patients with severe upper gastrointestinal bleeding (UGIB). Only 50% of patients with variceal bleeding stop bleeding spontaneously which is different from the more than 90% spontaneous cessation rate in patients with other forms of UGIB (6). Despite significant improvements in the early diagnosis and treatment of gastroesophageal variceal bleeding, the mortality rate of first variceal bleeding remains high and the long-term survival rate is less than 40% after one year with medical management alone.

Portal hypertension is responsible for the development of gastroesophageal varices. Portal hypertension is portal pressure gradient (PPG) between the portal vein and inferior vena cava above 5 mm Hg. PPG is assessed clinically by measuring the hepatic venous pressure gradient (HVPG) by hepatic vein catheterization, which is the difference between the wedged hepatic venous pressure and free hepatic venous pressure. HVPG more than 10, 12, and 20 mm Hg are responsible for the development of varices, variceal bleeding, and a greater risk of continued or recurrent bleeding, respectively (7).

Gastrointestinal Bleeding, Second Edition. Edited by Joseph J.Y. Sung, Ernst J. Kuipers and Alan N. Barkun. © 2012 Blackwell Publishing Ltd. Published 2012 by Blackwell Publishing Ltd.

Approximately 40% of patients with compensated cirrhosis have varices at the time of diagnosis. Their presence correlates with the severity of liver disease but the strongest predictor for development of varices in cirrhosis is an HVPG more than 10 mmHg (7, 8). Cirrhotic patients without EV but with an HVPG more than 10 mmHg have a double the risk of developing esophageal varices compared to those with an HVPG below this threshold value (7). The rate of formation of varices is approximately 5% per year (7). Once varices have developed, the overall incidence of variceal bleeding is approximately 25% at 2 years (9, 10). In the cases of active liver disease (such as alcoholic, viral hepatitis, or autoimmune types), abstinence from alcohol may result in improvement in liver disease, reductions in HVPG, and decreased size or disappearance of varices. Decrease in HVPG below 12 mmHg or decreases more than 15–20% from baseline value is usually accompanied by decrease in the size of the esophageal varices and lower risk of variceal bleeding (11). HVPG is the most accurate way to monitor the response to medical treatment to prevent first variceal bleed or rebleeding (7–10).

Prediction of cirrhotic patients at risk of variceal bleeding

Patients with liver cirrhosis and documented esophageal varices without prior variceal bleeding have a 25–40% chance of first variceal bleeding within two years of follow up when they do not receive effective prophylactic treatment (9, 10). Accurate identification of patients at highest risk of bleeding permits targeted use of preventive measures. Varices develop deep within the submucosa in the mid-esophagus, but become progressively more superficial in the distal esophagus. Thus, esophageal varices at the gastroesophageal junction have the thinnest coat of supporting tissue and are most likely to rupture and bleed.

Varices in direct continuity with the esophagus along the lesser and greater curves of the stomach are called gastroesophageal varices (GOV) types 1 and 2 respectively. Isolated gastric varices in the fundus (IGV1) occur less frequently than GOVs (10% versus 90%) but cause bleeding more often than either GOVs or isolated gastric varices at other loci in the stomach (IGV2).

Portal hypertensive gastropathy (PHG), a mosaic-like pattern of gastric mucosa with a characteristic pattern, is a common finding in patients with portal hypertension. A recent consensus statement of the Baveno III meeting on portal hypertension proposed a grading classification of PHG based on severity as "mild" or "severe"(12). Although the pathogenesis of PHG has not been clearly defined, a very close relationship exists between the severity of the portal hypertension and the development of PHG. Acute bleeding from PHG is often mild and self-limited. Currently, the only treatment that could be recommended for prophylaxis of bleeding from PHG is nonselective beta blockers (13).

Several clinical and physiologic factors are useful in predicting the risk of variceal bleeding in patients with cirrhosis. These include the location, size, and appearance of varices, their pressure and clinical features of the patient (4). Large variceal size is the most important predictor of bleeding (4). The endoscopic presence of red signs on the variceal wall and the severity of liver dysfunction also increase the risk of bleeding (4).

Size of varices

The risk of variceal bleeding correlates with the diameter of the varix. It is important to insufflate the esophagus while estimating variceal size. Varices are classified in three sizes – small, medium, or large (10, 14). Small varices are defined as minimally elevated vein above the esophageal mucosal surface. Medium varices are defined as tortuous veins occupying less than one-third of the esophageal lumen. Large varices are defined as those occupying more than one-third of the esophageal lumen. Medium and large are a high-risk group.

Appearance of varices

Several morphologic features of varices called "red signs" have been correlated with an increased risk of bleeding including diffuse erythema, red wale marks (longitudinal red streaks), cherry red spots (discrete red cherry-colored spots that are flat), and hematocystic spots (raised discrete red spots) (10).

Clinical features

Several clinical features of the patient are related to the risk of variceal bleeding including the degree of liver dysfunction and history of a previous variceal bleed (15). The Child-Pugh classification is an index of liver dysfunction in which a higher score is associated with a higher likelihood of variceal bleeding (Child-Pugh classes B and C are high risk groups). Previous variceal bleed predicts a high likelihood of a subsequent bleeding episode. As an example, while only one-third of all patients with cirrhosis experience variceal bleeding, over 70% experience further episodes of variceal bleeding after an index bleed.

Variceal pressure

Intravariceal pressure is a major predictive factor for variceal hemorrhage (16, 17). It is also a useful guide for studying the effect of pharmacotherapy of portal hypertension and a measure of the effects of transjugular intrahepatic portosystemic shunt (TIPS). HVPG is an alternative guide to accurately measure intravariceal pressure and widely accepted as the standard method for portal venous pressure determination. HVPG closely correlates with the directly measured portal venous pressure but it is invasive and inconvenient. Variceal pressure may be measured noninvasively with a pressure-sensitive endoscopic gauge or balloon technique (17).

A large multicenter, placebo-controlled, double-blinded trial failed to show benefit of nonselective beta blockers in the prevention of esophageal varix development (7). Thus, beta blockers are currently not recommended for preprimary prophylaxis. In these patients, follow-up endoscopies are recommended by the AASLD and other hepatology groups every 2–3 years to assess the possible development of esophageal varices (18, 19).

Primary prophylaxis of esophageal variceal bleeding (primary prevention)

Primary prophylaxis to prevent the first variceal bleeding is treatment of patients who never had previous variceal bleeding. The potential of preventing first variceal bleeding offers the promise of reducing mortality, morbidity, and associated health care costs. Endoscopic screening should be performed in the following subgroups of cirrhotics: all newly diagnosed cirrhotic patients and all other cirrhotics who are medically stable, willing to be treated prophylactically, and would benefit from medical or endoscopic therapies with exclusion of patients who have short life expectancy (10). The risk of first variceal bleeding is significantly related to the patient's Child–Pugh class, the size of the varices, the presence of red markings, and the HVPG or intravariceal pressure (10). Once a patient develops variceal bleeding, the risks of recurrent variceal bleeding and mortality increase. Therefore, a safe, effective, and cost-effective prophylactic treatment to prevent initial variceal bleeding could significantly reduce risks, complications, mortality and health-care costs associated with variceal bleeding.

Although the risk for first esophageal variceal bleeding is low in cirrhotic patients with absent or small varices, the size of the varices may change as the liver disease progresses and/or the portal pressure increases. Periodically, endoscopic screening should be repeated to determine whether esophageal varices are larger or increasing in risk (with red signs), but the optimum interval for endoscopic surveillance has not been determined. The American Association for the Study of Liver Diseases (AASLD) recommends repeating an esophagogastroduodenostomy (EGD) in 2–3 years and annually in compensated cirrhosis and decompensated cirrhosis, respectively (14, 19). Endoscopic ultrasound has also been used to study varices and to identify increased risk for bleeding, although it is unclear if this modality is superior to standard EGD (20). Esophageal capsule endoscopy is a promising technique, still evolving, which may also provide an accurate, less invasive alternative to EGD to screen for the presence of esophageal varices (21).

Nonselective beta blockers (propranolol, nadolol, and timolol) are the first treatment of choice in the primary prophylaxis of esophageal variceal bleeding by many hepatologists (14, 18) These drugs reduce portal pressure by causing beta blockade, which allows unopposed alpha adrenergic activity, thereby producing mesenteric arteriolar constriction that reduces portal venous flow, variceal blood flow, and the risk of initial bleeding (22). Nonselective beta blockers reduce the portal venous inflow by decreasing cardiac output via $\beta1$-adrenergic blockade and splanchnic blood flow via $\beta2$-adrenergic blockade. Furthermore, $\beta2$-adrenergic-receptor blockade is an important target in the reduction of portal pressure. Therefore, nonselective beta blockers have a greater portal hypotensive effect than selective beta blockers. Additionally, beta blockers may reduce the rate of progression from small to large varices (23). Long-term safety and efficacy of beta-blockers in preventing first esophageal varix hemorrhage are well established (24, 25). Beta blockers are the only drugs recommended for primary prophylaxis against a first variceal bleeding in patients with medium/large varices or small varices with red signs or advanced liver disease. In comparison to placebo, prophylactic beta blockers therapy decreased the risk of first esophageal variceal bleeding by 40–50% and the risk of death associated with gastrointestinal bleeding (26). Because of the portal pressure reducing effect of beta blockers, they are not only beneficial in decreasing variceal bleeding but may also attenuate the development of other complications of portal hypertension such as ascites, hepatorenal syndrome.(25) Beta blockers have been reported to be a cost-effective form of prophylactic therapy and are considered by most hepatologists to be the standard of care for prevention of first esophageal variceal bleeding (26). Carvedilol, a potent nonselective beta blocker with alpha-1 blockade, is also shown to be effective in preventing the first variceal bleed (27).

Ideally, the HVPG should be used to determine the efficacy of beta blockade as a reduction of HVPG to below 12 mmHg or by $> 10–20\%$ from baseline eliminates the risk of variceal bleeding (11). When these targets are achieved, the risk of variceal bleeding decreases to $< 10\%$. Furthermore, the time interval between the 2 HVPG measurements should be as short as possible, and an interval of less than 1 month is presently recommended (19). The acute hemodynamic response, propranolol administered intravenously and HVPG measurements repeated 20 minutes later, can also be used to predict the long-term response and outcome to beta blockade and to reduce the risk of first bleeding in primary prophylaxis (28).

In the absence of HVPG determination, the beta blocker dose is titrated based on increasing doses needed to produce a resting heart rate of 55 beats per minute, a 20% heart rate reduction from baseline or the development of side effects. Although tachyphylaxis to beta blockers can occur, beta blockers maintain their portal hypotensive effects in most patients during long-term administration. Nadolol and timolol are preferred because it can be given once daily. Beta blockers can decrease renal blood flow; thus, renal function should be monitored. In those patients in whom the pulse rate remains high despite large doses of beta blockers, measurement of the HVPG should be considered to guide further therapy. The adverse effects include bronchoconstriction, heart failure, and impotence. Patients with effective beta blockade do not require routine follow up endoscopy (14).

One of the major problems with estimating risk reduction by monitoring peripheral pulse and blood pressure is that these do not translate into HVPG reductions in a significant proportion of patients (10, 11). In several studies of both primary and secondary prophylaxis with beta blockers of patients who were maximally blocked peripherally, 50% or more failed to have HVPGs below 12 mm Hg or >10–20% reduction from baseline.

Nitrates – isosorbide mononitrate (ISMN) – also decrease portal pressure but are not currently recommended for primary prophylaxis. In patients who could not tolerate beta-blockers, there were no significant differences in the incidence of first esophageal variceal bleed or survival compared to placebo (29). The combination therapy with a beta blocker plus a nitrate had no significant benefit in preventing first bleeding or reducing mortality compared to treatment with a beta blocker alone (9).

Endoscopic variceal ligation

Endoscopic variceal ligation (EVL) reduces the risk for bleeding and improves survival compared with no treatment (30). Prophylactic banding reduced the rate of bleeding and bleed-related mortality as compared with beta blockers therapy but did not improve overall mortality (31, 32). A recent meta-analysis of trials of EVL versus beta blockers reported that EVL reduced the risk for first variceal bleeding by 43% with a number needed to treat (NNT) of 11 (33). EVL sessions are repeated at approximately 2–4 week intervals until varices are obliterated, which is achived in about 90% of patients after 2–4 sessions (31, 34).

There is a difference of opinion among hepatologists and endoscopists as to the preferred primary prophylactic treatment of high risk esophageal varices. Endoscopists favor EVL because more than 90% of all patients with high risk respond, whereas ≤60% of all selected patients treated with beta blockers alone either tolerate the drugs or reduce HVPG within the protective range (10, 11, 31). In contrast, as the first choice for primary prophylaxis, the AASLD and hepatologists favor beta blockers because of the general safety profile and cost-effectiveness (19).

EVL can also be used as primary therapy for those with contraindications to beta blockers or are intolerant of beta blockers. Patients who bled while receiving primary prophylaxis with beta blockers also should be treated with EVL. Variceal eradication is achieved in about 90% of patients (31, 33). Variceal recurrence is frequent, with 20–75% of patients requiring repeated EVL sessions (34). Minor complication of EVL, such as transient dysphagia and chest discomfort, are relatively frequent, being reported in 10–45% of patient (33).

In conclusion, prophylactic therapy with nonselective beta blocker is considered to be the standard of care by the AASLD for prevention of first esophageal variceal bleeding in high risk esophageal varices (19). In contrast, endoscopists recommend EVL for high risk varices because of overall efficacy, safety, and superiority to beta blockers in high risk varices (11, 30–33). Combining EVL plus beta blocker has not shown to be more beneficial of prevention of first time bleeding compared to EVL alone (35). AASLD also recommends nonselective beta blockers for patients with small varices who have criteria for increased risk of bleeding (Child-Pugh class B/C or presence of red signs on varices) (14). Nonselective beta blockers or EVL is used for patients with medium/large varices and EVL in patients with contraindications or intolerance or non-compliance to beta blockers (18). EVL can obviate the problems of daily drug compliance and prevent problems related to pharmacological treatment discontinuation.(36) The follow-up surveillance EGD is unnecessary for nonselective beta blocker user who has a significant HVPG decrease. For EVL, it should be repeated every 2–4 weeks until varix obliteration and then every 6 to 12 months to check for variceal recurrence. Nitrates, shunt therapy, or sclerotherapy should not be used in the primary prophylaxis of variceal bleeding (37).

Treatment of an active bleed

Initial resuscitation and prevention of complications

As an introduction to therapy for active variceal hemorrhage, current treatment options include medications (vasopressin and somatostatin and their analogs), balloon tamponade, endoscopy, TIPS, and surgery. TIPS and surgery are indicated in patients in whom variceal bleeding cannot be controlled or in whom bleeding recurs despite combined pharmacological and endoscopic therapy (see chapter "surgery and radiology").

The primary goals of medical and endoscopic management during the active bleeding episode are initial resuscitation, treatment of bleeding, and prevention and treatment of complications.

Initial resuscitation should follow the classic airway, breathing, circulation algorithms and is aimed at restoring an oxygen delivery to the tissues.

Airway protection should be provided in patients with altered respiratory or mental status, such as encephalopathic patients, since these patients are at risk for bronchial aspiration of gastric contents and blood. The restoration of the intravascular volume should be aggressively managed. Avoiding prolonged hypotension is particularly important to prevent infection and renal failure, which are associated with increased risk for rebleeding and death (38). Blood loss should be replaced by packed red blood cells (RBCs) and clotting factors should be replaced as needed. Platelet counts often drop within the first 48 hours after a severe bleed and may necessitate platelet transfusions if values below 50,000/mm^3 occur in an actively bleeding patient. Patients must be monitored carefully to avoid overtransfusion with volume overload, because of the risk of rebound portal hypertension and induction of variceal rebleeding. Patients with a prolonged prothrombin time (PT) that does not correct with fresh frozen plasma (FFP) may benefit from infusion of human recombinant factor VIIa. In one uncontrolled trial, a single 80 ug/kg dose of recombinant factor VIIa normalized the prothrombin time in all 10 patients within 30 minutes, with immediate control of bleeding in all patients (39). A multicenter placebo-controlled trial of recombinant factor VIIa failed to show a beneficial effect of recombinant factor VIIa over standard therapy (40). Because recombinant factor VIIa is expensive and confirmatory randomized studies and cost-effectiveness analyses are needed, its use should be reserved for patients with severe ongoing bleeding and irreversible coagulopathy.

Prevention and management of complications of variceal bleeding are important. Common complications are infection, hepatic encephalopathy, and renal failure. Up to 20% of cirrhotic patients who are hospitalized with GI bleeding have a bacterial infection at the time of admission to the hospital, and infection develops during the hospitalization in up to 50%.(41) The risk of infection is higher in patients with advanced disease (Child-Pugh class B or C) and in patients with repeated bleeding episodes (42). The most frequent infections are spontaneous bacterial peritonitis (50%), urinary tract infections (25%), and pneumonia (25%). Endotracheal intubation to protect the airway may be considered in patients with massive bleeding or with altered mental status to protect the airway and prevent aspiration pneumonia. A nasogastric (NG) tube can decompress the stomach and assist in clearing it of blood before emergency endoscopy. Patients with cirrhosis who present with UGIB should be given prophylactic antibiotics, before endoscopy. Multiple trials evaluating the effectiveness of prophylactic antibiotics in cirrhotic patients hospitalized for bleeding report reductions in infectious complications, rebleeding and mortality (43–45). Guidelines for antibiotics have been issued by the AASLD as short-term (maximum seven days) antibiotic prophylaxis (19). These should be instituted in any patient with cirrhosis and GI bleeding.(14) Oral norfloxacin (400 mg twice daily) or intravenous ciprofloxacin (in patients in whom oral administration is not possible, 400 mg every 12 hours) is the recommended antibiotic (14). Intravenous ceftriaxone (1 g/day) may be preferable in centers with a high prevalence of quinolone-resistant organisms or patients who have been receiving prophylactic norfloxacin for the prevention of spontaneous bacterial peritonitis (14). Hepatic encephalopathy should be managed with lactulose and reversible factors should be treated. The risk of renal failure can be minimized by appropriate volume replacement, and avoidance of nephrotoxic drugs.

Medical management of acute variceal bleeding

Pharmacological therapy should be initiated as soon as variceal bleeding is suspected and continued for 3–5 days after diagnosis is confirmed. Pharmacologic treatment in addition to endoscopic treatment is recommended. A previous meta-analysis showed that vasopressin with or without nitroglycerin, terlipressin, somatostatin, or octreotide were as effective as sclerotherapy for controlling variceal bleeding and caused fewer adverse events (46).

As a somewhat older pharmacologic treatment, intravenous vasopressin (0.4 unit bolus followed by 0.4 to 1.0 units/min as an infusion) has been recommended. It constricts mesenteric arterioles and decreases portal venous inflow, thereby reducing portal pressures. Vasopressin can achieve initial hemostasis in 60–80% of patients, but has only marginal effects on early rebleeding episodes and does not improve survival from active variceal bleeding. However, the benefit of bleeding cessation may be counterbalanced by enhanced mortality due to extrasplanchnic vasoconstrictive properties and resultant ischemia of myocardium, brain, bowel and/or limb. These complications were responsible for drug withdrawal in 25% of cases.(2) Patients in whom vasopressin is still utilized despite the concerns described above should receive it in combination with intravenous nitroglycerin (10–50 μg/min) (47–49).

Terlipressin is a synthetic analog of vasopressin that is a longer biologic half-life and possesses far fewer side effects. It has been used in Europe and other countries with good results in past studies. The clinical efficacy of terlipressin versus placebo has been reported in seven randomized controlled trials (RCTs), and a meta-analysis showed that terlipressin significantly reduced failure to control bleeding and mortality (50). Terlipressin was the only pharmacologic treatment associated with a reduction in mortality compared with placebo. Terlipressin was as effective as sclerotherapy for control of bleeding, rebleeding, and mortality (34% relative risk reduction in mortality) (51). A study comparing the acute hemodynamic effects of terlipressin to octreotide in stable cirrhotic patients reported a sustained effect of terlipressin on portal pressure and blood flow compared with only a transient effect from octreotide, suggesting that terlipressin might have more sustained hemodynamic effects in patients with bleeding varices (52). The efficacy of terlipressin was similar to octreotide as an adjuvant therapy for the control of esophageal variceal bleed and in-hospital survival (53). The longer half-life allows the intravenous administration of the terlipressin in bolus dosing, 2 mg every 4–6 hours until 24 hours free from bleeding is achieved (54).

Somatostatin (250 µg bolus followed by 250 µg/h by intravenous infusion for 5 days) inhibits the release of vasodilator hormones, indirectly causing splanchnic vasoconstriction and decreased portal inflow. The higher dose can be suggested for those who continue to bleed despite the 250 µg/h infusion (55). It causes selective splanchnic vasoconstriction and lower portal pressure without causing the cardiac complications of vasopressin. Severe side effects are rare, and minor side effects, such as nausea, vomiting, and hyperglycemia, occur in about 30% (56). Somatostatin (and octreotide) has fewer serious complications than vasopressin or terlipressin. Somatostatin was also reported to be more effective in controlling variceal bleeding than placebo or vasopressin. Several RCTs have shown its efficacy in the control of bleeding; however, somatostatin did not reduce mortality (9). It has a short half-life and disappears within minutes of a bolus infusion. In contrast, octreotide (50 µg bolus followed by 50 µg/h by intravenous infusion for five days) is a long-acting analog of somatostatin. Somatostatin or octreotide are as effective as sclerotherapy alone for acute management of variceal bleeding (46). However, combined therapy (octreotide or somatostatin and endoscopic treatment) is more effective than sclerotherapy or endoscopic variceal band ligation (EVL) alone (57). Somatostatin plus EVL combination therapy was associated with significantly better survival and control of bleeding at five days (57). Given the potential ability of octreotide to control acute variceal bleeding and its low toxicity, octreotide appears to be the pharmacologic drug of choice as an initial pharmacologic treatment and as an adjunct to endoscopic therapy for the treatment of acute or active variceal bleeding.

Balloon tamponade

Balloon tamponade of varices is seldom used anymore to control variceal bleeding. It may be used for short-term hemostasis to stabilize a patient with massive bleeding prior to definitive therapy. Three types of tamponade balloons are available. The Sengstaken–Blakemore tube has gastric and esophageal balloons, with a single gastric suction port. The Minnesota tube is a modified Sengstaken-Blakemore tube with an esophageal suction port added, above the esophageal balloon. The Linton–Nicholas tube has a single large gastric balloon (600 cc) and aspiration ports in the stomach and esophagus. Balloon tamponade provides initial control of bleeding in

30–98% of cases, but variceal rebleeding recurs soon after the balloon is deflated in 21–60% of patients (58–60). The major problem with tamponade balloons is a 30% rate of serious complications, such as aspiration pneumonia, esophageal rupture, and airway obstruction (58). It can also cause pressure necrosis of the mucosa if the balloon remains inflated for more than 24–48 hours. Patients should have endotracheal intubation before placement of a tamponade balloon to minimize the risk of pulmonary complications. Clinical studies have not shown a significant difference in efficacy between vasopressin administration and balloon tamponade. However, both may be associated with serious complications.

Endoscopic therapy

Variceal bleeding is best diagnosed by upper endoscopy, which shows active bleeding from a varix, a platelet plug or "white nipple" sign on a varix, clots over a varix, or varices without other potential etiologies of UGIB. Endoscopic therapy (EVL and sclerotherapy) is currently the definitive treatment of choice for active variceal bleeding with an efficacy of 80–90% (61). A combination of somatostatin or octreotide and sclerotherapy or band ligation is more effective than sclerotherapy or band ligation alone (46, 57). EVL involves placing small elastic bands around varices in the distal 5–7 cm of the esophagus. EVL is at least as effective as sclerotherapy for achieving hemostasis and for prevention of early rebleeding. Sclerotherapy involves injection of a sclerosant solution into or around the varices using a freehand technique. In the setting of active spurting bleeding, it is often more convenient to perform sclerotherapy acutely because it is faster, provides better vision, and is more effective than EVL for acute hemostasis with active bleeding. Once active bleeding is controlled by sclerotherapy, EVL is recommended during the same endoscopy session for treatment of all esophageal variceal columns, to prevent early rebleeding. The experience and expertise of the endoscopist should dictate the selection of the specific modality. EVL can also be used in patients who fail sclerotherapy or in whom bleeding is slowed enough to perform EVL.

Both EVL and sclerotherapy have the potential to worsen PHG or cause enlargement of gastric varices following obliteration of esophageal varices. In initial reports, the rate of complications was significantly lower with EVL than sclerotherapy (63–65). In a meta-analysis, a much lower rate of esophageal stricture was reported with band ligation (64). Rebleeding episodes from esophageal varices can be managed with additional sessions of endoscopic treatment.

Emergent endoscopic treatment fails to control bleeding in 10–20% of patients. A second attempt at endoscopic hemostasis can be made but more definitive therapy must be instituted immediately, such as with portosystemic shunt (TIPS or surgery).

Bleeding gastric varices are a difficult therapeutic problem because most nonsurgical treatments are ineffective, except for cyanoacrylate. This tissue adhesive is still investigational in the U.S. and not widely utilized. Also, when isolated gastric varices occur from splenic vein thrombosis, splenectomy is the treatment of choice. Endoscopy is important diagnostically to confirm the site of bleeding. Gastric varices treated with sclerotherapy or rubber band ligation (RBL) often rebleed despite initially successful endoscopic therapy. TIPS should be considered in patients in whom bleeding cannot be controlled or recurs despite combined pharmacological and endoscopic therapy.

Endoscopic sclerotherapy

Endoscopic variceal sclerotherapy involves injecting a sclerosant into or adjacent to esophageal varices. Endoscopic sclerotherapy controls bleeding in acutely 80–90% of patients and decreases the risk for early bleeding, although an improvement in patient survival has never been shown (9). The most commonly used sclerosants are ethanolamine oleate, sodium tetradecyl sulfate, sodium morrhuate, and ethanol. The outcome is similar regardless of the type of sclerosant used (62). Cyanoacrylate is a glue that effectively stops bleeding, but it is difficult to use, can damage the endoscope and is not approved by the US Food and Drug Administration (FDA). Various techniques are used, with a goal of achieving initial hemostasis and then performing sclerotherapy on a weekly basis until all varices are obliterated. The frequency of complications increases when sclerotherapy is performed weekly, while injections at two- to three-week intervals take longer to achieve variceal obliteration. Esophageal varices are much more amenable than gastric varices to eradication with endoscopic therapy. Once varices are obliterated, surveillance endoscopy should be undertaken every six months for the first year and annually thereafter.

Prospective, randomized trials have shown mixed results but suggest improved immediate hemostasis and a reduction in acute rebleeding with sclerotherapy compared with medical therapy alone for bleeding esophageal varices (63, 64). Complications of endoscopic variceal sclerotherapy include esophageal ulcers, which can bleed or perforate, esophageal strictures, mediastinitis, pleural effusions, aspiration pneumonia, acute respiratory distress syndrome, chest pain, fever, and bacteremia. EVL is the preferred endoscopic therapy for variceal bleeding because of fewer complications and more rapid obliteration than sclerotherapy (65, 66). Endoscopic sclerotherapy can be used in the acute setting if EVL proves technically difficult (18). Combination of somatostatin or octreotide and sclerotherapy or EVL is more effective than sclerotherapy or EVL alone (57).

Endoscopic variceal ligation

The technique of EVL is attachment of a device loaded with rubber bands to the tip of the endoscope. Esophageal varices are suctioned into the device and then the rubber band is deployed around its base by pulling on a trip wire. Devices used for band ligation allow up to 10 bands to be placed without the need to remove the endoscope to re-load the banding device. Application of bands is started at the gastroesophageal junction (GEJ) and progresses upwards for approximately 5–7 cm (10, 34). The varices subsequently undergo thrombosis, sloughing, and fibrosis. EVL is as effective as sclerotherapy in achieving initial hemostasis, reducing the rate of rebleeding, overall mortality, and death from bleeding from esophageal varices (66). EVL is associated with fewer local complications, especially esophageal strictures, and requires fewer endoscopic treatment sessions than sclerotherapy (65). EVL causes fewer ulcers that have severe secondary bleeding than sclerotherapy (67). Therefore, by consensus, EVL is the preferred form of endoscopic therapy, especially of primary or secondary prophylaxis or treatment of non-actively bleeding esophageal varices.(14) Band ligation, however, may be more technically difficult to perform than sclerotherapy during active variceal bleeding. Recurrent bleeding, in-hospital and 30-day mortality were lower in the combined EVL and pharmacologic agents group compared to EVL alone (68). Baveno IV consensus recommended both drug therapy and performing EVL after initial resuscitation (18).

Rescue therapies

Despite urgent endoscopic and/or pharmacologic therapy, variceal bleeding cannot be controlled or recurs in about 10–20% of patients. An elevated HVPG of more than 20 mmHg has been shown to be predictive of treatment failure.(69) Shunt therapy, either as shunt surgery or TIPS, has clinical efficacy as salvage therapy.(70) TIPS produces hemostasis in over 90% of cases (71, 72). TIPS is effective in the short term control of bleeding gastroesophageal varices.(73) Randomized trials that compared TIPS with endoscopic sclerotherapy also suggest that TIPS is more effective for the long term prevention of rebleeding (74). TIPS-related complications include procedural complications (in about 10%) and later TIPS dysfunction or stenosis (75). The most frequent complication encountered is that of worsening encephalopathy, which occurs in about 20–25% of patients following TIPS placement (76). The rate of TIPS occlusion is up to 80% within one year (76). The surgical options currently used to treat variceal bleeding are either surgical shunts or non-shunt procedures (such as devascularization). When compared with sclerotherapy, surgical shunts decrease the rebleeding rate significantly but do not improve survival. (77, 78) Surgical shunts may be associated with hepatic encephalopathy and can make future liver transplantation technically more difficult. Because both procedures (TIPS versus surgical therapy) have similar outcomes, the choice is dependent on available local expertise.

Prevention of recurrent variceal bleeding (secondary prevention)

The incidence of early rebleeding after untreated esophageal variceal hemorrhage is about 20% within the first six weeks (with the greatest risk within the first 48 to 72 hours), and over 50% of all early rebleeding episodes occur within the first 10 days (1). The risk of bleeding and of death in patients who survive 6 weeks is similar to that in cirrhotic patients of equivalent severity who have never bled.

The median rebleeding rate in untreated individuals is approximately 60% within 1–2 years of the index bleeding, with a mortality of 33% (9, 79). The prevention of recurrent variceal bleeding remains the cornerstone of management and "secondary prophylaxis" should be instituted after the initial episode. Risk factors for rebleeding include ascites, low serum albumin, severe coagulopathies, and high HVPG. Available treatments for preventing variceal rebleeding include endoscopic therapy, pharmacological treatments, TIPS and surgery and orthotopic liver transplant (OLT). EVL plus pharmacotherapy is the standard treatment (14).

Endoscopic sclerotherapy

Endoscopic sclerotherapy of esophageal varices compared to placebo decreases both the risk of rebleeding (40–50% vs 70%) and death (30–60% vs 50–75%).(80, 81) Recurrence of esophageal varices occurs in nearly 40% of patient within 1 year from eradication. Due to complications of sclerotherapy and ease of application of EVL, endoscopic sclerotherapy has been largely replaced by EVL. There is no evidence that the addition of sclerotherapy to EVL changes clinically relevant outcomes (variceal rebleeding, death, time to variceal obliteration) in the secondary prophylaxis of esophageal variceal bleeding (82, 83). Moreover, combination EVL and sclerotherapy caused more esophageal strictures than EBL alone (82, 83).

EVL

Compared with sclerotherapy of esophageal varices, ligation reduced the rebleeding rate, the mortality rate, the rate of death due to rebleeding, and the development of esophageal strictures (61). Variceal obliteration was achieved in similar proportions with both techniques but the number of treatments necessary to achieve obliteration was lower with ligation (61).

These data suggest that EVL should be the initial procedure of choice for prevention of recurrent variceal bleeding. Secondary prophylaxis with EVL involves repeated ligation of esophageal varices until obliteration followed by regular surveillance for recurrence. Small varices are not optimally treated by EVL. *EVL may also be associated with a higher rate of recurrence of varices subsequently.* Combining initial EVL with a session of sclerotherapy used for eradication of small residual varices offers the benefit of reducing variceal recurrence while minimizing complications. Adding beta blockers to EVL reduces the risk of rebleeding and esophageal variceal recurrence (84, 85). AASLD recommends combination of non-selective beta blockers plus EVL for secondary prophylaxis of variceal bleeding (14).

Nonselective beta blockers

Meta-analyses suggest that the risk of rebleeding is decreased by approximately 40% while the risk of death is decreased by 20%. The addition of isosorbide mononitrate to beta blockers appears to enhance the protective effect of beta blockers alone for the prevention of recurrent variceal bleeding but offers no survival advantage and reduces the tolerability of therapy (86). A meta-analysis reported that a combination of endoscopic (sclerotherapy or banding) and drug therapy reduces variceal rebleeding in cirrhosis more than either therapy alone (87). Combining beta blockers with EVL is more effective at preventing rebleeding than band ligation alone or beta blockers alone, so that combination therapy is now recommended for secondary prophylaxis of esophageal variceal bleeding (84, 85, 88).

TIPS

TIPS is used primarily as a salvage therapy for Child-Pugh class A or B patients with recurrent bleeding despite an adequate trial of endoscopic therapy (at least two sessions of endoscopic treatment performed no more than 2 weeks apart) and pharmacologic treatment. TIPS is better than either the combination of isosorbide mononitrate and beta blockers or endoscopic therapy in the prevention of variceal rebleeding and provides a survival benefit, but TIPS increases rate of developing encephalopathy (89, 90). The potential benefit of TIPS is greater in patients with a high HVPG. TIPS can reduce the increased portal pressure by creating a communication between the hepatic vein and the portal vein. It has been reported that bleeding was controlled in 90% of the patients and the 30-day survival rate was 63% (72). The obstruction and re-intervention rates are markedly decreased with the use of polytetrafluoroethylene-covered stents (91).

Shunt surgery

Surgical options are principally used in Child-Pugh class A patients with continued bleeding despite endoscopic and/or pharmacotherapy. A previous Cochrane review reported that shunt therapy in contrast to endoscopic therapy significantly reduced the rebleeding rate, but significantly increased the incidences of both acute and chronic hepatic encephalopathy (92).

OLT

OLT is the only treatment which definitively corrects the portal hypertension. All patients with Child-Pugh class B or C cirrhosis should be evaluated for possible transplantation. A previously placed TIPS can be removed with the explant at the time of transplant.

Guidelines

AASLD has issued guidelines for secondary prevention of recurrent variceal bleeding and they recommend a combination nonselective beta blockers and EVL (14). EVL should be repeated every 1–2 weeks until obliteration with the first surveillance EGD performed one to three months after obliteration and then every 6–12 months to check for variceal recurrence. TIPS should be considered in patients who are Child-Pugh class A or B and experience recurrent variceal bleeding despite combination pharmacological and endoscopic therapy. Patients who are liver transplant candidates should be referred to a transplant center.

Summary

- Screening esophagogastroduodenoscopy (EGD) for the diagnosis of esophageal and gastric varices is recommended when the diagnosis of cirrhosis is made.In patients who have compensated cirrhosis and no varices on the initial EGD, it should be repeated in 2–3 years. For decompensated cirrhotic patients, EGD should be done at that time and repeated annually.
- In patients with cirrhosis and small varices that have not bled but have criteria for increased risk of hemorrhage (Child-Pugh class B/C or presence of red signs), nonselective beta blockers should be used for the prevention of first variceal bleeding. Nonselective beta blockers or endoscopic variceal ligation (EVL) is used for patients with medium/large varices.
- If a patient is placed on a nonselective blocker and responds well with decreased HVPG, follow-up surveillance EGD is unnecessary. If a patient is treated with EVL, the first surveillance EGD should be performed

1–3 months after obliteration and then every 6–12 months to check for variceal recurrence.

- Short-term antibiotic prophylaxis should be instituted in any patient with cirrhosis and gastrointestinal bleeding.
- For active variceal bleeding, pharmacological therapy (terlipressin or somatostatin or its analogues) should be initiated as soon as variceal bleeding is suspected and continued for 3–5 days after diagnosis is confirmed. EGD should be used to make the diagnosis and to treat variceal hemorrhage.
- TIPS is indicated in patients in whom variceal bleeding cannot be controlled or in whom bleeding recurs despite combined pharmacological and endoscopic therapy.
- Combination of nonselective beta blockers plus EVL is the best option for secondary prophylaxis of variceal bleeding.
- TIPS should be considered in patients who are Child-Pugh A or B who experience recurrent variceal bleeding despite combination pharmacological and endoscopic therapy. Surgical shunt can be considered in Child-Pugh A patients.

Conclusions

For the prophylaxis of first esophageal variceal bleeding, the AASLD recommends nonselective beta blockers. However, EVL is favored by gastrointestinal endoscopists for high risk varices. EVL should also be offered to those patients with contraindications or those who cannot tolerate beta blockers. Patients surviving a first episode of variceal bleeding have a high risk of recurrent bleeding and should receive active treatments for the prevention of rebleeding. The combination of both nonselective beta blockers and EVL is the best choice in the prevention of rebleeding. TIPS and surgery are the rescue therapy for failures of medical and endoscopic treatment.

References

1. D'Amico G, De Franchis R. Upper digestive bleeding in cirrhosis. Post-therapeutic outcome and prognostic indicators. Hepatology 2003;38:599–612.
2. D'Amico G, Garcia-Tsao G, Pagliaro L. Natural history and prognostic indicators of survival in cirrhosis: a systematic review of 118 studies. J Hepatol 2006;44:217–31.
3. D'Amico G, Luca A. Natural history. Clinical-haemodynamic correlations. Prediction of the risk of bleeding. Baillieres Clin Gastroenterol 1997;11:243–56.
4. North Italian Endoscopic Club for the Study and Treatment of Esophageal Varices. Prediction of the first variceal hemorrhage in patients with cirrhosis of the liver and esophageal varices. A prospective multicenter study. N Engl J Med 1988;319:983–9.

5. Graham DY, Smith JL. The course of patients after variceal hemorrhage. Gastroenterology 1981;80:800–9.
6. Toubia N, Sanyal AJ. Portal hypertension and variceal hemorrhage. Med Clin North Am 2008;92:551–74.
7. Groszmann RJ, Garcia-Tsao G, Bosch J, et al. Beta-blockers to prevent gastroesophageal varices in patients with cirrhosis. N Engl J Med 2005;24;353:2254–2261.
8. de Franchis R, Primignani M. Natural history of portal hypertension in patients with cirrhosis. Clin Liver Dis 2001;5:645–63.
9. D'Amico G, Pagliaro L, Bosch J. Pharmacological treatment of portal hypertension: an evidence-based approach. Semin Liver Dis 1999;19:475–505.
10. Jensen DM. Endoscopic screening for varices in cirrhosis: findings, implications, and outcomes. Gastroenterology 2002;122:1620–1630.
11. D'Amico G, Garcia-Pagan JC, Luca A, et al. Hepatic vein pressure gradient reduction and prevention of variceal bleeding in cirrhosis: a systematic review. Gastroenterology 2006;131:1611–1624.
12. de Franchis R. Updating consensus in portal hypertension: report of the Baveno III Consensus Workshop on definitions, methodology and therapeutic strategies in portal hypertension. J Hepatol 2000;33:846–52.
13. Perez-Ayuso RM, Pique JM, Bosch J, et al. Propranolol in prevention of recurrent bleeding from severe portal hypertensive gastropathy in cirrhosis. Lancet 1991; 337:1431–1434.
14. Garcia-Tsao G, Sanyal AJ, Grace ND, et al. Prevention and management of gastroesophageal varices and variceal hemorrhage in cirrhosis. Hepatology 2007;46:922–38.
15. de Franchis R, Primignani M. Why do varices bleed? Gastroenterol Clin North Am 1992;21:85–101.
16. Nevens F, Bustami R, Scheys I, et al. Variceal pressure is a factor predicting the risk of a first variceal bleeding: a prospective cohort study in cirrhotic patients. Hepatology 1998;27:15–19.
17. Tandon RK, Saikia N. Measuring intravariceal pressure. Gastrointest Endosc 2009;70:414–6.
18. de Franchis R. Evolving consensus in portal hypertension. Report of the Baveno IV consensus workshop on methodology of diagnosis and therapy in portal hypertension. J Hepatol 2005;43:167–76.
19. Garcia-Tsao G, Bosch J, Groszmann RJ. Portal hypertension and variceal bleeding – unresolved issues. Summary of an American Association for the study of liver diseases and European Association for the study of the liver single-topic conference. Hepatology 2008;47:1764–1772.
20. Rigau J, Bosch J, Bordas JM, et al. Endoscopic measurement of variceal pressure in cirrhosis: correlation with portal pressure and variceal hemorrhage. Gastroenterology 1989;96:873–80.
21. Eisen GM, Eliakim R, Zaman A, et al. The accuracy of PillCam ESO capsule endoscopy versus conventional upper endoscopy for the diagnosis of esophageal varices: a prospective three-center pilot study. Endoscopy 2006;38:31–5.
22. The PROVA Study Group. Prophylaxis of first hemorrhage from esophageal varices by sclerotherapy, propranolol or both in cirrhotic patients: a randomized multicenter trial. The PROVA Study Group. Hepatology 1991;14:1016–1024.
23. Merkel C, Marin R, Angeli P, et al. A placebo-controlled clinical trial of nadolol in the prophylaxis of growth of small esophageal varices in cirrhosis. Gastroenterology 2004;127:476–84.

24. Turnes J, Garcia-Pagan JC, Abraldes JG, et al. Pharmacological reduction of portal pressure and long-term risk of first variceal bleeding in patients with cirrhosis. Am J Gastroenterol 2006;101:506–12.

25. Abraczinskas DR, Ookubo R, Grace ND, et al. Propranolol for the prevention of first esophageal variceal hemorrhage: a lifetime commitment? Hepatology 2001; 34:1096–1102.

26. Poynard T, Cales P, Pasta L, et al. Beta-adrenergic-antagonist drugs in the prevention of gastrointestinal bleeding in patients with cirrhosis and esophageal varices. An analysis of data and prognostic factors in 589 patients from four randomized clinical trials. Franco-Italian Multicenter Study Group. N Engl J Med 1991; 30; 324:1532–1538.

27. Tripathi D, Ferguson JW, Kochar N, et al. Randomized controlled trial of carvedilol versus variceal band ligation for the prevention of the first variceal bleed. Hepatology 2009;50; 825–33.

28. Villanueva C, Aracil C, Colomo A, et al. Acute hemodynamic response to beta-blockers and prediction of long-term outcome in primary prophylaxis of variceal bleeding. Gastroenterology 2009;137:119–28.

29. Garcia-Pagan JC, Villanueva C, Vila MC, et al. Isosorbide mononitrate in the prevention of first variceal bleed in patients who cannot receive beta-blockers. Gastroenterology 2001;121:908–14.

30. Sarin SK, Lamba GS, Kumar M, et al. Comparison of endoscopic ligation and propranolol for the primary prevention of variceal bleeding. N Engl J Med 1999;340:988–93.

31. Jutabha R, Jensen DM, Martin P, et al. Randomized study comparing banding and propranolol to prevent initial variceal hemorrhage in cirrhotics with high-risk esophageal varices. Gastroenterology 2005;128:870–81.

32. Imperiale TF, Chalasani N. A meta-analysis of endoscopic variceal ligation for primary prophylaxis of esophageal variceal bleeding. Hepatology 2001;33: 802–7.

33. Khuroo MS, Khuroo NS, Farahat KL, et al. Meta-analysis: endoscopic variceal ligation for primary prophylaxis of oesophageal variceal bleeding. Aliment Pharmacol Ther 2005;21:347–61.

34. Garcia-Pagan JC, Bosch J. Endoscopic band ligation in the treatment of portal hypertension. Nat Clin Pract Gastroenterol Hepatol 2005;2:526–35.

35. Sarin SK, Wadhawan M, Agarwal SR, et al. Endoscopic variceal ligation plus propranolol versus endoscopic variceal ligation alone in primary prophylaxis of variceal bleeding. Am J Gastroenterol 2005;100:797–804.

36. Tripathi D, Graham C, Hayes PC. Variceal band ligation versus beta-blockers for primary prevention of variceal bleeding: a meta-analysis. Eur J Gastroenterol Hepatol 2007;19:835–45.

37. The Veterans Affairs Cooperative Variceal Sclerotherapy Group. Prophylactic sclerotherapy for esophageal varices in men with alcoholic liver disease. A randomized, single-blind, multicenter clinical trial. The Veterans Affairs Cooperative Variceal Sclerotherapy Group. N Engl J Med 1991;324:1779–1784.

38. Cardenas A, Gines P, Uriz, et al. Renal failure after upper gastrointestinal bleeding in cirrhosis: incidence, clinical course, predictive factors, and short-term prognosis. Hepatology 2001;34:671–6.

39. Ejlersen E, Melsen T, Ingerslev J, et al. Recombinant activated factor VII (rFVIIa) acutely normalizes prothrombin time in patients with cirrhosis during bleeding from oesophageal varices. Scand J Gastroenterol 2001;36:1081–1085.

40. Bosch J, Thabut D, Bendtsen F, et al. Recombinant factor VIIa for upper gastrointestinal bleeding in patients with cirrhosis: a randomized, double-blind trial. Gastroenterology 2004;127:1123–1130.

41. Soares-Weiser K, Brezis M, Tur-Kaspa R, et al. Antibiotic prophylaxis for cirrhotic patients with gastrointestinal bleeding. 2002: CD002907.

42. Caly WR, Strauss E. A prospective study of bacterial infections in patients with cirrhosis. J Hepatol 1993;18:353–8.

43. Hou MC, Lin HC, Liu TT, et al. Antibiotic prophylaxis after endoscopic therapy prevents rebleeding in acute variceal hemorrhage: a randomized trial. Hepatology 2004;39:746–53.

44. Bernard B, Grange JD, Khac EN, et al. Antibiotic prophylaxis for the prevention of bacterial infections in cirrhotic patients with gastrointestinal bleeding: a meta-analysis. Hepatology 1999;29:1655–1661.

45. Soares-Weiser K, Brezis M, Tur-Kaspa R, et al. Antibiotic prophylaxis of bacterial infections in cirrhotic inpatients: a meta-analysis of randomized controlled trials. Scand J Gastroenterol 2003;38:193–200.

46. D'Amico G, Pietrosi G, Tarantino I, et al. Emergency sclerotherapy versus vasoactive drugs for variceal bleeding in cirrhosis: a Cochrane meta-analysis. Gastroenterology 2003;124:1277–1291.

47. Groszmann RJ, Kravetz D, Bosch J, et al. Nitroglycerin improves the hemodynamic response to vasopressin in portal hypertension. Hepatology 1982;2:757–62.

48. Gimson AE, Westaby D, Hegarty J, et al. A randomized trial of vasopressin and vasopressin plus nitroglycerin in the control of acute variceal hemorrhage. Hepatology 1986;6:410–3.

49. Tsai YT, Lay CS, Lai KH, et al. Controlled trial of vasopressin plus nitroglycerin vs. vasopressin alone in the treatment of bleeding esophageal varices. Hepatology 1986;6:406–9.

50. Ioannou GN, Doust J, Rockey DC. Systematic review: terlipressin in acute oesophageal variceal haemorrhage. Aliment Pharmacol Ther 2003;17:53–64.

51. Krag A, Borup T, Moller S, et al. Efficacy and safety of terlipressin in cirrhotic patients with variceal bleeding or hepatorenal syndrome. Adv Ther 2008;25: 1105–1140.

52. Baik SK, Jeong PH, Ji SW, et al. Acute hemodynamic effects of octreotide and terlipressin in patients with cirrhosis: a randomized comparison. Am J Gastroenterol 2005;100:631–5.

53. Abid S, Jafri W, Hamid S, Salih M, Azam Z, Mumtaz K, et al. Terlipressin vs. octreotide in bleeding esophageal varices as an adjuvant therapy with endoscopic band ligation: a randomized double-blind placebo-controlled trial. Am J Gastroenterol 2009;104:617–23.

54. Sass DA, Chopra KB. Portal hypertension and variceal hemorrhage. Med Clin North Am 2009;93:837–53, vii–viii.

55. Cirera I, Feu F, Luca A, et al. Effects of bolus injections and continuous infusions of somatostatin and placebo in patients with cirrhosis: a double-blind hemodynamic investigation. Hepatology 1995;22:106–11.

56. Moitinho E, Planas R, Banares R, Albillos A, Ruiz-del-Arbol L, Galvez C, et al. Multicenter randomized controlled trial comparing different schedules of somatostatin in the treatment of acute variceal bleeding. J Hepatol 2001;35:712–18.

57. Banares R, Albillos A, Rincon D, et al. Endoscopic treatment versus endoscopic plus pharmacologic treatment for acute variceal bleeding: a meta-analysis. Hepatology 2002;35:609–15.

58. Pinto-Marques P, Romaozinho JM, Ferreira M, et al. Esophageal perforation – associated risk with balloon tamponade after endoscopic therapy. Myth or reality? Hepatogastroenterology 2006;53:536–9.

59. Avgerinos A, Armonis A. Balloon tamponade technique and efficacy in variceal haemorrhage. Scand J Gastroenterol Suppl 1994;207:11–16.

60. Pitcher JL. Safety and effectiveness of the modified Sengstaken-Blakemore tube: a prospective study. Gastroenterology 1971;61:291–8.

61. de Franchis R, Primignani M. Endoscopic treatments for portal hypertension. Semin Liver Dis 1999;19:439–55.

62. Sarin SK, Kumar A. Sclerosants for variceal sclerotherapy: a critical appraisal. Am J Gastroenterol 1990;85:641–9.

63. Larson AW, Cohen H, Zweiban B, et al. Acute esophageal variceal sclerotherapy. Results of a prospective randomized controlled trial. JAMA 1986;255:497–500.

64. The Copenhagen Esophageal Varices Sclerotherapy Project. Sclerotherapy after first variceal hemorrhage in cirrhosis. A randomized multicenter trial. The Copenhagen Esophageal Varices Sclerotherapy Project. N Engl J Med 1984;311:1594–1600.

65. Laine L, el-Newihi HM, Migikovsky B, et al. Endoscopic ligation compared with sclerotherapy for the treatment of bleeding esophageal varices. Ann Intern Med 1993;119:1–7.

66. Laine L, Cook D. Endoscopic ligation compared with sclerotherapy for treatment of esophageal variceal bleeding. A meta-analysis. Ann Intern Med 1995;123:280–7.

67. Stiegmann GV, Goff JS, Michaletz-Onody PA, et al. Endoscopic sclerotherapy as compared with endoscopic ligation for bleeding esophageal varices. N Engl J Med 1992;326:1527–32.

68. Sung JJ, Chung SC, Yung MY, et al. Prospective randomised study of effect of octreotide on rebleeding from oesophageal varices after endoscopic ligation. Lancet 1995; 23–30; 346:1666–1669.

69. Moitinho E, Escorsell A, Bandi JC, et al. Prognostic value of early measurements of portal pressure in acute variceal bleeding. Gastroenterology 1999;117:626–31.

70. Henderson JM. Salvage therapies for refractory variceal hemorrhage. Clin Liver Dis 2001;5:709–25.

71. Sanyal AJ, Freedman AM, Luketic VA, et al. Transjugular intrahepatic portosystemic shunts for patients with active variceal hemorrhage unresponsive to sclerotherapy. Gastroenterology 1996;111:138–46.

72. Ochs A. Transjugular intrahepatic portosystemic shunt. Dig Dis 2005;23:56–64.

73. Ring EJ, Lake JR, Roberts JP, et al. Using transjugular intrahepatic portosystemic shunts to control variceal bleeding before liver transplantation. Ann Intern Med 1992;116:304–9.

74. Cello JP, Ring EJ, Olcott EW, et al. Endoscopic sclerotherapy compared with percutaneous transjugular intrahepatic portosystemic shunt after initial sclerotherapy in patients with acute variceal hemorrhage. A randomized, controlled trial. Ann Intern Med 1997;126:858–65.

75. Freedman AM, Sanyal AJ, Tisnado J, et al. Complications of transjugular intrahepatic portosystemic shunt: a comprehensive review. Radiographics 1993;13:1185–1210.

76. Boyer TD. Transjugular intrahepatic portosystemic shunt: current status. Gastroenterology 2003;124:1700–1710.

77. Cello JP, Grendell JH, Crass RA, et al. Endoscopic sclerotherapy versus portacaval shunt in patient with severe cirrhosis and acute variceal hemorrhage. Long-term follow-up. N Engl J Med 1987;316:11–15.

78. Planas R, Boix J, Broggi M, et al. Portacaval shunt versus endoscopic sclerotherapy in the elective treatment of variceal hemorrhage. Gastroenterology 1991;100: 1078–86.

79. Sharara AI, Rockey DC. Gastroesophageal variceal hemorrhage. N Engl J Med 2001;345:669–81.

80. Soderlund C, Ihre T. Endoscopic sclerotherapy v. conservative management of bleeding oesophageal varices. A 5-year prospective controlled trial of emergency and long-term treatment. Acta Chir Scand 1985;151:449–56.

81. MacDougall BR, Westaby D, Theodossi A, et al. Increased long-term survival in variceal haemorrhage using injection sclerotherapy. Results of a controlled trial. Lancet 1982;1:124–7.

82. Singh P, Pooran N, Indaram A, et al. Combined ligation and sclerotherapy versus ligation alone for secondary prophylaxis of esophageal variceal bleeding: a meta-analysis. Am J Gastroenterol 2009;97:623–9.

83. Karsan HA, Morton SC, Shekelle PG, et al. Combination endoscopic band ligation and sclerotherapy compared with endoscopic band ligation alone for the secondary prophylaxis of esophageal variceal hemorrhage: a meta-analysis. Dig Dis Sci 2005;50:399–406.

84. Lo GH, Lai KH, Cheng JS, et al. Endoscopic variceal ligation plus nadolol and sucralfate compared with ligation alone for the prevention of variceal rebleeding: a prospective, randomized trial. Hepatology 2000;32:461–5.

85. de la Pena J, Brullet E, Sanchez-Hernandez E, et al. Variceal ligation plus nadolol compared with ligation for prophylaxis of variceal rebleeding: a multicenter trial. Hepatology 2005;41:572–8.

86. Gournay J, Masliah C, Martin T, et al. Isosorbide mononitrate and propranolol compared with propranolol alone for the prevention of variceal rebleeding. Hepatology 2000;31:1239–1245.

87. Gonzalez R, Zamora J, Gomez-Camarero J, et al. Meta-analysis: Combination endoscopic and drug therapy to prevent variceal rebleeding in cirrhosis. Ann Intern Med 2008;149:109–22.

88. Lo GH, Chen WC, Chan HH, et al. A randomized, controlled trial of banding ligation plus drug therapy versus drug therapy alone in the prevention of esophageal variceal rebleeding. J Gastroenterol Hepatol 2009 Jun; 24:982–7.

89. Escorsell A, Banares R, Garcia-Pagan JC, et al. TIPS versus drug therapy in preventing variceal rebleeding in advanced cirrhosis: a randomized controlled trial. Hepatology 2002;35:385–92.

90. Burroughs AK, Vangeli M. Transjugular intrahepatic portosystemic shunt versus endoscopic therapy: randomized trials for secondary prophylaxis of variceal bleeding: an updated meta-analysis. Scand J Gastroenterol 2002;37:249–52.

91. Bureau C, Garcia-Pagan JC, Otal P, et al. Improved clinical outcome using polytetra-fluoroethylene-coated stents for TIPS: results of a randomized study. Gastroenterology 2004;126:469–75.

92. Khan S, Tudur Smith C, Williamson P, et al. Portosystemic shunts versus endoscopic therapy for variceal rebleeding in patients with cirrhosis. Cochrane Database Syst Rev 2006: CD000553.

CHAPTER 7

Variceal Bleeding: Surgery and Radiology

Dennis M. Jensen, Thomas O.G. Kovacs & Disaya Chavalitdhamrong

CURE Digestive Diseases Research Center, David Geffen School of Medicine at UCLA and Divisions of Digestive Diseases, UCLA Medical Center and West Los Angeles VA Medical Center, Los AngelesCA, USA

Introduction

Endoscopic and pharmacologic treatments are first-line therapy for active variceal bleeding, and both primary and secondary prophylaxis (see Chapter 6). For 5–20% of patients who continue to have bleeding or rebleeding with these therapies, portal pressure decompression is rescue therapy. Three options for portal pressure decompression are transjugular intrahepatic portal systemic shunt (TIPS), surgical shunt, or orthotopic liver transplantation (OLT). This chapter focuses on these options.

TIPS has a major role in patients who are poor-risk candidates for surgery. TIPS involves creating a low-resistance channel between the hepatic vein and the intrahepatic portion of the portal vein (usually the right branch) with interventional radiology techniques. A tract is kept patent by deployment of an expandable metal stent, thereby allowing blood to shunt to the systemic circulation. While TIPS avoids the risks of general anesthesia and surgery, it is often associated with stent stenosis (80–100%) and hepatic encephalopathy and requires close follow-up. In contrast, the risks of shunt surgery are more "up-front" and those who survive surgery do not need to be followed as closely for shunt failure or stenosis.

The American Association for the Study of Liver Diseases (AASLD) recommends that TIPS and surgical shunt are now considered to be equal efficacy in control of active variceal bleeding and in the prevention of variceal rebleeding (1).– Patients who have poor access to medical services may also be better served by surgical shunt therapy. On the other hand, TIPS may be a useful temporizing measure in those awaiting liver transplantation.

Gastrointestinal Bleeding, Second Edition. Edited by Joseph J.Y. Sung, Ernst J. Kuipers and Alan N. Barkun. © 2012 Blackwell Publishing Ltd. Published 2012 by Blackwell Publishing Ltd.

Bleeding from gastric varices is difficult to control endoscopically. However, in countries where cyanoacrylated glue is available, this is usually effective for the endoscopic control of active gastric variceal hemorrhage. In most countries, the initial treatment is pharmacologic and the traditional treatment is surgical portal decompression. Clinical trials have shown that TIPS can also be effective (2, 3). TIPS may be less effective than shunt surgery in patients with bleeding gastric varices who have spontaneous splenorenal collaterals. Flow through the collaterals, which feed the gastric varices, often persists after TIPS, and the gastric varices may not disappear even after an adequate TIPS shunt is created (4). Where surgical expertise is available, ligation of the splenorenal collateral and portal decompression are the treatments of choice in such cases. Balloon-occluded retrograde transvenous obliteration has also been increasingly reported but it is not widely used at present.

Ectopic varices can develop at sites other than the stomach and esophagus, such as in surgical anastomosis in patients with portal hypertension. Endoscopic treatment is usually unsuccessful in these cases, and traditional treatment is surgical portal decompression and/or segmental resection of the gut segment with the varices. In selected cases, the bleeding can also be controlled by TIPS. In spite of potential limitations of TIPS for ectopic varices and bleeding, the AASLD recommends TIPS as the preferred initial approach for secondary prevention of rebleeding in patients with bleeding from ectopic varices (1).

Patients with Budd-Chiari syndrome who failed to improved with anticoagulation is now recommended to use TIPS, preferably with a covered stent (5).

TIPS

TIPS is a shunt between the hepatic vein and the intrahepatic portion of the portal vein using angiographic techniques (Figs 7.1–7.4). The stent keeps the tract patent and allows blood to return to the systemic circulation. TIPS is used to treat portal hypertension mainly for active and recurrent variceal bleeding, with failure of endoscopic and medical therapy. TIPS has also been reported as a therapy for refractory ascites, hepatorenal syndrome, Budd-Chiari syndrome, hepatic veno-occlusive disease, hepatic hydrothorax, portal hypertensive gastropathy, protein losing enteropathy due to portal hypertension, and preoperative treatment prior to abdominal surgery in portal hypertensive patients. It is contraindicated in pulmonary hypertension, hepatopumonary syndrome, and polycystic liver disease.

TIPS placement usually is carried out under sedation by an interventional radiologist. The hepatic vein is cannulated through a transjugular approach to the portal vein. A guidewire is then passed to connect the hepatic vein and a branch of the portal vein. Following dilation of the tract, a stent is

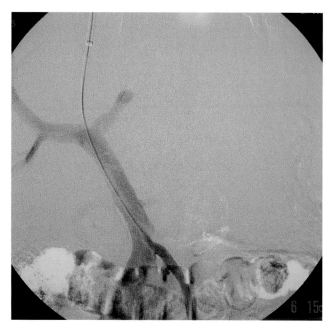

Figure 7.1 A needle catheter was passed via the transjugular route into the hepatic vein (Courtesy of Elavin Petplook, MD.)

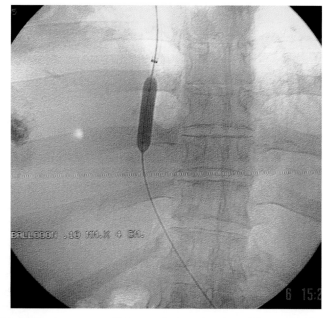

Figure 7.2 Guidewire was passed between the hepatic vein and the portal vein. A balloon catheter is inflated to dilate the tract (Courtesy of Elavin Petplook, MD.)

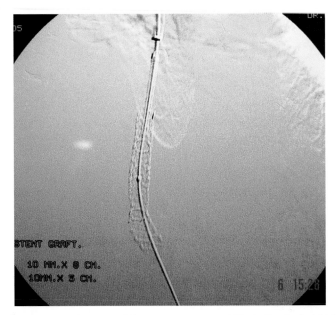

Figure 7.3 Deployment of the stent (Courtesy of Elavin Petplook, MD.)

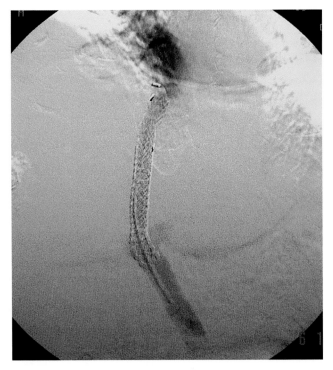

Figure 7.4 Stent in its final position (Courtesy of Elavin Petplook, MD.)

placed and dilated to reduce the portocaval pressure gradient to below 12 mmHg. Coil embolization can be added to occlude the vessels feeding the varices. The stents most commonly used for a TIPS are the Wall-stent and the Palmaz stent. Use of expanded polytetrafluoroethylene (PTFE)-covered stents is now preferred. A meta-analysis shows that the use of PTFE-covered stents improves shunt patency without increasing the risk of hepatic encephalopathy and there is a trend towards better survival (6). The lower risk of shunt dysfunction and perhaps improved outcomes using covered as opposed to bare stents are the basis for this AASLD 2009 guidelines (1).

Surgical shunt

Surgical shunts are used as a salvage therapy when pharmacologic and endoscopic therapy fails in patients with Childs-Pugh class A or B cirrhosis. There are two basic types of operations: portasystemic shunts and non-shunt operations.

Shunt operations are categorized as selective shunts (which preserve some sinusoidal perfusion, decompress gastroesophageal varices but maintain portal hypertension) such as distal splenorenal shunts, partial shunts (which reduce portal hypertension to approximately 12 mmHg) such as side-to-side calibrated portacaval shunt, and total portasystemic shunts (which divert all the portal flow to the systemic circulation) such as portacaval shunts. With selective shunts, portal hypertension is maintained in the superior mesenteric vein and portal vein and these may exacerbate ascites formation. Therefore, a portacaval shunt is preferred in patients with marked ascites.

Non-shunt operations (devascularization procedures) have the components of splenectomy, gastric and esophageal devascularization, and esophageal transection. They are indicated in patients who are not candidates for a shunt operation such as those with extensive portal vein thrombosis or are unable to shunt. The advantage of these procedures is that they do not accelerate liver failure or encephalopathy. The disadvantage is that portal hypertension remains and this accounts for high rate of rebleeding.

Primary prophylaxis of first esophageal variceal bleed

Only about one-third of patients with esophageal varices will experience variceal bleeding during their lifetimes. Pharmacologic treatment with nonselective beta blockers can decrease the frequency of first variceal hemorrhage with relatively little morbidity and expense, in patients able to tolerate the medications long-term. In comparison, TIPS is a much more expensive, invasive procedure and causes significantly more morbidity and mortality. TIPS also requires closer follow-up due to the high incidence of shunt stenosis and recurrent portal hypertension. Thus, TIPS is not indicated for the primary prophylaxis to prevent first esophageal variceal hemorrhage, because of the risk of increasing morbidity. mortality, and cost (1).

Rescue therapies for acute variceal bleeding

Despite optimal urgent endoscopic and pharmacologic therapy by experienced endoscopists, severe esophageal variceal bleeding cannot be controlled or recurs in about 5–20% of patients. An elevated hepatic venous pressure gradient (HVPG) of more than 20 mmHg has been shown to be predictive of such treatment failures (7). Shunt therapy, either TIPS or shunt surgery, is clinically effective as salvage therapy (8). Because both procedures have similar acute outcomes, the choice of TIPS or shunt surgery is dependent on available local expertise. Early use of TIPS for acute variceal bleeding (within 96 hours after admission) has been reported to significantly reduce treatment failure and mortality compared to vasoactive drugs plus endoscopic therapy (9).– TIPS provides initial hemostasis in over 90% of cases (3, 10). TIPS is effective for the short term control of bleeding from gastroesophageal varices (11).

TIPS-related complications include procedural complications and later TIPS dysfunction or stenosis (12). The most frequent TIPS complication is worsening encephalopathy, which occurs in 20–25% of patients following TIPS placement (13). The role of TIPS in acute variceal hemorrhage is as rescue therapy (1). This is due to TIPS related complications and burden of diagnostic and therapeutic endovascular maneuvers to ensure stent patency along with regular follow ups (1). TIPS insertion can be successfully completed in more than 90% of cases (4, 14). Morbidity of TIPS placement in the emergency setting is 10-fold higher than for elective TIPS placement (1). Early performance of TIPS in patients with a HVPG >20 mmHg was associated with a better outcome than in those with lower HVPGs (15). For recurrent or active esophageal variceal bleeding, TIPS can provide long-term definitive hemostasis, varying from 70% to 90% (16). However, no benefit in survival has been shown. PTFE-covered stents improve TIPS patency and decrease the number of clinical relapses and re-interventions without increasing the risk of encephalopathy (17).

Compared to sclerotherapy, surgical shunts significantly decrease the rebleeding rate but do not improve survival (18, 19). However, surgical shunts can make future liver transplantation technically more difficult. After shunt surgery, the risk of encephalopathy is high (40–60%), which can be reduced to about 10% by more selective shunts, such as the distal splenorenal shunt (20). After shunt surgery, the veins may need some adaptation before the portal pressure drops. Therefore recurrent variceal bleeding may recur in the first several weeks, but this should be managed by medical or endoscopic therapies (21). Mortality within 30 days of shunt surgery is high and due to the severity of the underlying liver disease (e.g. Child-Pugh grade of cirrhosis) (22). Mortality can exceed 50% in Child-Pugh class C patients (22).

A few studies have compared TIPS to surgery in the management of refractory bleeding in patients who are good surgical candidates. One study compared TIPS with a surgical H-graft shunt in patients with bleeding varices who had failed nonoperative management. TIPS treated patients had more interventions, experienced more episodes of severe rebleeding, as well as had more irreversible shunt occlusions, liver transplantation, and deaths (23). While TIPS was less expensive initially, the costs escalated over time due to repeated hospitalizations for gastrointestinal bleeding and correction of TIPS stenosis (24).

Prevention of recurrent variceal bleeding (secondary prophylaxis)

Long-term pharmacologic therapy with nonselective beta blockers and repeated endoscopy sessions with band ligation or sclerotherapy is not successful in all patients. TIPS is used primarily as a salvage therapy for Child-Pugh class A or B patients with recurrent bleeding who failed an adequate trial of endoscopic (at least 2–3 sessions of endoscopic treatment performed no more than two weeks apart) and pharmacologic treatment (usually a simultaneous beta blocker). TIPS was reported to be superior to combination of beta blockers and isosorbide mononitrate or endoscopic therapy in the prevention of variceal rebleeding (25–28). However, TIPS was more expensive and had an increased risk of encephalopathy, and there was no survival benefit (25–29).

The benefit of TIPS was greater in patients with an elevated HVPG. It has been reported that bleeding could be controlled in 90% of the patients and the 30-day survival rate was 63% (10). A recent meta-analysis of TIPS versus endoscopic therapy showed that TIPS decreased the incidence of variceal rebleeding and deaths due to rebleeding but increased the rate of post-treatment encephalopathy, while the hospitalization days and death rates due to all causes were similar (30). The superiority of TIPS for prevention of rebleeding is offset by its failure to improve survival, its increasing morbidity due to the development of liver failure and encephalopathy, and the frequent occurrence of TIPS stenosis. For these reasons, TIPS is regarded as a salvage therapy for those patients who bleed despite adequate medical and endoscopic treatment (1).

Advanced age, liver failure, large shunt diameter, and a history of encephalopathy prior to TIPS are all risk factors for worsening encephalopathy after TIPS (31, 32). Variceal bleeding is unlikely to recur as long as the TIPS remains patent, and the HVPG is below 12 mg Hg. The usual cause of variceal rebleeding after TIPS is the recurrence of portal hypertension. This may result from TIPS thrombosis, stent retraction and kinking, stent stenosis, or the development of right heart failure (4). TIPS thrombosis is the most common cause of recurrent portal hypertension and usually occurs within the first month (4).

TIPS was compared with the distal splenorenal shunt (DSRS) in Child-Pugh class A and B patients with esophageal varix bleeding (33). No significant differences in rebleeding rate, incidence of hepatic encephalopathy, liver transplantation or mortality were reported (33). These results were obtained with a significant higher reintervention rate in the TIPS group than in the DSRS group. However, a multicenter randomized controlled trial reported much lower obstruction and reintervention rates with the use of PTFE-covered stents (17). TIPS was associated with lower rates of recurrent bleeding and ascites without increased the incidence of encephalopathy, as observed with bare stents (17). These results suggest that the small disadvantage of TIPS versus surgical shunt would be overcome by the use of PTFE-covered stents (17, 34). In conclusion, TIPS may be more cost effective than DSRS whereas TIPS is equal to DSRS in the prevention of variceal rebleeding in patients who are medical failures (35).

Surgical options are principally used in Child-Pugh class A patients. A previous Cochrane review reported that shunt therapy in contrast to endoscopic therapy significantly reduced rebleeding, but with a significantly increased incidence of acute and chronic hepatic encephalopathy (36). A randomized trial of emergency portacaval shunt compared to sclerotherapy reported that portacaval shunt permanently stopped variceal bleeding, rarely became occluded, was accomplished with a low incidence of portasystemic encephalopathy (PSE), and produced greater long term survival (37). The choice of therapy should be based on the local expertise in each technique, the possibility of achieving an adequate follow-up of the patient as well as the logistics of promptly intervening if needed.

Successful OLT is the only definite treatment which corrects the portal hypertension. Patients with Child-Pugh class B or C cirrhosis should be evaluated for transplantation. A previously placed TIPS can be removed with the explant at the time of transplant.

Complications of TIPS

TIPS is associated with a number of complications, and some may be fatal. Complications of TIPS are listed in Box 7.1. The direct procedural mortality rate is less than 2% and the 30-day mortality rate ranges from 4% to 45% (12). The technical complications associated with insertion of TIPS can occur at various stages of the procedure. Complications may start early in the TIPS procedure. In addition to inadvertent carotid artery or tracheal puncture, the most common complication is the development of cardiac arrhythmias as the catheter passes through the heart (12). Serious arrhythmias, such as atrial fibrillation, conduction defects (nodal or infranodal), ventricular tachycardia, and complete heart block in patients with a preexisting left bundle branch block, can occur (38). Using a Check Flow II introducer, with a relatively stiff sheath, which prevents buckling of the catheter in the right heart can help minimize these arrhythmias. The main complication related to creation of the intrahepatic tract is traversal of the liver capsule and creation of a tract between the shunt or the portal vein and the hepatic artery or bile ducts. The reported incidence of capsule traversal is approximately 33% but the development of clinically obvious hemoperitoneum is relatively rare (12). This complication is most likely to occur when the liver is

---

Box 7.1 Complications of TIPS

Procedure related
  - Shunt displacement
  - Inadequately deployed shunt
  - Laceration of vessels
  - Arrhythmia
  - Hemobilia
  - Extrahepatic puncture of the portal vein with hemoperitomeum
  - TIPS-biliary fistula
  - TIPS-arterial fistula
  - Hepatic infarction
  - Rupture of liver or inferior vena cava
Sepsis
Portasystemic encephalopathy
TIPS dysfunction
  - Occlusion
  - Stenosis
  - Thrombosis
Prosthesis related
  - Hemolytic anemia
  - Migration of stent
  - Misplacement of stent
  - Kinking
  - Infective endotipsitis

small, hard, and displaced upward by tense ascites or when the portal vein is thrombosed and replaced by collaterals. This complication can be prevented by a large volume paracentesis and evaluation of portal vein patency by Doppler sonography or mesenteric angiography prior to the TIPS procedure. A complication of portal vein manipulation can be extrahepatic puncture of the portal vein with exsanguinating hemorrhage after attempts to dilate the site of portal vein puncture (12).

Up to 80% of patients experience some degree of TIPS stenosis within the first year (4, 13, 16). By two years, virtually all surviving patients develop TIPS stenosis (4). Extensive thrombosis of the TIPS, the portal vein, or the splenic vein occur in 3 to 12% of patients after TIPS (12). TIPS created with expanded PTFE-covered stent have better three-month primary patency rates and better 3-month and 12-month clinical success rates compared with those created with bare stents (34). Once thrombosis occurs, treatment options include thrombolysis, anticoagulation, or suction thrombectomy (39). In those who are candidates, liver transplantation is the optimal definitive treatment. Angiography is the gold standard for assessment of shunt patency and is required for treatment of shunt stenosis (4). However, it is limited by its invasive nature and cost. Doppler ultrasonography is a noninvasive alternative method to monitor shunt patency with relative insensitivity in detecting stent stenosis. Early detection of TIPS dysfunction requires periodic Doppler ultrasound examination (40). Due to the lack of the sensitivity of Doppler ultrasound for identification of TIPS stenosis, AASLD recommends performing catheterization of the TIPS or upper endoscopy (to detect resultant varices) at one year (1). A commonly used follow-up regimen is angiography at 6 and 12 months after TIPS and annually thereafter for the first three years (4). The propensity for development of stent stenosis decreases after four years (4). Echo-enhanced Doppler sonography and helical CT angiography have shown promise (41, 42). TIPS stenosis responds well to dilation and placement of additional stents in series with the preexisting stents to shore up the dilated stents. TIPS stenosis is an important cause of recurrent portal hypertension and variceal bleeding. It is therefore mandatory to periodically monitor TIPS patency. PTFE-covered stents have significantly improved TIPS patency (17, 45). The need for follow-up and interventions has been reduced significantly as a result of improved shunt patency (17, 45).

TIPS-associated hemolytic anemia occurs in approximately 10% of patients which presents within 7 to 14 days after stent placement, but this spontaneously resolves within 8 to 12 weeks in the majority of patients (44). Most patients have a minor reduction in hemoglobin concentration, but severe anemia can occur. Hemolysis results from injury to red cells from shear stress or direct mechanical trauma in the shunt. TIPS infections can occur weeks to months after TIPS placement. The organisms are predominantly of enteric origin (45).

Complications related to portasystemic shunting

The main complication due to shunting of blood from the portal to systemic circulation is the development of PSE. Patients undergoing TIPS can also develop focal neurologic deficits compatible with shunt myelopathy (46). PSE is a very frequent complication, and certainly constitutes one of the major drawbacks of TIPS. It is potentially the most disabling and limiting complication to patients and should be considered before selecting TIPS as treatment. The one-year incidence of PSE ranges from 35% to 55% and is similar to that reported after surgical shunt (16, 47, 48). Twenty-five per cent of TIPS recipients experience de novo PSE or worsening of prior PSE (15). PSE usually becomes clinically apparent 2–3 weeks after TIPS insertion (32). In 90% of cases, PSE develops within the first three months of TIPS insertion at which time the stent is fully patent, and portal pressure is <12mm Hg (16). In a typical clinical course after TIPS, progressive stent stenosis or other dysfunction contributes to the improvement of PSE and eventual disappearance of PSE (4). Up to 5% of cases require endovascular treatment for PSE with diameter reducing stents or TIPS intentional occlusion (49, 50). The shunt diameter can be reduced mechanically in specially designed stents.(49). Risk factors are age >65 years, Child-Pugh class C, prior PSE, high diameter stent (>10 mm), and low portasystemic pressure gradient (<5 mmHg) (16, 32, 51, 52). Pharmacologic prophylaxis during the first month after TIPS was not beneficial in a controlled trial (53). When PSE develops after TIPS, a search for precipitating factors which can be reversed is mandatory. PSE responds to medical treatment in the majority of patients (32). PSE after TIPS with PTFE-covered stent is not decreased (54). OLT is the treatment of choice for refractory PSE.

Orthotopic liver transplantation

OLT has emerged over the past several decades as a viable treatment option for patients with fulminant hepatic failure and end-stage liver disease. Successful OLT corrects both liver dysfunction and portal hypertension but does not always cure the underlying liver disease. OLT has significantly improved survival of patients with bleeding varices and Child-Pugh class C cirrhosis. The indication for liver transplantation, however, is end-stage liver disease (as monitored by high MELD scores) rather than variceal bleeding. In high-risk patients, the need for OLT should be discussed before the performance of an elective TIPS (1). The presence of TIPS does not affect operative mortality or blood transfusion requirements in patients having transplantation (55), but may increase the technical difficulty of the surgery (56, 57). An early referral to a transplant center should be the standard of care. The selection of a transplant candidate is a risk-benefit analysis, in which co-morbidities and the inherent risks of surgery, recurrent disease, and long-term immunosuppression must be weighed against the potential benefits of transplantation.

Summary

- Transjugular intrahepatic portasystemic shunt (TIPS) and shunt surgery are effective in controlling acute bleeding from varices that is refractory to medical and endoscopic therapy.
- TIPS stenosis is common. TIPS surveillance by catheterization of the TIPS or upper endoscopy (to detect esophageal varices) should be performed for recurrent UGI bleeding or at one year after TIPS and annually.
- In patients with good liver function, either a TIPS or a shunt surgery are appropriate choices for control of active variceal bleeding and the prevention of rebleeding in patients who have failed medical and endoscopic therapy. In patients with poor liver function, TIPS is preferred to surgical therapy for control of active variceal bleeding and in the prevention of rebleeding in patients who have failed medical and endoscopic therapy
- Portasystemic encephalopathy is a common complication of portosystemic shunting (surgical or TIPS). The identification of variables associated with an increased risk of encephalopathy may be useful in the selection of appropriate candidates.
- Successful orthotopic liver transplantation corrects both liver dysfunction and portal hypertension.

Conclusion

TIPS and surgical shunting effectively decrease portal pressure especially in patients with HVPG >20 mm Hg. Through this effect, shunting has gained a major role in the salvage therapy for Child-Pugh class A or B patients with active or recurrent variceal bleeding despite standard endoscopic and pharmacologic treatments. TIPS is a non-surgical procedure which achieves the desired hemodynamic goal in more than 90% of cases, in experienced hands. TIPS does not require general anesthesia and is associated with very low procedure-related mortality. However, PSE and stent dysfunction are the major drawbacks. Newly developed covered-stents, which have lower stenosis rates, might expand the currently accepted recommendations for TIPS use. Surgery is an option in patients with failures of endoscopic treatment and impossibility to perform TIPS. OLT corrects both liver dysfunction and portal hypertension and therefore is a therapeutic option for patients with severe end-stage liver disease and refractory variceal bleeding.

References

1. Boyer TD, Haskal ZJ. The Role of Transjugular Intrahepatic Portosystemic Shunt (TIPS) in the Management of Portal Hypertension: update 2009. Hepatology 51(1):306.
2. Chau TN, Patch D, Chan YW, Nagral A, Dick R, Burroughs AK. "Salvage" transjugular intrahepatic portosystemic shunts: gastric fundal compared with esophageal variceal bleeding. Gastroenterology 1998;114(5):981–7.
3. Sanyal AJ, Freedman AM, Luketic VA, Purdum PP, Shiffman ML, Tisnado J, et al. Transjugular intrahepatic portosystemic shunts for patients with active variceal hemorrhage unresponsive to sclerotherapy. Gastroenterology 1996;111(1):138–46.
4. Sanyal AJ, Freedman AM, Luketic VA, Purdum PP, 3rd, Shiffman ML, DeMeo J, et al. The natural history of portal hypertension after transjugular intrahepatic portosystemic shunts. Gastroenterology 1997;112(3):889–98.
5. Garcia-Pagan JC, Heydtmann M, Raffa S, Plessier A, Murad S, Fabris F, et al. TIPS for Budd-Chiari syndrome: long-term results and prognostics factors in 124 patients. Gastroenterology 2008;135(3):808–15.
6. Yang Z, Han G, Wu Q, Ye X, Jin Z, Yin Z, et al. Patency and clinical outcomes of transjugular intrahepatic portosystemic shunt with polytetrafluoroethylene-covered stents versus bare stents: a meta-analysis. J Gastroenterol Hepatol 25(11): 1718–2725.
7. Moitinho E, Escorsell A, Bandi JC, Salmeron JM, Garcia-Pagan JC, Rodes J, et al. Prognostic value of early measurements of portal pressure in acute variceal bleeding. Gastroenterology 1999;117(3):626–31.
8. Henderson JM. Salvage therapies for refractory variceal hemorrhage. Clin Liver Dis 2001;5: 709–25.
9. Garcia-Pagan JC, Caca K, Bureau C, Laleman W, Appenrodt B, Luca A, et al. Early use of TIPS in patients with cirrhosis and variceal bleeding. N Engl J Med.; 362 (25).2370–2379.
10. Ochs A. Transjugular intrahepatic portosystemic shunt. Dig Dis 2005;23(1):56–64.
11. Ring EJ, Lake JR, Roberts JP, Gordon RL, LaBerge JM, Read AE, et al. Using transjugular intrahepatic portosystemic shunts to control variceal bleeding before liver transplantation. Ann Intern Med 1992;116(4):304–9.
12. Freedman AM, Sanyal AJ, Tisnado J, Cole PE, Shiffman ML, Luketic VA, et al. Complications of transjugular intrahepatic portosystemic shunt: a comprehensive review. Radiographics 1993;13(6):1185–1210.
13. Boyer TD, Henderson JM, Heerey AM, Arrigain S, Konig V, Connor J, et al. Cost of preventing variceal rebleeding with transjugular intrahepatic portal systemic shunt and distal splenorenal shunt. J Hepatol 2008;48(3):407–14.

14. Rossle M, Haag K, Ochs A, Sellinger M, Noldge G, Perarnau JM, et al. The transjugular intrahepatic portosystemic stent-shunt procedure for variceal bleeding. N Engl J Med 1994;330(3):165–71.

15. Monescillo A, Martinez-Lagares F, Ruiz-del-Arbol L, Sierra A, Guevara C, Jimenez E, et al. Influence of portal hypertension and its early decompression by TIPS placement on the outcome of variceal bleeding. Hepatology 2004;40 (4):793–801.

16. Colombato L. The role of transjugular intrahepatic portosystemic shunt (TIPS) in the management of portal hypertension. J Clin Gastroenterol 2007; 41 Suppl 3: S344–51.

17. Bureau C, Garcia-Pagan JC, Otal P, et al. Improved clinical outcome using polytetra-fluoroethylene-coated stents for TIPS: results of a randomized study. Gastroenterology 2004;126: 469–75.

18. Cello JP, Grendell JH, Crass RA, Weber TE, Trunkey DD. Endoscopic sclerotherapy versus portacaval shunt in patient with severe cirrhosis and acute variceal hemorrhage. Long-term follow-up. N Engl J Med 1987;316(1):11–15.

19. Planas R, Boix J, Broggi M, Cabre E, Gomes-Vieira MC, Morillas R, et al. Portacaval shunt versus endoscopic sclerotherapy in the elective treatment of variceal hemorrhage. Gastroenterology 1991;100(4):1078–1086.

20. Rikkers LF. The changing spectrum of treatment for variceal bleeding. Ann Surg 1998;228: 536–46.

21. Henderson JM. Role of distal splenorenal shunt for long-term management of variceal bleeding. World J Surg 1994;18: 205–10.

22. Stipa S, Balducci G, Ziparo V, Stipa F, Lucandri G. Total shunting and elective management of variceal bleeding. World J Surg 1994;18(2):200–4.

23. Rosemurgy AS, Serafini FM, Zweibel BR, Black TJ, Kudryk BT, Nord HJ, et al. Transjugular intrahepatic portosystemic shunt vs. small-diameter prosthetic H-graft portacaval shunt: extended follow-up of an expanded randomized prospective trial. J Gastrointest Surg 2000;4(6):589–97.

24. Rosemurgy AS, 2nd, Bloomston M, Zervos EE, Goode FSE, Pencev D, Zweibel B, et al. Transjugular intrahepatic portosystemic shunt versus H-graft portacaval shunt in the management of bleeding varices: a cost-benefit analysis. Surgery 1997;122(4):794–9; discussion 9–800.

25. Escorsell A, Banares R, Garcia-Pagan JC, Gilabert R, Moitinho E, Piqueras B, et al. TIPS versus drug therapy in preventing variceal rebleeding in advanced cirrhosis: a randomized controlled trial. Hepatology 2002;35(2):385–92.

26. Burroughs AK, Vangeli M. Transjugular intrahepatic portosystemic shunt versus endoscopic therapy: randomized trials for secondary prophylaxis of variceal bleeding: an updated meta-analysis. Scand J Gastroenterol 2002;37(3):249–52.

27. Papatheodoridis GV, Goulis J, Leandro G, Patch D, Burroughs AK. Transjugular intrahepatic portosystemic shunt compared with endoscopic treatment for prevention of variceal rebleeding: A meta-analysis. Hepatology 1999;30(3):612–22.

28. D'Amico G, Pagliaro L, Bosch J. The treatment of portal hypertension: a meta-analytic review. Hepatology 1995;22(1):332–54.

29. Jalan R, Forrest EH, Stanley AJ, Redhead DN, Forbes J, Dillon JF, et al. A randomized trial comparing transjugular intrahepatic portosystemic stent-shunt with variceal band ligation in the prevention of rebleeding from esophageal varices. Hepatology 1997;26(5):1115–1122.

30. Zheng M, Chen Y, Bai J, Zeng Q, You J, Jin R, et al. Transjugular intrahepatic portosystemic shunt versus endoscopic therapy in the secondary prophylaxis of

variceal rebleeding in cirrhotic patients: meta-analysis update. J Clin Gastroenterol 2008;42(5):507–16.

31. Sanyal AJ, Freedman AM, Shiffman ML, Purdum PP, 3rd, Luketic VA, Cheatham AK. Portosystemic encephalopathy after transjugular intrahepatic portosystemic shunt: results of a prospective controlled study. Hepatology 1994;20(1 Pt 1):46–55.

32. Pomier-Layrargues G. TIPS and hepatic encephalopathy. Semin Liver Dis 1996; 16(3):315–20.

33. Henderson JM, Boyer TD, Kutner MH, et al. Distal splenorenal shunt versus transjugular intrahepatic portal systematic shunt for variceal bleeding: a randomized trial. Gastroenterology 2006;130: 1643–1651.

34. Jung HS, Kalva SP, Greenfield AJ, Waltman AC, Walker TG, Athanasoulis CA, et al. TIPS: comparison of shunt patency and clinical outcomes between bare stents and expanded polytetrafluoroethylene stent-grafts. J Vasc Interv Radiol 2009;20(2):180–5.

35. Boyer TD, Henderson JM, Heerey AM, Arrigain S, Konig V, Connor J, et al. Cost of preventing variceal rebleeding with transjugular intrahepatic portal systemic shunt and distal splenorenal shunt. J Hepatol 2008;48(3):407–14.

36. Khan S, Tudur Smith C, Williamson P, Sutton R. Portosystemic shunts versus endoscopic therapy for variceal rebleeding in patients with cirrhosis. Cochrane Database Syst Rev 2006 (4):CD000553.

37. Orloff MJ, Isenberg JI, Wheeler HO, Haynes KS, Jinich-Brook H, Rapier R, et al. Randomized trial of emergency endoscopic sclerotherapy versus emergency portacaval shunt for acutely bleeding esophageal varices in cirrhosis. J Am Coll Surg 2009 Jul; 209(1):25–40.

38. Pidlich J, Peck-Radosavljevic M, Kranz A, Wildling R, Winkelbauer FW, Lammer J, et al. Transjugular intrahepatic portosystemic shunt and cardiac arrhythmias. J Clin Gastroenterol 1998;26(1):39–43.

39. Raat H, Stockx L, Ranschaert E, Nevens F, Wilms G, Baert AL. Percutaneous hydrodynamic thrombectomy of acute thrombosis in transjugular intrahepatic portosystemic shunt (TIPS): a feasibility study in five patients. Cardiovasc Intervent Radiol 1997;20(3):180–3.

40. Lafortune M, Martinet JP, Denys A, Patriquin H, Dauzat M, Dufresne MP, et al. Short- and long-term hemodynamic effects of transjugular intrahepatic portosystemic shunts: a Doppler/manometric correlative study. AJR Am J Roentgenol 1995 Apr; 164(4):997–1002.

41. Uggowitzer MM, Kugler C, Machan L, Hausegger KA, Groell R, Quehenberger F, et al. Value of echo-enhanced Doppler sonography in evaluation of transjugular intrahepatic portosystemic shunts. AJR Am J Roentgenol 1998;170(4):1041–1046.

42. Chopra S, Dodd GD, 3rd, Chintapalli KN, Rhim H, Encarnacion CE, Palmaz JC, et al. Transjugular intrahepatic portosystemic shunt: accuracy of helical CT angiography in the detection of shunt abnormalities. Radiology 2000;215(1):115–22.

43. Cura M, Cura A, Suri R, El-Merhi F, Lopera J, Kroma G. Causes of TIPS dysfunction. AJR Am J Roentgenol 2008;191(6):1751–7.

44. Sanyal AJ, Freedman AM, Purdum PP, Shiffman ML, Luketic VA. The hematologic consequences of transjugular intrahepatic portosystemic shunts. Hepatology 1996; 23(1):32–9.

45. Sanyal AJ, Reddy KR. Vegetative infection of transjugular intrahepatic portosystemic shunts. Gastroenterology 1998;115(1):110–15.

46. Wang MQ, Dake MD, Cui ZP, Wang ZQ, Gao YA. Portal-systemic myelopathy after transjugular intrahepatic portosystemic shunt creation: report of four cases. J Vasc Interv Radiol 2001;12(7):879–81.

47. Mutchnick MG, Lerner E, Conn HO. Portal-systemic encephalopathy and portacaval anastomosis: a prospective, controlled investigation. Gastroenterology 1974;66(5): 1005–1019.

48. Grace ND, Conn HO, Resnick RH, Groszmann RJ, Atterbury CE, Wright SC, et al. Distal splenorenal vs. portal-systemic shunts after hemorrhage from varices: a randomized controlled trial. Hepatology 1988;8(6):1475–81.

49. Hauenstein KH, Haag K, Ochs A, Langer M, Rossle M. The reducing stent: treatment for transjugular intrahepatic portosystemic shunt-induced refractory hepatic encephalopathy and liver failure. Radiology 1995;194(1):175–9.

50. Maleux G, Verslype C, Heye S, Wilms G, Marchal G, Nevens F. Endovascular shunt reduction in the management of transjugular portosystemic shunt-induced hepatic encephalopathy: preliminary experience with reduction stents and stent-grafts. AJR Am J Roentgenol 2007;188(3):659–64.

51. Rossle M, Piotraschke J. Transjugular intrahepatic portosystemic shunt and hepatic encephalopathy. Dig Dis 1996;14Suppl 1: 12–19.

52. Somberg KA, Riegler JL, LaBerge JM, Doherty-Simor MM, Bachetti P, Roberts JP, et al. Hepatic encephalopathy after transjugular intrahepatic portosystemic shunts: incidence and risk factors. Am J Gastroenterol 1995;90(4):549–55.

53. Riggio O, Masini A, Efrati C, Nicolao F, Angeloni S, Salvatori FM, et al. Pharmacological prophylaxis of hepatic encephalopathy after transjugular intrahepatic portosystemic shunt: a randomized controlled study. J Hepatol 2005;42(5):674–9.

54. Riggio O, Angeloni S, Salvatori FM, De Santis A, Cerini F, Farcomeni A, et al. Incidence, natural history, and risk factors of hepatic encephalopathy after transjugular intrahepatic portosystemic shunt with polytetrafluoroethylene-covered stent grafts. Am J Gastroenterol 2008;103(11):2738–3746.

55. Somberg KA, Lombardero MS, Lawlor SM, Ascher NL, Lake JR, Wiesner RH, et al. A controlled analysis of the transjugular intrahepatic portosystemic shunt in liver transplant recipients. The National Institute of Diabetes and Digestive and Kidney Diseases (NIDDK) Liver Transplantation Database. Transplantation 1997 27;63(8): 1074–1079.

56. Tripathi D, Therapondos G, Redhead DN, Madhavan KK, Hayes PC. Transjugular intrahepatic portosystemic stent-shunt and its effects on orthotopic liver transplantation. Eur J Gastroenterol Hepatol 2002;14(8):827–32.

57. Guerrini GP, Pleguezuelo M, Maimone S, Calvaruso V, Xirouchakis E, Patch D, et al. Impact of tips preliver transplantation for the outcome posttransplantation. Am J Transplant 2009;9(1):192–200.

CHAPTER 8

Other Causes of Upper Gastrointestinal Bleeding

I. Lisanne Holster[1] & Ernst J. Kuipers[1,2]
[1]Department of Gastroenterology and Hepatology, Rotterdam, the Netherlands
[2]Department of Internal Medicine, Erasmus MC University Medical Centre, Rotterdam, the Netherlands

Upper gastrointestinal bleeding can be classified into several different categories, according to etiology and pathophysiology. The commonest causes of upper gastrointestinal (GI) bleeding, as reported in several endoscopic studies, are variceal bleeding and peptic ulcer bleeding (1–3). These two main causes have been discussed in the previous chapters, yet the list of differential diagnoses of bleeding of the upper gastrointestinal tract is much longer (Box 8.1). Although less common than variceal and peptic ulcer bleeding, these other causes are met frequently. A retrospective study from Sweden reported that the incidence of peptic ulcer bleeding had decreased over a 20-year period from 62 to 32 per 100,000 per year, the incidence of non-ulcer, non-variceal upper gastrointestinal bleeding had remained stable at 30 per 100,000 per year (4). These data are in line with the results of a UK study on 5,004 patients presenting with upper GI bleeding. Peptic ulcer and varices were present in 36 and 11% patients; the remainder of bleeds was related to other causes (5). In a similar Dutch study on 769 patients with upper GI bleeding, 47% had non-ulcer non-variceal bleeding (3). The main causes of non-ulcer, non-variceal bleeding are gastroduodenal erosions and esophagitis. This chapter deals with the spectrum and variety of causes of non-variceal non-ulcer upper GI bleeding.

Erosive causes of upper gastrointestinal bleeding

An erosion is a breach of the epithelial surface that does not extend beyond the muscularis mucosa and has a diameter ≤ 5 mm. Erosions can occur throughout the gastrointestinal tract. Causes of upper gastrointestinal erosions can be divided into direct toxic, mechanic and inflammatory etiology.

Gastrointestinal Bleeding, Second Edition. Edited by Joseph J.Y. Sung, Ernst J. Kuipers and Alan N. Barkun. © 2012 Blackwell Publishing Ltd.
Published 2012 by Blackwell Publishing Ltd.

Box 8.1 Etiology of non-variceal, non-peptic ulcer upper gastrointestinal bleeding

EROSIVE
- Drug induced
- Mechanic (e.g. Cameron lesions)
- Inflammatory (esophagitis/gastritis/duodenitis)

VASCULAR
- Angiodysplasia
- Dieulafoy lesion
- Vasoenteric fistula
- Portal hypertensive gastropathy
- Gastric antral vascular ectasia
- Hereditary vascular anomalies
- Vasculitides and systemic disorders
- Ischemia

NEOPLASTIC
- Polyp (adenomatous/hyperplastic/fundic gland/hamartomatous)
- Adeno-/squamous cell carcinoma
- Lymphoma
- Mesenchymal neoplasm

- Kaposi's sarcoma
- Melanoma
- Neuroendocrine tumor
- Metastatic tumor

TRAUMATIC OR IATROGENIC
- Mallory-Weiss tear
- Intramural hematoma
- Boerhaave's Syndrome
- Foreign body/toxic substance ingestion
- Post-endoscopy intervention
- Post-surgical intervention

MISCELLANEOUS
- Hemobilia
- Hemosuccus pancreaticus
- Bleeding diathesis
- Nasopharyngeal lesion

Erosions are a common finding during upper endoscopy. In a random sample of the adult population of two Swedish municipalities, 1,001 subjects underwent upper endoscopy. Esophageal erosions were found in 16% of the population (6). Based on a validated questionnaire, two-thirds of subjects with esophageal erosions reported gastrointestinal symptoms. The erosions were often seen in combination with gastro-esophageal reflux disease. In a similarly designed study in Italy, endoscopic abnormalities were found in 23% of the subjects. Esophagitis was found in 11.8% and peptic ulcer in 5.9% of individuals, whereas 5.3% had gastroduodenal erosions (7). A large population-based study in China among 1,022 randomly selected volunteers who underwent a gastroscopy, reported a much higher prevalence of gastroduodenal erosions (49.9%) (8). The majority (77.3%) of these individuals with erosive lesions were asymptomatic. Duodenal erosions were more prevalent among men.

Drug induced erosion

Mucosal erosions caused by direct toxic effects of drugs are more frequently seen since aging populations are naturally burdened with chronic diseases and polypharmacy. Non-steroidal anti-inflammatory drugs (NSAIDs) and aspirin are considered the main cause of erosive disease in Western patients (9). NSAIDs can produce a spectrum of mucosal damage. Intramucosal petechial hemorrhage can occur within two hours of initial ingestion. Superficial and hemorrhagic erosions, gastroduodenitis and ulceration may develop with continued exposure (10). In an endoscopic study of 187 patients using low dose aspirin for at least three months without gastroprotective agents, erosions were found in 63% of subjects (11). A similar study in asymptomatic patients using aspirin with gastroprotective agents reported the presence of erosions in 34% (12).

Other notorious mucosal damage causing drugs are selective serotonin reuptake inhibitors (SSRIs), and corticosteroids. Both classes of drugs are associated with peptic ulcer bleeds as well as non-ulcer, non-variceal bleeds. In a large case-control study from Sweden, current use of SSRIs was associated with an odds ratio of 1.67 (95% CI 1.46–1.92) for upper gastrointestinal bleeding (13). These bleeds are related both to overt ulcer disease, as well as gastroduodenal erosions.

Nitrogen-containing bisphosphonates, mainly used for the treatment of osteoporosis, can also cause mucosal irritation of the upper GI tract and even ulceration, bleeding and perforation. A review on the adverse effect of bisphosphonates showed little or no increased risk of gastrointestinal complications if bisphosphonates were administered properly and discontinued promptly if esophageal symptoms developed (14). However, proper administration requires that bisophosphonate tablets are taken in the morning with sufficient water and the patient remaining upright and fasting for at least 30 minutes after bisphosponate intake. These precautions are often not adhered to. Other classes of drugs which can lead to erosions and ulceration are potassium tablets, some antibiotics (e.g. Erythromycin, Nalidixin acid, Sulfonamides and derivatives) and chemotherapy as well as radiation therapy (10).

Mechanical erosions

A common cause of mechanical erosive disease is hiatal hernia. Larger hiatal hernia can give rise to development of linear erosions and ulcers or so-called Cameron lesions within the stomach at the impression of the diaphragm (Fig. 8.1) (15). They predominantly occur along the smaller curvature, and their exact etiology is unknown. They most likely occur as a result of the combination of chronic mechanical trauma (e.g. rubbing of the mucosal folds at the level of the diaphragm during respiratory excursions) and acid injury. Local ischemia has been suggested to contribute to this process, H. pylori does not appear to play a role.

Cameron lesions are found in about 5% of the patients with hiatal hernia undergoing upper endoscopy, two thirds of these patients have multiple

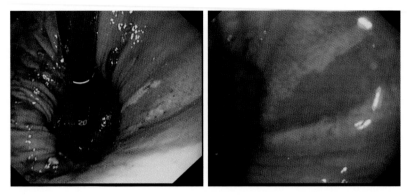

Figure 8.1 Cameron lesions showing as white mucosal breaks at the 1 to 3 o'clock position in a large hiatal hernia with the endoscope in retroflexion. Some red spots indicate minor bleeding

lesions (16). Their prevalence rises with the size of the hernia. They have been reported to occur in 10–20% of patients with a hernia ≥5 cm (17). Usually they are seen accidentally, although they may cause acute or chronic gastrointestinal bleeding and iron deficiency anemia. This was already illustrated by the first description of lesions in 1986 by Cameron and Higgins (15). They reported on 109 patients with hiatal hernia, half of whom had anemia. Cameron lesions were found in 24% of those anaemic patients. Since then, Cameron lesions have been associated with chronic bleeding leading to anemia, but also with acute bleeding. The treatment of choice is acid suppression, generally with excellent outcome. Acute bleeds sometimes require endoscopic treatment such as of a visible vessel, for the treatment is similar to the approach of other gastroduodenal ulcers. Cameron lesions are a well known cause of missed diagnoses in patients with upper GI bleeding undergoing endoscopy. Patients with larger hiatal hernia and signs of anemia or bleeding should therefore be adequately inspected including endoscopy in retroversion to optimize the inspection of the hernia.

Inflammatory erosions

Erosive esophago-gastro-duodenitis, an acute or chronic inflammation of the lining of the esophagus, stomach and/or duodenum, has many possible causes. Acute causes are associated with excessive alcohol consumption and the use of drugs (see before) (18). Chronic causes include gastro-esophageal reflux disease and *H. pylori* infection (Fig. 8.2) (19, 20). Infection with *H. pylori* causes chronic inflammation of the gastric mucosa, which may slowly progress via atrophic gastritis, intestinal metaplasia, and dysplasia to gastric adenocarcinoma (21).

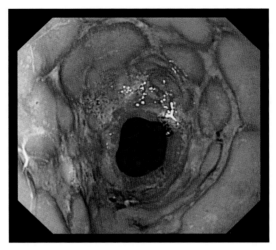

Figure 8.2 Reflux oesophagitis in the presence of hiatal herniation

In most cross-sectional studies of patients with upper gastrointestinal bleeding, erosive disease is reported as underlying cause in 8% to 34% percent of cases (Table 8.1) (1, 3, 22–24).

However, in a 17-year follow-up study of 117 patients with gastric erosions without peptic ulcer disease, no clinical history of gastrointestinal bleeding during the follow-up and no difference in haemoglobin level

Table 8.1 Proportional distribution of causes of upper gastrointestinal bleeding in various studies.

	Czernichow (1)	Paspatis (24)	Van Leerdam (3)	Di Fiore (22)	Theocharis (23)
Country	France	Greece	The Netherlands	France	Greece
Year of report	1996	1998–1999	2000	2000	2005
No. of patients	2133	353	769	453	353
Peptic ulcer	37	49	46	31	67
Gastric	NR	21	NR	NR	32
Duodenal	NR	27	NR	NR	33
Erosive disease	12	31	20*	16**	8***
Esophagitis	12	3	NR	11	NR
Esophageal/gastric varices	14	4	7	20	6
Mallory-Weiss tear	7	NR	NR	8	4
Malignancy	3	3	5	2	8
Other diagnosis	7	3	8	NR	2
No cause identified	8	7	14	11	5

NR: not reported
*Including esophageal ulcers, esophagitis, gastritis, bulbitis and erosions
**Including gastritis
***Gastroduodenitis

compared with the group patients without erosions was seen (19). This indicates that gastroduodenal erosions infrequently cause clinically significant blood loss. This is supported, for instance, by data from cohort studies of long-term aspirin users, showing the common occurrence of gastroduodenal erosions, but a low incidence of clinically overt bleeding. A systematic review of literature data reported an annual incidence of any major bleeding in 1 per 769 low-dose aspirin users (25).

Treatment and prevention of (bleeding from) erosions depends upon the cause. Most cases respond well to proton pump inhibitor (PPI) therapy, leading to healing of erosions and normalization of haemoglobin levels. The offending agent should be discontinued whenever possible and, if present, *H. pylori* should be eradicated. Some patients require surgical therapy, such as correction of a hiatal hernia for recurrent bleeding from Cameron lesions (17).

Angiodysplasia

Angiodysplasia is defined as a sharply delineated vascular lesion within the mucosa, with a typical red appearance, with flat or slightly raised surface (Fig. 8.3). The lesions are often multiple and frequently seen in the colon, but may also involve the upper gastrointestinal tract and small bowel. They are generally believed to be acquired, since the peak of diagnosis lies in the fifth and sixth decade of life. The exact causes of angiodysplasia are unknown (26). Associations with renal insufficiency and cardiac valve disease have been reported, but it is unknown whether these associations

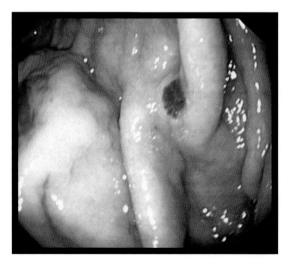

Figure 8.3 Angiodysplasias of the gastric corpus, presenting as marked red spots within the mucosa

are in any way causal (27, 28). An explanation is that the lesions are actually not more common in patients with renal and cardiac disease, but are instead detected more frequently because of the increased risk of bleeding in these patients.

Patients with angiodysplasia can present with chronic anemia, as well as with acute gastrointestinal bleeding with melena and seldom hematemesis. In a study from the USA evaluating 727 patients with end-stage renal disease and acute upper gastrointestinal bleeding, 1.3% bled from an angiodysplastic lesion (29). The current standard of endoscopic treatment of bleeding angiodysplasias consists of coagulation therapy. Although this is associated with a high success rate for treatment of individual lesions, patients may during follow-up often present with recurrent anemia or overt bleeding due to incomplete treatment of multiple lesions, or due to occurrence of renewed lesions. This may require repeat endoscopy, often also including colonoscopy and sometimes enteroscopy.

In a Dutch study of 132 patients who underwent balloon-assisted enteroscopy for reasons of recurrent or persistent anemia without a focus on gastroduodenoscopy and ileocolonoscopy, angiodysplasia or vascular malformation was found in 40 patients (30%). Twenty-two percent of patients initially treated for angiodysplasia suffered from rebleeding after initial improvement. In all but one patient, persistent angiodysplasias and/or vessel malformations were seen, requiring repeated therapy. This repeated therapy resulted in improvement in 58% (30).

In this context, systemic medical therapy may play an adjuvant or even primary role (31). The best-studied pharmacological agents are estrogen and progesterone, but their effects remain controversial. A Spanish multicenter, randomized controlled trial compared ethinylestradiol (0.01 mg) plus norethisterone (2 mg) with placebo for a minimum period of one year. No difference in bleeding episodes and transfusion requirements was found between both treatment arms (32).

Another potential effective drug is somatostatin analogues such as octreotide. A recent meta-analysis including a total of 62 patients of three studies showed a beneficial effect of octreotide on the need for transfusion in patients with angiodysplastic lesions (33). The weighted mean difference in transfusion requirements before starting therapy and after treatment initiation was -2.2 (95% CI -3.9 to -0.5). Although less widely studied, thalidomide may be a promising drug where other therapies failed to stop the bleeding (34, 35). In a pilot study, seven patients with chronic angiodysplastic bleeding were treated with thalidomide in a starting dose of 50 mg/day, increased if tolerated with 50 mg/day every week up to 200 mg daily. Therapy was then continued for six months. Four patients discontinued treatment within 3–8 weeks because of side effects and required the same amount of blood transfusions as pre-study. In contrast the other three patients did not require any transfusion during the six months of therapy (36).

Dieulafoy lesion

A Dieulafoy lesion consists of a dilated tortuous artery with a diameter up to 3 mm that protrudes through the mucosa (Fig. 8.4). These lesions most commonly occur in the proximal stomach along the lesser curve, but they are incidentally seen in the esophagus (37), small intestine and colon (38). Dieulafoy lesions may cause massive gastrointestinal hemorrhage by rupture of the artery, accounting for 1–6% of cases of acute non-variceal upper gastrointestinal bleeding (39). Rupture occurs probably by a combination of factors like straining of the vascular wall during peristalsis, morphologic changes of the artery, and peptic digestion (39, 40). The high prevalence of co-morbidity (90%) and correlated drug-use in patients with Dieulafoy lesions is likely to play an additional role in the process of vessel rupture (39).

Dieulafoy lesions can easily be missed during endoscopy, because the mucosal break is usually minor, may be hidden from view due to blood remnants, and because the bleed can be intermittent. This may give rise to a typical pattern of repeated acute severe bleeding with shock, yet failure to identify the source of the bleed during endoscopy. This requires adequate full inspection of the gastric mucosa, with removal of blood remnants if necessary, combined with proper insufflation and sometimes change in position of the patient if needed for a full view, in particular in the presence of large clots. In rare cases, endoscopic ultrasound may help to identify the lesion. Endoscopic treatment is the first choice in bleeding Dieulafoy lesions (41) and is able to achieve hemostasis in more than 90% of cases (39). Treatment is usually performed with clipping or banding of the lesion. Overall mortality rates due to bleeding Dieulafoy lesions are up to

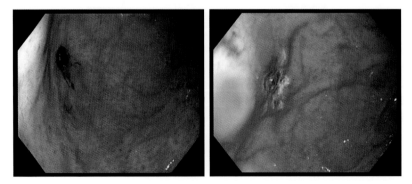

Figure 8.4 Dieulafoy lesion in the fundus before and after treatment with argon plasma coagulation

20% (39) and associated with advanced age and co-morbidity rather than directly to exsanguination (40).

Vasoenteric fistula

A fistula developing between an abdominal vessel and the gastrointestinal tract is an uncommon but severe, life threatening cause of gastrointestinal bleeding. The diagnosis can be difficult as bleeding may occur intermittently and the actual lesion is often small. Most lesions arise from the aorta, in particular in the presence of an aneurysm (so-called primary fistulas) or an aortic prosthesis (secondary fistula). Secondary aortoduodenal fistulas are far more frequent. Primary aortoduodenal fistulas are most frequently caused by infrarenal aneurysms of the abdominal aorta. Other reported causes are the primary or metastatic tumors, ingested foreign bodies puncturing the luminal wall into a major adjacent artery, radiation therapy, diverticulitis, and perforating ulcers. (42). About three-quarters of aortoenteric fistulas communicate with the duodenum, usually the horizontal part. In rare cases, a duodenocaval fistula may occur, of which some 40 cases have been described in the literature, among others after ingestion of a fish bone and after surgery (43). Fistulas to vascular bypasses or prostheses, such as a mesocaval shunt, may also give rise to bleeding (Fig. 8.5). An early contrast-enhanced computed tomography is indicated in cases suspected of vasoenteric fistula, rather than an endoscopy, which is inferior in detecting these lesions. However, endoscopy is relevant for exclusion of other causes of acute gastrointestinal hemorrhage (44). Without operative management

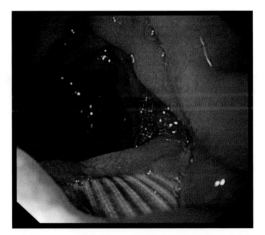

Figure 8.5 Appearance of a mesocaval shunt eroding into the duodenum in a patient presenting with intermittent severe upper GI bleeding 27 years after bypass surgery for reasons of portal hypertension

the mortality rate of bleeding due to vasoenteric fistula is nearly 100%. Open surgery is the option of choice in most patients. Endovascular aortic repair (EVAR) may be an option in fragile patients and can be used as a bridging procedure to definitive repair (42, 45, 46).

Portal hypertensive gastropathy

Portal hypertensive gastropathy or congestive gastropathy refers to changes in the gastric mucosa in patients with portal hypertension. Gastroscopy classically reveals a mosaic like pattern of the mucosa, resembling a snake-skin (Fig. 8.6) (47). These endoscopic findings correspond to dilated mucosal capillaries without inflammation. Similar mucosal changes can be seen in the small bowel and colon of patients with portal hypertension, named portal hypertensive enteropathy (48) and portal hypertensive colopathy (49), respectively. Bleeding from these conditions usually occurs as slow, diffuse oozing, but it may also be acute (and even) massive.

A recent review (50) reported prevalence of portal hypertensive gastropathy ranging from 20% to 98% in various series of patients with liver cirrhosis. This wide range in prevalence was likely related to a combination of factors including patient selection, absence of uniform diagnostic criteria and classification, and differences in inter- and intra-observer interpretation of endoscopic lesions.

Portal hypertensive gastropathy is often seen in the presence of esophageal or gastric varices. The degree of portal hypertension needed for development of portal hypertensive gastropathy remains controversial

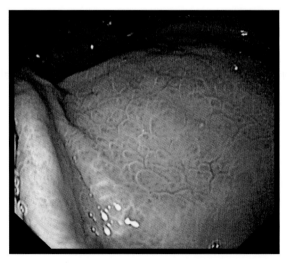

Figure 8.6 Portal hypertensive gastropathy

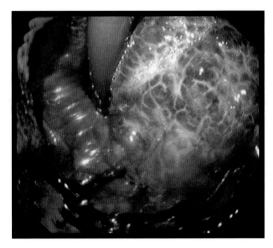

Figure 8.7 Severe acute portal hypertensive gastropathy after TIPS closure

(50). *Helicobacter pylori* infection is unlikely to be involved in the pathogenesis (51).

As portal hypertension is a key factor in etiology, treatment in portal hypertensive gastropathy aims to reduce portal venous pressure. This may be accomplished by a variety of measures including non-selective B-blockers, somatostatin and octreotide, surgical portocaval shunts, and TIPS (52).

A similar pattern of vascular disease can in rare cases be observed when there is acute, severe venous outflow obstruction of stomach and/or duodenum, for instance due to a severe right-sided cardiac decompensation, or in case of thrombosis (Fig. 8.7).

Gastric antral vascular ectasia

Gastric antral vascular ectasia (GAVE) is often confused with portal hypertensive gastropathy. Although GAVE is closely related to portal hypertension, it can also appear in the absence of portal hypertension. It is also called "Watermelon Stomach" because of linear red stripes, separated by normal mucosa, giving the appearance of a watermelon (Fig. 8.8).

GAVE have been associated with several auto-immune diseases (e.g. Sjögren's Syndrome, Addison's disease, and systemic sclerosis), renal failure and bone marrow transplantation (53–56). GAVE generally does not respond to treatments which reduce portal pressure. The first-line treatment of actively bleeding GAVE as well as recurrent bleeding from GAVE therefore is endoscopic ablation of the lesion (52). This is usually done by means of argon plasma coagulation. In a series of 20 patients with GAVE-related bleeding and liver cirrhosis treated with argon plasma coagulation, GAVE

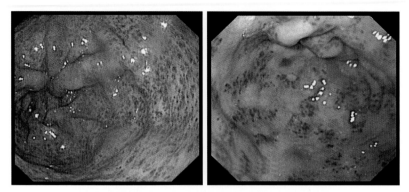

Figure 8.8 Gastric antral vascular ectasia

eradication was achieved after a median of 3 sessions per patient. Thirty percent of patients had relapse of GAVE after a mean of 7.7 months. These patients were successfully retreated with argon plasma coagulation (57).

Hereditary vascular anomalies

A wide variety of hereditary and congenital vascular anomalies can cause upper gastrointestinal bleeding. These include hereditary haemorrhagic telangiectasia (58), pseudoxanthoma elasticum (59), Ehlers-Danlos Syndrome (60), and Blue Rubber Bleb Naevus Syndrome (61, 62) (Table 8.2). Together, these syndromes are rare causes of upper gastrointestinal bleeding.

Hereditary haemorrhagic telangiectasia (HHT), also known as Osler-Weber-Rendu Syndrome is an autosomal dominant disorder of the fibro-vascular tissue. It is characterized by teleangiectasias and arteriovenous malformations of skin, mucosa (Fig. 8.9) and viscera. There are two different phenotypes, HHT1 and HHT2 with respectively mutations of endoglin and Activin A receptor like kinase-1 genes (63). In a study on 25 patients with HHT, teleangiectasias were found in 92% of the patients throughout the gastrointestinal tract, with lesions observed in 67% of patients at gastro-duodenoscopy, in 76% at videocapsule endoscopy, and in 32% at colonoscopy. Large teleangiectasias in small intestine and colon appear to occur predominantly in HHT1. Hepatic arteriovenous malformations are mainly found in HHT2 (63). Recurrent gastrointestinal bleeding occurs in up to one third of the patients. This bleeding can be severe. A study of hereditary haemorrhagic teleangiectasia families in Denmark documented that 25% of patients of 60 years and older suffered from severe gastrointestinal bleeding, defined as requiring at least 6 units of blood within six months (64). Curative options are limited. The use of photocoagulation using bipolar electrocoagulation, argon plasma coagulation, or laser techniques is useful

Table 8.2 Hereditary vascular anomalies related to gastrointestinal bleeding.

Disease	Original reporter(s)	Prevalence	Heredity	Pathophysiology	Gastrointestinal manifestations
Hereditary hemorrhagic telangiectasia	Osler-Weber-Rendu	1:5,000–8,000	Autosomal dominant	Diverse, depending on the mutation	Iron deficiency anemia or acute bleeding
Pseudoxanthoma elasticum	Grönblad-Strandberg	1:25,000–100,000	Autosomal recessive (80%) also autosomal dominant and sporadic	Progressive calcification and fragmentation of elastic fibers	Gastrointestinal bleeding
Cutis hyperelastica	Ehlers-Danlos	1:5,000–10,000	Autosomal dominant or recessive depending on type	Defect in the synthesis of collagen	Perforation and massive bleeding
Blue Rubber Bleb Naevus Syndrome	Bean	Extremely rare	Usually sporadic, seldom autosomal dominant	Venous malformations	Massive or occult hemorrhage and iron deficiency anemia

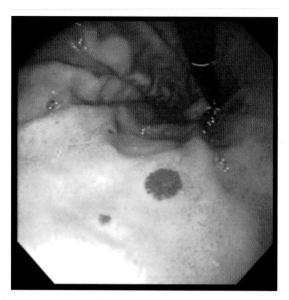

Figure 8.9 Vascular anomaly in the stomach of a patient with Osler-Weber-Rendu
Syndrome

for control of bleeding in the short term. Medical treatment with progesterone and oestrogen has shown to be beneficial in reducing the incidence of
rebleeding (65).

Pseudoxanthoma elasticum (Grönblad–Strandberg Syndrome) is an autosomal recessive disease characterized by progressive calcification and frag-
mentation of elastic fibers (66). Patients typically develop ocular, cutaneous
and cardiovascular manifestations but the gastrointestinal tract may also be
affected. The principal symptom is gastrointestinal bleeding (59). Ehlers-
Danlos Syndrome is also a hereditary connective tissue disorder. The classic
manifestations are skin hyper-extensibility and generalized joint hypermo-
bility. Less known is the fact that these patients are also prone to gastrointestinal catastrophes such as perforation and massive bleeding (60).

Blue Rubber Bleb Naevus Syndrome is a very rare vascular anomaly
syndrome consisting of multifocal venous malformations. The venous
malformations can occur in any tissue. However, lesions of the gastrointestinal tract appear to be more clinically relevant than skin or soft tissue
lesions, since chronic continuous bleeding, leading to anemia, or massive
sudden hemorrhage can occur. Therapies are not widely studied. Anti-
angiogenetic agents, octreotide, argon photo coagulation, and endoscopic
band ligation have not shown durable beneficial effect. Serious chronic
bleedings can be effectively treated by aggressive resection of the venous
malformations (67).

Vasculitides and systemic disorders

In rare cases, upper gastrointestinal bleeding is caused by vasculitis, in particular as part of Henoch-Schönlein purpura, Behçet's disease, polyarteritis nodosa, Churg-Strauss Syndrome, Wegener granulomatosis, or microscopic polyangiitis (68–71). Furthermore, gastrointestinal vasculitis has also been described in giant cell arteritis, Takayasu's disease, Buerger's disease, lupus vasculitis, mixed connective tissue disease, and rheumatoid arthritis (71, 72). Bleeding lesions due to these vascular conditions may occur from the upper nasopharynx throughout the gastrointestinal tract, even in rare cases giving rise to bleeding from other sites such as hemobilia when vasculitis affects the bile ducts or gall bladder (72). The bleeding focus can usually be diagnosed by gastroduodenoscopy, in some cases additional procedures such as enteroscopy or ERCP are required. Lesions may typically be very topical, affecting sharply demarcated areas, yet arising at multiple sites. With transmural involvement of the bowel such as in Churg-Strauss vasculitis, lesions may not only give rise to bleeding, but also to perforation. Endoscopic biopsy specimens of the affected area may reveal ulceration and inflammation, but are often insufficient to demonstrate the underlying vasculitis. This is more likely to be found in full thickness biopsy specimens, such as can be obtained when surgery is needed for complicated disease. Diagnosis of the underlying disease is more adequately done by full assessment for systemic disease, including targeted auto-immune serology, urine sediment and measurement of renal function, thorax X-ray, and others. Treatment mostly starts with corticosteroids and immune suppressives, together with PPIs in patients with upper GI lesions.

Ischemia of the digestive tract

Acute gastric ischemia (Fig. 8.10) is uncommon because of the stomach's rich vascular supply. Nevertheless it is important to recognize, since progression to necrosis can lead to perforation and sepsis. Cases reported in the literature include arterial thrombosis of mesenteric vessels, gastric volvulus or hiatus hernias, acute necrotizing gastritis, ingestion of caustic substances, therapeutic embolizations, postoperative complications and acute gastric dilatation related to eating disorders, trauma, acute pancreatitis, and diabetic ketoacidosis (73, 74). It may also occur in case of stenosis of the celiac trunk and insufficient collateral circulation (75). Gastrointestinal bleeding due to ischemia has been described in a few case reports (76, 77).

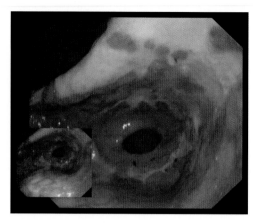

Figure 8.10 Gastric ulceration due to ischemia in the presence of severe stenosis of the celiac trunk and upper mesenteric artery

Neoplastic lesions

Neoplastic lesions of the upper GI tract account for 2–8% of the cases of gastrointestinal bleeding (Table 8.1) (1, 3, 22–24). These lesions include benign polyps as well as malignancies, among which gastric adenocarcinomas are the most prevalent among patients presenting with upper GI bleeding.

Polyps

Polyps of the gastrointestinal tract can be either sporadic or arise as part of a hereditary polyposis syndrome. In the upper gastrointestinal tract, the stomach and proximal duodenum are the most frequently affected sites. Most of these polyps are asymptomatic, but some may give rise to bleeding, typically occult. This in particular occurs from larger or ulcerated polyps (78). In a large endoscopic study of 987 patients with anemia, hyperplastic polyps of the stomach were found in 1.4% of cases (79).

Polyps can be grossly divided into fundic gland polyps, hyperplastic polyps (Fig. 8.11), adenomatous polyps, and hamartomas (80). Fundic gland polyps typically affect the acid secreting proximal compartment of the stomach. They either occur as part of a hereditary syndrome, in particular familial adenomatous polyposis, or sporadic. The vast majority, if not all sporadic fundic gland polyps occur in long-term users of protonpump inhibitors. This is thought to be due to a blocking of the glandular flow by swelling and intraluminal protrusion of parietal cells with blocked secretory function. This explains why these lesions only arise in the corpus, have a somewhat transparent, soft fluid-filled appearance, and can show regression after

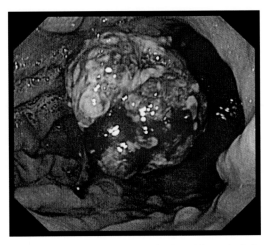

Figure 8.11 Hyperplastic polyp of the gastric body, with marked signs of bleeding

withdrawal of PPI therapy. They usually are discovered by chance, and do not require therapy. In some cases, however, the polyps may become large (>1–2 cm) and may give rise to blood loss. In those cases, the only existing therapies are endoscopic removal of the largest polyps. The clinical indication for PPI therapy should then also be reconsidered, but routine withdrawal of PPI therapy is not indicated. Malignant degeneration of these PPI-associated sporadic fundic gland polyps has hardly ever been described. There is therefore no evidence that these patients require any surveillance. This does not pertain to patients with familial adenomatous polyposis (FAP), when diagnosed with PPI-unrelated fundic gland polyps. These fundic gland polyps do have malignant potential and should be surveyed together with other polypoid lesions which may arise in stomach and duodenum of these patients (81).

Hyperplastic polyps in particular occur sporadically. Gastroduodenal adenomas can also occur sporadically, as well as against a background of a familial polyp syndrome, in particular including FAP, and to a lesser extent Lynch Syndrome, and Peutz-Jeghers Syndrome (82). In FAP, the adenomas in particular arise in the proximal duodenum. In Lynch and Peutz-Jeghers Syndrome, there may be predominance for gastric lesions. Sporadic adenomas of the duodenum are associated with a risk for co-existent colorectal adenomas. In a study on 49 cases (M/F 27/22, mean age 63 yrs, range 29–88) with sporadic duodenal adenoma, 47% was found to have colorectal adenoma on colonoscopy (83). The discovery of all these upper gastrointestinal polyps lies in the identification of hereditary cancer syndromes, surveillance and early detection of progression to malignancy, and treatment of complications such as bleeding. Bleeding lesions are best treated by endoscopic removal of the polypoid lesion.

Adeno- and squamous cell carcinoma

Gastric and esophageal cancer are the second and sixth leading cause of cancer mortality worldwide respectively (84). Most gastric cancers are adenocarcinomas. In the esophagus, squamous cell carcinoma is still the most common type worldwide, although the incidence of esophageal adenocarcinomas has risen rapidly in the past three decades and has become the predominant esophageal malignancy in the United States and northern Europe. Major risk factors for esophageal adenocarcinoma are obesity, gastro-esophageal reflux and its resultant Barrett's esophagus (85).

Most patients with esophageal cancer have complaints of dysphagia (74%) or odynophagia (17%) at time of diagnosis. Weight loss is common, and (if more than 10% of body weight) associated with poor prognosis (86). Bleeding is an infrequent first presentation of esophageal cancer, but is more common during the course of disease if curative surgery cannot be performed. Adenocarcinomas of the stomach (Fig. 8.12) more often bleed as initial presentation (87). A North American study (87) of 42 patients with severe upper gastrointestinal bleeding due to upper gastrointestinal cancer showed that most presented at an advanced stage presumably with larger ulcerating tumor masses. Bleeding was the initial presentation of the tumor in half of the cases. Endoscopic hemostasis was initially effective in all cases. However, severe bleeding from gastrointestinal tumors was correlated with a poor one-year survival. In contrast to the success of endoscopic therapy in this case series, endoscopy offers little treatment options in case of diffusely bleeding cancers. Surgery is the mainstay of therapy for cure of gastro-esophageal carcinomas, nowadays mostly combined with perioperative

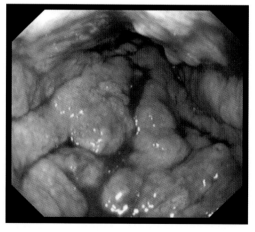

Figure 8.12 Invasive gastric adenocarcinoma circumferentially affecting the stomach wall, and giving rise to diffuse bleeding

chemotherapy or chemoradiation (88). In patients with bleeding cancers for whom surgery is no option, short-term radiotherapy or angiography with embolization of the supplying vessel are alternative treatment options. In a retrospective study of 30 patients with gastric cancer bleeding, 73% responded to radiotherapy, with a three-month rebleeding rate of 60%. Twelve patients received concurrent chemoradiotherapy and had a significant lower rebleeding rate (17.5%) (89). In another retrospective study, 23 patients with gastric cancer bleeding underwent transcatheter arterial embolization. The overall clinical success rate was 52%, with a one-month rebleeding rate of 8% (90). Bleeding of the cancer or surrounding mucosa may also occur as a result of the radio- and/or chemotherapy. These bleeding episodes are often difficult to manage because of their diffuse character and vulnerability of the mucosa, and primarily require supportive measures and temporary or permanent withdrawal of therapy.

Lymphoma

Upper gastrointestinal lymphomas in particular occur in the stomach. They are almost invariably associated with *H. pylori*. Most are low-grade, marginal zone B-cell lymphomas confined to the mucosa and submucosa (stage IE) (Fig. 8.13). Fifty-five to 78% of these lesions show partial or complete remission after *H. pylori* eradication as monotherapy (91). The recognition of the association between these lymphomas and *H. pylori*, the increased use of diagnostic upper GI endoscopy, and improved knowledge on the appearance and biology of these lymphomas led a decade ago first to a rise in gastric lymphoma incidence. This incidence is now decreasing as a result of decreasing *H. pylori* prevalence (92). Nevertheless, gastric lymphomas still make up for 30% or more of all primary gastrointestinal lymphomas. Some 5% of all GI lymphomas are small bowel lymphomas, in particular T-cell lymphomas associated with long-existing celiac disease (93, 94).

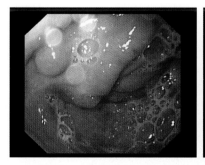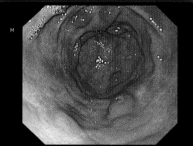

Figure 8.13 Marginal zone B-cell lymphoma

Data on the incidence of bleeding of these tumors are scarce. In a small study of 14 patients with primary gastrointestinal NK-/T-cell lymphoma, gastrointestinal bleeding was the most frequent presenting symptom (42% of cases). Unfortunately, the disease was at an advanced stage at the time of diagnosis in all cases (95). Likewise, gastric marginal zone lymphomas may present as ulcerative disease giving rise to bleeding, either acute or chronic. In these cases, endoscopic treatment may be feasible if the bleeding is focal. Successful endoscopic treatment should be followed by PPI therapy, and full workup of the lesion followed by individualized therapy depending on the histology and transmural depth of the lesion, and the presence of extra-gastric local or distant disease. Therapeutic options primarily consist of *H. pylori* eradication. For more advanced and high-grade lesions as well as those which do not respond adequately to *H. pylori* eradication, CHOP chemotherapy and radiotherapy, as well as surgery, all form alternatives. *H. pylori* eradication as monotherapy is in particular indicated for low-grade lesions confined to the (sub-) mucosa, stage IE. More advanced lesions usually require additional therapy. This is also true for lesions which carry a specific chromosomal rearrangement, the API2-MALT mutation as the presence of this mutation is a predictor for poor response to *H. pylori* eradication. In a systematic review of 1,408 cases, only 22% of patients with this mutation responded to *H. pylori* eradication (91). Other gastrointestinal lymphomas such as small bowel T-cell lymphomas are primarily treated with chemotherapy.

Mesenchymal tumors

Like many other organ systems, the gastrointestinal tract is the origin of a wide range of mesenchymal or stromal neoplasms. The most common group consists of neoplasms that are collectively referred to as gastrointestinal stromal tumors (GISTs) (Figs 8.14, 8.15). Less frequent mesenchymal neoplasms include leiomyomas/leiomyosarcomas, lipomas/liposarcomas, Schwannomas and peripheral nerve sheath tumors. They are classified upon their morphologic and immunophenotypic profile.

GISTs are most frequent observed in the stomach, although they are estimated to account only for 1 to 3 percent of all gastric neoplasms (96). They are characterised by the presence of KIT mutations as well as mutations in platelet-derived growth factor receptor alpha tyrosine kinases (97). The most common presentation of GISTs is gastrointestinal bleeding, which may be either acute or chronic. Patients can also present with abdominal pain caused by tumor rupture, internal bleeding, or gastrointestinal obstruction. Smaller GISTs are often coincidentally found during endoscopy. About 20–25% of gastric and 40–50% of small intestinal GISTs are malignant.

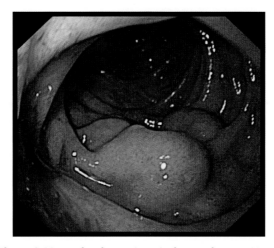

Figure 8.14 Duodenal gastrointestinal stromal tumor (GIST)

Common metastatic sites are the abdominal cavity and liver, but bones, soft tissues, skin and seldom lymph nodes and lungs may also be affected. Long-term clinical follow-up is needed since metastases can occur more than 15 years after initial diagnosis (98).

Leiomyoma is the most common esophageal mesenchymal tumor (99). They are slowly growing benign intramural tumors. Most patients are asymptomatic and lesions are often found accidentally during endoscopy. However, with increasing size of the lesion, symptoms like dysphagia, retrosternal pain and regurgitation can occur. Ulcerated leiomyomas may

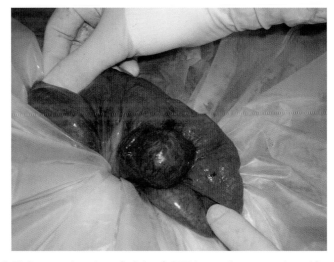

Figure 8.15 Peroperative view of a jejunal GIST in a patient presenting with repeated episodes of melena

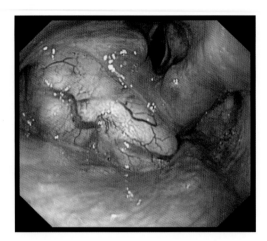

Figure 8.16 Liposarcoma of the esophagus

occasionally present with bleeding. Although smaller lesions are often followed by means of endoscopy with endoscopic ultrasound, bleeding lesions require treatment both because of the bleeding and the risk of malignant degeneration which increases with size. Treatment usually consists of surgical or endoscopic resection. The latter is done by means of endoscopic submucosal dissection. Malignant transformation is extremely rare in leiomyoma. Malignant leiomyosarcomas grow much faster and occur at older age (100).

Gastrointestinal lipomas account for 4% of benign gastrointestinal tumors (101). The majority are located in the colon (60–75%), followed by small bowel (20–25%) and stomach (5%). They are usually asymptomatic, but can cause the same symptoms as leiomyomas. Larger lesions most frequently present with gastrointestinal hemorrhage (in over 50% of cases) (102).

Liposarcomas are extremely rare in the gastrointestinal tract. Less than 20 cases, mainly esophageal liposarcomas (Fig. 8.16), have been reported in the world literature (103). Treatment of bleeding lesions is the same as for leiomyomas and GISTs.

Kaposi's sarcoma

Kaposi's sarcoma is a low grade vascular tumor associated with human herpesvirus-8 infection (Fig. 8.17). It is the most common HIV-related gastrointestinal tumor and seen in about 40% of AIDS patients. The incidence of Kaposi sarcoma has decreased significantly since the availability of HAART therapy. Kaposi sarcomas are usually asymptomatic, but gastrointestinal hemorrhage has been reported. (78). Possible therapies

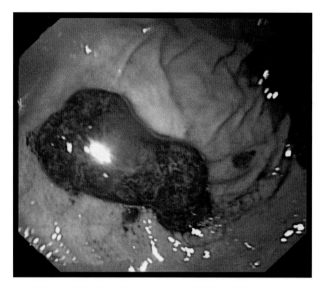

Figure 8.17 Kaposi's sarcoma in a HIV positive patient

for bleeding from Kaposi's sarcomas are injection therapy, heat coagulation, sclerotherapy, radiotherapy, systemic chemotherapy, surgical excision and angiographic embolization (104).

Primary malignant melanoma

Although most malignant melanomas of the gastrointestinal tract are of metastatic origin, primary malignant melanomas do occur in the gastrointestinal tract, in particular in the esophagus, small bowel, rectum and anus. They tend to be more aggressive and are associated with worse outcome than metastatic melanoma lesions of the gastrointestinal tract (105). Initial presentation with gastrointestinal bleed is rare and has only been described in case reports (106, 107). Treatment of bleeding depends on the location and situation of the tumor, and angiographic embolization is one of the treatment options of first choice, as it is for other malignant bleeding lesions.

Neuroendocrine tumor

The gastrointestinal tract is the largest neuroendocrine system in the body. The majority of neuroendocrine tumors (NET) arise from the gastrointestinal and pulmonary system (108). NETs comprised 0.8% of all gastrointestinal tumors in an English population based cancer registry between 1971 and 2006. Their incidence is rising. Of primary gastrointestinal NETs 38% arose in the appendix, 29% in the small intestine, 13% in the colon 13%, 12% in the stomach and 8% in the rectum (109). NETs can occur sporadically or as part of a syndrome (e.g. Zollinger-Ellison and multiple endocrine neoplasia type 1 (MEN1)). Most gastroentero-pancreatic neuroendocrine tumors are asymptomatic and discovered coincidentally upon imaging or surgery for unrelated reasons. About 10% of neuroendocrine tumors secrete excessive levels of hormones, most notably serotonin, causing flushing, wheezing, diarrhea, abdominal cramping and peripheral edema. In rare cases, hemorrhage is the presenting symptom (110). As is the case with other malignant tumors, primary diagnosis and treatment for bleeding lesions consists of endoscopy, if needed, followed by secondary intervention, in particular angiographic embolization.

Metastatic tumor

Metastatic tumors to the gastrointestinal tract are very rare in comparison to primary malignancies. Malignancies which are known to metastasize to the gastrointestinal tract are malignant melanoma, breast cancer, lung, and renal cancer. Disseminated lymphoma can also affect the gastrointestinal tract. Furthermore, primary gastrointestinal malignancies such as esophageal cancers may sometimes also give rise to metastases elsewhere in the tract, although local transmural growth such as from airways and mediastinum to the esophagus and from the colon to the stomach is more common. The relative frequencies of these tumors are not well defined, given the fact that the reported series are small. For instance, two series from the United States and Japan on respectively 67 and 389 cases with metastatic tumors in the stomach found a range of primary tumors, mostly coming the lungs, skin (melanoma), and breast (111, 112).

A typical sign both on radiological and endoscopic imaging of metastatic disease is the so-called bull's eyes sign, corresponding to the clinical appearance of a submucosal tumor with central ulceration (Fig. 8.18). Another characteristic is the presence of multiple lesions, present in about 35% of cases (112). Bleeding from the ulcerative lesion may be the first presenting sign; these bleeds are often diffuse from vulnerable tissue and thus offer limited options for endoscopic treatment. Endoscopy remains the first tool in management, to assess the source of the bleed and look for treatment options. The appearance of the lesion is typical for malignant disease. In patients with a known primary tumor, the association is usually readily made. In patients with an unknown primary, further investigation has to reveal the source of the metastasis. In both cases, histology may be needed to confirm the source or to guide further evaluation. Depending on the severity

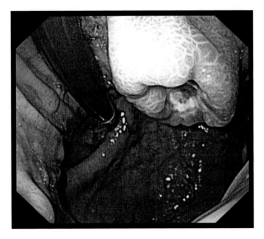

Figure 8.18 Metastasis of malignant melanoma in the stomach with central ulceration (bull's eyes sign)

of the bleed, histology is either obtained at the first endoscopy, or postponed till a more severe bleed is adequately managed.

Traumatic or iatrogenic bleeding

Mallory-Weiss tear

A Mallory-Weiss tear is a mucosal laceration at the gastro-esophageal junction or gastric cardia usually caused by retching or forceful vomiting (Fig. 8.19). This condition was first described in 1929 by G. K. Mallory and S. Weiss (113). A typical presentation is with the occurrence of hematemesis after first having vomited without blood. Mallory-Weiss lesions are a common cause of upper gastrointestinal bleeding, several epidemiological studies reported these lesions as the bleeding source in 2% to 8% of patients

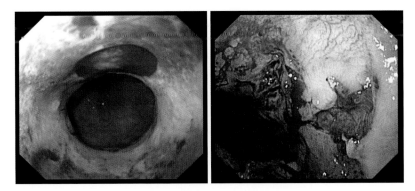

Figure 8.19 Mallory-Weiss tear

Table 8.3 Treatment of Mallory-Weiss lesions in randomized controlled trials.

Treatment options	Llach (118) 2001		Huang (120) 2002		Park (122) 2004		Cho (119) 2008		Lecleire (121) 2009	
Year of publication	EEI*	NET	EHP	EEI	EBL	EEI	EBL	EHP	EBL	EHP + EEI
Patients per arm	32	31	18	17	17	17	20	21	29	27
Primary hemostasis	100%	NR	100%	100%	100%	94.1%	100%	100%	100%	100%
Rebleeding	6.2%	25.8%	6%	6%	0%	0%	10%	6%	0%	18%

NR: not reported

EEI: Endoscopic epinephrine injection

NET: No endoscopic therapy

EHP: Endoscopic hemoclip placement

EBL: Endoscopic band ligation

*and polidocanol

presenting with acute upper gastrointestinal bleeding (1, 5, 22, 23, 114). In a large UK audit including 5,004 patients undergoing endoscopy for upper GI bleeding, Mallory-Weiss lesions were the only bleeding source in 2.1% of cases, and were overall present in 4.3% of cases (5). Many factors have been associated with the development of Mallory-Weiss lesions, including alcohol use, use of aspirin and coumarines, paroxysms of coughing, pregnancy, heavy lifting, straining, seizure, blunt abdominal trauma, colonic lavage and cardiopulmonary resuscitation (115). It is best diagnosed with upper endoscopy, but is also reported as a complication in <0.1% of diagnostic endoscopies (116). The amount of blood loss is usually mild. In a retrospective study in the USA of 73 patients with Mallory-Weiss lesions, 20% needed blood transfusion of >6 units, 11% had further bleeding, 3% underwent surgery and 3% died (117). The management of Mallory-Weiss lesions is thus mostly supportive because about 90% of lesions spontaneously stop bleeding (114, 117). A minority of cases requires endoscopic treatment. In a French series of 218 patients with Mallory-Weiss bleeding, 56 (26%) had active bleeding on endoscopy. In other series, this proportion ranged from 5 to 44% (114, 118). Various studies have looked at optimal endoscopic treatment (Table 8.3). In a series of randomised controlled trials, rebleeding rates after only supportive therapy were much higher than after any form of endoscopic therapy. Endoscopic epinephrine injection, endoscopic hemoclip placement, and endoscopic band ligation were equivalent for primary haemostasis. Rebleeding rates after band ligation and hemoclip placement were similar in a randomized Korean trial, but significantly lower after band ligation in a French trial (118–122). It is unknown whether prescription of a proton-pump inhibitor accelerates healing.

Intramural hematoma

Intramural hematoma of the upper GI tract can occur spontaneously, or on minor or larger trauma, such as improper swallowing of pills, food impaction, strained vomiting, or endoscopic intervention including endoscopic biopsy, esophageal dilatation, and variceal injection therapy (123). Conditions that impair haemostasis, such as use of coumarins, are considered risk factors. It typically appears as a bulging, purplish lesion with a smooth, normal overlying mucosa, occupying most of the lumen (Fig. 8.20) (115). The condition predominantly occurs in the esophagus, where it is considered an intermediate stage in the spectrum from Mallory-Weiss tear to Boerhaave's Syndrome. It may however also affect other parts of the gastrointestinal tract such as the duodenum. Most lesions resolve completely within a few weeks, with conservative treatment (124), in some cases the hematoma may break through to the lumen, giving rise to overt blood loss (Fig. 8.21).

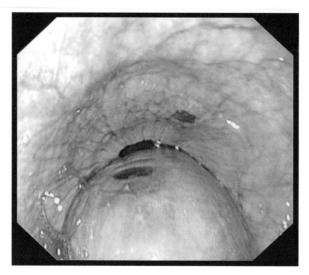

Figure 8.20 Endoscopic view of esophageal hematoma appearing as purplish lesion bulging into the lumen

Boerhaave's Syndrome and other causes of transmural perforation

Boerhaave's Syndrome is a rupture of the esophagus caused by a rapid rise in intraluminal pressure in the distal esophagus combined with negative intrathoracic pressure caused by straining or vomiting. Other causes of benign esophageal perforation include endoscopic and surgical handling and foreign body impaction (125). A diagnosis of esophageal perforation is usually readily made by chest X-ray and thorax CT showing signs of

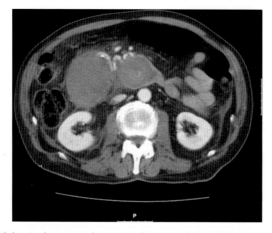

Figure 8.21 Abdominal computed tomography scan of the abdomen revealing a large hematoma in the duodenal wall. This patient developed melena, three days after presentation with signs of Gastric Outlet Syndrome, due to ruptured hematoma

mediastinal air and fluid, and often pleural effusion, with leakage of contrast. In some cases, bleeding may be an accompanying symptom. Endoscopy has a role in the diagnosis of small lesions, as well as in the treatment of bleeding and closure of the perforation. This can be done by means of placement of a self-expandable metal stent, which is appearing as a good alternative to conventional surgical therapy (125).

Foreign body and toxic substance ingestion

Ingestion of foreign bodies and toxic substance can be both accidental and intentional. They are mainly seen in children and persons attempting suicide. Caustic injury can be caused by a range of alkaline (e.g. $NaOH$, KOH, NH_3), as well acidic agents (e.g. HCl, H_2SO_4), and by neutral substances such as phenol, formaldehyde, iodine, and concentrated hydrogen peroxide. The ingestion of strong alkali results in liquefaction necrosis, which is associated with deep tissue penetration and may result in perforation (126). Acidic agents cause more superficial coagulation necrosis with scarring that may limit the extent of the injury (127). Induction of emesis and caustic neutralization with acids are both contraindicated, and empiric use of antibiotics has no proven benefit. Early prophylactic esophageal stenting is under investigation (128). Bleeding may occur as a result of widespread ulceration. Endoscopy has a role in evaluation of tissue damage, but often has little to offer in terms of treatment of bleeding. More severe bleeding is, however, rare.

Upper gastrointestinal mucosal injury is also seen after foreign body ingestion. In children, these often include toy particles, coins, and other smaller things. Potentially more harmful are batteries, and magnets. Leaking batteries can lead to local mucosal damage. When two or more magnets (present in toys as well as certain children's jewellery such as earrings) are swallowed, they can attach to each other within the gut. If this occurs with interpositioning of gut wall, ulceration can occur. Both leakage and pressure adhesion can lead to local ulceration, bleeding and perforation (129). In adults, foreign bodies often include partial dentures, toothpicks, needles, and indigestible parts of the meal, like fish and other animal bones (Box 8.2). Hemorrhage is the second most frequent complication after foreign body ingestion (130). It can occur as a result of local pressure, or puncture of the mucosa with sometimes fistula formation to a larger vessel (131). Endoscopy has a role in removal of the foreign body if needed, and in diagnosis and treatment of the source of a bleed.

Post-Endoscopy bleeding

Bleeding is one of the most common complications of upper gastrointestinal endoscopy, in particular intervention endoscopy. Higher risk procedures include endoscopic mucosal resection (EMR) and submucosal dissection (ESD), as well as endoscopic polypectomy.

Box 8.2 Frequently ingested foreign bodies associated with gastrointestinal hemorrhage

Metallic	**Liquids**
• Coins	• Alkalis (e.g. NaOH, KOH, NH$_3$)
• Batteries	• Acids (e.g. HCl, H$_2$SO$_4$)
• Magnets	• Other caustics (e.g. phenol, formaldehyde, iodine,
• Wires	concentrated hydrogen peroxide)
• Needles	• Alcohol
Indigestible food parts	**Other**
• Fish bones	• Denture/dental bridges
• Other animal bones	• Toothpicks

In a series of 273 gastric low-grade dysplastic lesions removed by EMR, bleeding rate was 6.2% (132). In a large study of 468 subjects with gastric non-invasive adenocarcinoma, post-ESD bleeding occurred in 5.5% of cases (133). Bleeding reported after endoscopic gastroduodenal polypectomy occurred in less than 1% (134, 135). Most of these bleeds occur during the initial procedure and can be dealt directly. Polypectomy bleeds are often clipped, whereas mucosal resection bleeds can be well treated by treatment of the small bleeding vessels by means of brief grasping and coagulation with a hot biopsy forceps. Lower risk interventions include dilation with balloon, bougies, or needle knife (136, 137). In a series of 985 balloon dilations for achalasia, only 2 episodes of bleeding were noted (136).

Post-Surgery bleeding

Gastrointestinal bleeding is an infrequent well-known major complication of abdominal surgery. Notorious surgical procedures are oesophagectomy, (partial or total) gastrectomy, pancreaticoduodenectomy and bariatric surgery (138). Bariatric procedures at risk include: gastric band placement, sleeve gastrectomy, Roux-en-Y gastric bypass and biliopancreatic diversion. Immediate postoperative bleeding is usually from staple lines, from the site of the anastomosis, or from poor haemostasis at the time of surgery. Late bleeding can occur due to erosions and ulcerations in the gastric remnant, at the site of the gastric band and at anastomoses (139).

Miscellaneous causes of bleeding

Hemobilia

Haemobilia or bleeding from the hepatobiliary tract is a rare cause of gastrointestinal bleeding. It either occurs as a result of an intrabiliary lesion, or when there is a fistula between a vessel of the splanchnic circulation and the intrahepatic or extrahepatic biliary system. The causes include iatrogenic and accidental trauma (e.g. liverbiopsy (140), percutaneous transhepatic cholangiography, cholecystectomy (141), TIPS, endoscopic biliary biopsies/stenting, angioembolization and blunt abdominal trauma), gallstones, cholecystitis, hepatic or bile duct tumors, hepatic artery aneurysms and hepatic abscesses. In an older series of 196 with hemobilia, 137 were secondary to accidental trauma, and 59 cases resulted from iatrogenic causes (142). Since then, the incidence of iatrogenic hemobilia has increased with the rise of percutaneous liver procedures. In a more recent review on 222 cases with hemobilia, 65% was iatrogenic, while accidental trauma accounted for only 6%. Other causes were inflammation (13%), vascular malformations (9%), malignancy (7%) and other (1%) (143). In rare cases, bleeding may occur due to a fistula to the portal system or a hepatic vein, either due to trauma, malignancy, endoscopy or surgery. In most cases, these bleeds are self-limiting and do not require intervention other than preventing biliary obstruction due to clots. In rare cases, a connection between the biliary ducts and a hepatic vein can lead to rapid onset of extreme jaundice (144).

Symptoms of hemobilia can be diverse. The classic triad of jaundice, biliary colic and upper gastrointestinal bleeding was in the most recent series only observed in 22% of the patients (143). Endoscopic retrograde cholangiography (ERCP) is helpful to confirm diagnosis and the underlying cause, and can also be of help in clearance of the biliary tree, with stenting if necessary to reduce the risk of renewed obstruction (Fig. 8.22). Most bleeds are self-limiting. In the previously mentioned review 43% of cases were managed conservatively, whereas 36% were treated by transarterial

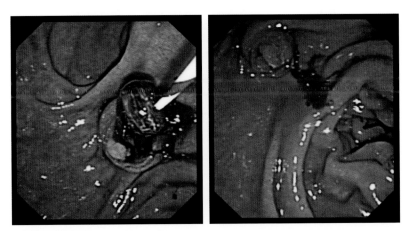

Figure 8.22 Hemobilia due to an aneurysm of the right hepatic artery in a patient with primary sclerosing cholangitis

embolisation (TAE). Surgery was indicated when laparotomy was performed for other reasons and after failure of TAE (143).

Hemosuccus pancreaticus

Hemosuccus pancreaticus, previously known as Wirsungorrhage, is caused by a bleeding source in the pancreas, pancreatic duct or adjacent structures, such as the splenic artery connecting to the pancreatic duct (145). It is another rare cause of upper gastrointestinal bleeding and has been estimated to occur in about 1 per 500–1,500 cases of upper GI bleeding. Hemosuccus pancreaticus predominantly occurs in men (sex ratio: 7:1) (146, 147), and is most often due to pancreatic pseudoaneurysms resulting of acute or chronic pancreatitis (146–148). It is also reported sporadically caused by pancreatic tumors (149), true splenic artery aneurysms (150) and after therapeutic endoscopy of the pancreas or pancreatic duct, including pancreatic stone removal, pseudocyst drainage, pancreatic duct sphincterotomy, or pancreatic duct stenting (Fig. 8.23) (151). Pseudoaneurysms can occur as a complication of pancreatitis, when a pseudocyst erodes a neighbouring artery, resulting in hemorrhage into the pancreatic duct.

In two retrospective studies, including a total of 40 patients, the most frequent complaints at presentation were maelena, hematochezia, hematemesis, and epigastric pain. Less reported was presence of a pulsating epigastric mass with a thrill at auscultation (146, 147). Patients may also develop symptoms of nausea and vomiting, weight loss and jaundice (when the bleed also leads to obstruction of the common bile duct).

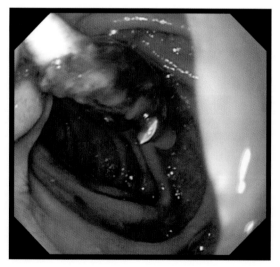

Figure 8.23 Hemosuccus pancreaticus (here seen in the form of an adhered clot on the endoprothesis in the pancreatic duct) in a patient with chronic pancreatitis

In a recent report including 31 patients with hemosuccus pancreaticus, the presence of duodenal blood was observed during upper GI endoscopy in only half of the patients (147). This underlines that the diagnosis is not always easy to establish, mainly due to the hidden and intermittent nature of the bleeding. A side-viewing duodenoscope can be helpful to localize the bleeding. Other diagnostic tools are abdominal ultrasonography and abdominal computed tomography and CT-angiography. Conventional angiography may be used to visualize the celiac axis, and in particular the gastroduodenal and splenic arteries, to determine the bleeding focus. This technique may also be used to terminate the bleeding. Selective arterial embolization is successful in 50% of the patients, while surgery is often necessary in emergency situations or after failure to control the bleeding by arterial embolization (147). Surgical procedures include distal pancreatectomy and splenectomy, central pancreatectomy, intracystic ligation of blood vessel and aneurysmal ligation of bypass graft, depending on the nature of the bleeding.

Bleeding diathesis

Bleeding diathesis is an unusual susceptibility to bleeding mostly due to a coagulopathy (e.g. von Willebrand disease, and hemophilia). Bleeding diathesis as a cause of upper gastrointestinal bleeding should be considered in presence of other relating symptoms of prolonged bleeding and rebleeding. Bleeding can occur from minute lesions, and may often require repeated endoscopy in the acute setting to determine the source of the bleed and treat accordingly. Further treatment primarily consists of correction of coagulopathy if possible.

Bleeding from the posterior nasopharynx

Bleeding from the posterior nasopharynx can sometimes be mistaken for a gastrointestinal bleeding. Presentation can be similar with maelena and/or hematemesis. In the absence of another bleeding focus, this diagnosis should be anticipated and should lead to a careful examination of the nose and nasopharynx (152).

Conclusion

Peptic ulcers and esophago-gastric varices are by far the most common causes of severe upper gastrointestinal bleeding. Nevertheless, 27–49 percent of upper GI bleeds is due to other causes, which include a range of conditions (1, 3, 22–24). Upper gastrointestinal endoscopy is the same as for peptic ulcer and varices the mainstay for diagnosis and treatment. The medical history with focus on items such as symptoms, timing of onset of the bleed in relation to other parameters such as a meal or vomiting, drug use, and previous interventions provide important clues for a diagnosis and therapeutic approach.

References

1. Czernichow P, Hochain P, Nousbaum JB, Raymond JM, Rudelli A, Dupas JL, et al. Epidemiology and course of acute upper gastro-intestinal haemorrhage in four French geographical areas. Eur J Gastroenterol Hepatol 2000;12(2):175–81.
2. Enestvedt BK, Gralnek IM, Mattek N, Lieberman DA, Eisen G. An evaluation of endoscopic indications and findings related to nonvariceal upper-GI hemorrhage in a large multicenter consortium. Gastrointest Endosc 2008;67(3):422–9.
3. van Leerdam ME, Vreeburg EM, Rauws EA, Geraedts AA, Tijssen JG, Reitsma JB, et al. Acute upper GI bleeding: did anything change? Time trend analysis of incidence and outcome of acute upper GI bleeding between 1993/1994 and 2000. Am J Gastroenterol 2003;98(7):1494–1499.
4. Ahsberg K, Hoglund P, Kim WH, von Holstein CS. Impact of aspirin, NSAIDs, warfarin, corticosteroids and SSRIs on the site and outcome of non-variceal upper and lower gastrointestinal bleeding. Scand J Gastroenterol 2010;45: 1401–1415.
5. Hearnshaw SA, Logan RF, Lowe D, Travis SP, Murphy MF, Palmer KR. Use of endoscopy for management of acute upper gastrointestinal bleeding in the UK: results of a nationwide audit. Gut 2010;59(8):1022–1029.
6. Ronkainen J, Aro P, Storskrubb T, Johansson SE, Lind T, Bolling-Sternevald E, et al. High prevalence of gastroesophageal reflux symptoms and esophagitis with or without symptoms in the general adult Swedish population: a Kalixanda study report. Scand J Gastroenterol 2005;40(3):275–85.
7. Zagari RM, Law GR, Fuccio L, Pozzato P, Forman D, Bazzoli F. Dyspeptic symptoms and endoscopic findings in the community: the Loiano-Monghidoro study. Am J Gastroenterol 2010;105(3):565–71.
8. Ma X, Zhao Y, Wang R, Yan X, Li Z, Zou D, et al. Epidemiology of gastroduodenal erosions in the general population: endoscopic results of the systematic investigation of gastrointestinal diseases in China (SILC). Scand J Gastroenterol 2010;45: 1416–1423.
9. Cryer B, Feldman M. Effects of very low dose daily, long-term aspirin therapy on gastric, duodenal, and rectal prostaglandin levels and on mucosal injury in healthy humans. Gastroenterology 1999;117(1):17–25.
10. Gore RM, Levine MS, Ghahremani GG. Drug-induced disorders of the stomach and duodenum. Abdom Imaging 1999;24(1):9–16.
11. Yeomans ND, Lanas AI, Talley NJ, Thomson AB, Daneshjoo R, Eriksson B, et al. Prevalence and incidence of gastroduodenal ulcers during treatment with vascular protective doses of aspirin. Aliment Pharmacol Ther 2005;22(9):795–801.
12. Tamura A, Murakami K, Kadota J, Investigators O-GS. Prevalence and independent factors for gastroduodenal ulcers/erosions in asymptomatic patients taking low-dose aspirin and gastroprotective agents: the OITA-GF study. QJM 2010;104: 133–9.
13. Dall M, Schaffalitzky de Muckadell OB, Lassen AT, Hansen JM, Hallas J. An association between selective serotonin reuptake inhibitor use and serious upper gastrointestinal bleeding. Clin Gastroenterol Hepatol 2009;7(12):1314–1321.

14. Papapetrou PD. Bisphosphonate-associated adverse events. Hormones (Athens) 2009;8(2):96–110.
15. Cameron AJ, Higgins JA. Linear gastric erosion. A lesion associated with large diaphragmatic hernia and chronic blood loss anemia. Gastroenterology 1986; 91(2):338–42.
16. Weston AP. Hiatal hernia with cameron ulcers and erosions. Gastrointest Endosc Clin N Am 1996;6(4):671–9.
17. Maganty K, Smith RL. Cameron lesions: unusual cause of gastrointestinal bleeding and anemia. Digestion 2008;77(3–4):214–7.
18. Sugawa C, Lucas CE, Rosenberg BF, Riddle JM, Walt AJ. Differential topography of acute erosive gastritis due to trauma or sepsis, ethanol and aspirin. Gastrointest Endosc 1973;19(3):127–30.
19. Toljamo KT, Niemela SE, Karttunen TJ, Karvonen AL, Lehtola JK. Clinical significance and outcome of gastric mucosal erosions: a long-term follow-up study. Dig Dis Sci 2006;51(3):543–7.
20. Morris A, Nicholson G. Ingestion of Campylobacter pyloridis causes gastritis and raised fasting gastric pH. Am J Gastroenterol 1987;82(3):192–9.
21. Kuipers EJ. Review article: exploring the link between Helicobacter pylori and gastric cancer. Aliment Pharmacol Ther 1999;13Suppl 1: 3–11.
22. Di Fiore F, Lecleire S, Merle V, Herve S, Duhamel C, Dupas JL, et al. Changes in characteristics and outcome of acute upper gastrointestinal haemorrhage: a comparison of epidemiology and practices between 1996 and 2000 in a multicentre French study. Eur J Gastroenterol Hepatol 2005;17(6):641–7.
23. Theocharis GJ, Thomopoulos KC, Sakellaropoulos G, Katsakoulis E, Nikolopoulou V. Changing trends in the epidemiology and clinical outcome of acute upper gastrointestinal bleeding in a defined geographical area in Greece. J Clin Gastroenterol 2008;42(2):128–33.
24. Paspatis GA, Matrella E, Kapsoritakis A, Leontithis C, Papanikolaou N, Chlouverakis GJ, et al. An epidemiological study of acute upper gastrointestinal bleeding in Crete, Greece. Eur J Gastroenterol Hepatol 2000;12(11):1215–1220.
25. McQuaid KR, Laine L. Systematic review and meta-analysis of adverse events of low-dose aspirin and clopidogrel in randomized controlled trials. Am J Med 2006; 119(8):624–38.
26. Gilmore PR. Angiodysplasia of the upper gastrointestinal tract. J Clin Gastroenterol 1988;10(4):386–94.
27. Kaaroud H, Fatma LB, Beji S, Boubaker K, Hedri H, Hamida FB, et al. Gastrointestinal angiodysplasia in chronic renal failure. Saudi J Kidney Dis Transpl 2008;19(5): 809–12.
28. Mishra PK, Kovac J, de Caestecker J, Fancourt G, Logtens E, Spyt T. Intestinal angiodysplasia and aortic valve stenosis: let's not close the book on this association. Eur J Cardiothorac Surg 2009;35(4):628–34.
29. Chalasani N, Cotsonis G, Wilcox CM. Upper gastrointestinal bleeding in patients with chronic renal failure: role of vascular ectasia. Am J Gastroenterol 1996; 91(11):2329–2332.
30. Godeschalk MF, Mensink PB, van Buuren HR, Kuipers EJ. Primary balloon-assisted enteroscopy in patients with obscure gastrointestinal bleeding: findings and outcome of therapy. J Clin Gastroenterol 2010;44(9):e195–200.
31. Almadi M, Ghali PM, Constantin A, Galipeau J, Szilagyi A. Recurrent obscure gastrointestinal bleeding: dilemmas and success with pharmacological therapies. Case series and review. Can J Gastroenterol 2009;23(9):625–31.

32. Junquera F, Feu F, Papo M, Videla S, Armengol JR, Bordas JM, et al. A multicenter, randomized, clinical trial of hormonal therapy in the prevention of rebleeding from gastrointestinal angiodysplasia. Gastroenterology 2001;121(5):1073–1079.

33. Brown C, Subramanian V, Wilcox CM, Peter S. Somatostatin analogues in the treatment of recurrent bleeding from gastrointestinal vascular malformations: an overview and systematic review of prospective observational studies. Dig Dis Sci 2010;55(8):2129–2134.

34. Dabak V, Kuriakose P, Kamboj G, Shurafa M. A pilot study of thalidomide in recurrent GI bleeding due to angiodysplasias. Dig Dis Sci 2008;53(6):1632–1635.

35. de Koning DB, Drenth JP, Friederich P, Nagengast FM. [Thalidomide for the treatment of recurrent gastrointestinal blood loss due to intestinal angiodysplasias] Thalidomide als behandeling bij recidiverend gastro-intestinaal bloedverlies op basis van intestinale angiodysplasieen. Ned Tijdschr Geneeskd 2006;150(36):1994–1997.

36. Kamalaporn P, Saravanan R, Cirocco M, May G, Kortan P, Kandel G, et al. Thalidomide for the treatment of chronic gastrointestinal bleeding from angiodysplasias: a case series. Eur J Gastroenterol Hepatol 2009;21(12):1347–1350.

37. Ertekin C, Barbaros U, Taviloglu K, Guloglu R, Kasoglu A. Dieulafoy's lesion of esophagus. Surg Endosc 2002;16(1):219.

38. Moreira-Pinto J, Raposo C, Teixeira da Silva V, Curado J, Barbosa E, Honavar M, et al. Jejunal Dieulafoy's lesion: case report and literature review. Pediatr Surg Int 2009;25 (7):641–2.

39. Lee YT, Walmsley RS, Leong RW, Sung JJ. Dieulafoy's lesion. Gastrointest Endosc 2003;58(2):236–43.

40. Lara LF, Sreenarasimhaiah J, Tang SJ, Afonso BB, Rockey DC. Dieulafoy Lesions of the GI Tract: Localization and Therapeutic Outcomes. Dig Dis Sci 2010;55: 3436–3441.

41. Yanar H, Dolay K, Ertekin C, Taviloglu K, Ozcinar B, Guloglu R, et al. An infrequent cause of upper gastrointestinal tract bleeding: "Dieulafoy's lesion". Hepatogastroenterology 2007;54(76):1013–1017.

42. Lozano FS, Munoz-Bellvis L, San Norberto E, Garcia-Plaza A, Gonzalez-Porras Jr. Primary aortoduodenal fistula: new case reports and a review of the literature. J Gastrointest Surg 2008;12(9):1561–1565.

43. Brandao D, Canedo A, Maia M, Ferreira J, Vaz G. Duodenocaval fistula as a result of a fish bone perforation. J Vasc Surg 2010;51(5):1276–1278.

44. Khan MF, Novak D, Anain P, McDonald J. Primary aortoduodenal fistula: a rare cause of upper GI bleeding. Gastrointest Endosc 2009;70(6):1271–1272.

45. Brountzos EN, Vasdekis S, Kostopanagiotou G, Danias N, Alexopoulou E, Petropoulou K, et al. Endovascular treatment of a bleeding secondary aorto-enteric fistula. A case report with 1-year follow-up. Cardiovasc Intervent Radiol 2007; 30(5):1037–1041.

46. Lonn L, Dias N, Veith Schroeder T, Resch T. Is EVAR the treatment of choice for aortoenteric fistula? J Cardiovasc Surg (Torino) 2010;51(3):319–27.

47. Thuluvath PJ, Yoo HY. Portal Hypertensive gastropathy. Am J Gastroenterol 2002; 97(12):2973–2978.

48. Higaki N, Matsui H, Imaoka H, Ikeda Y, Murakami H, Hiasa Y, et al. Characteristic endoscopic features of portal hypertensive enteropathy. J Gastroenterol 2008; 43(5):327–31.

49. Bini EJ, Lascarides CE, Micale PL, Weinshel EH. Mucosal abnormalities of the colon in patients with portal hypertension: an endoscopic study. Gastrointest Endosc 2000;52(4):511–16.

50. Cubillas R, Rockey DC. Portal hypertensive gastropathy: a review. Liver Int 2010; 30(8):1094–1102.
51. Balan KK, Jones AT, Roberts NB, Pearson JP, Critchley M, Jenkins SA. The effects of Helicobacter pylori colonization on gastric function and the incidence of portal hypertensive gastropathy in patients with cirrhosis of the liver. Am J Gastroenterol 1996;91(7):1400–1406.
52. Garcia N, Sanyal AJ. Portal Hypertensive Gastropathy and Gastric Antral Vascular Ectasia. Curr Treat Options Gastroenterol 2001;4(2):163–71.
53. Goel A, Christian CL. Gastric antral vascular ectasia (watermelon stomach) in a patient with Sjogren's syndrome. J Rheumatol 2003;30(5):1090–1092.
54. Viiala CH, Kaye JM, Hurley DM, Kaushik SP. Watermelon stomach arising in association with Addison's disease. J Clin Gastroenterol 2001;33(2):173.
55. Ingraham KM, O'Brien MS, Shenin M, Derk CT, Steen VD. Gastric antral vascular ectasia in systemic sclerosis: demographics and disease predictors. J Rheumatol 2010;37(3):603–7.
56. Burak KW, Lee SS, Beck PL. Portal hypertensive gastropathy and gastric antral vascular ectasia (GAVE) syndrome. Gut 2001;49(6):866–72.
57. Fuccio L, Zagari RM, Serrani M, Eusebi LH, Grilli D, Cennamo V, et al. Endoscopic argon plasma coagulation for the treatment of gastric antral vascular ectasia-related bleeding in patients with liver cirrhosis. Digestion 2009;79(3):143–50.
58. Lee HE, Sagong C, Yeo KY, Ko JY, Kim JS, Yu HJ. A case of hereditary hemorrhagic telangiectasia. Ann Dermatol 2009;21(2):206–8.
59. Goral V, Demir D, Tuzun Y, Keklikci U, Buyukbayram H, Bayan K, et al. Pseudoxantoma elasticum, as a repetitive upper gastrointestinal hemorrhage cause in a pregnant woman. World J Gastroenterol 2007;13(28):3897–3899.
60. Solomon JA, Abrams L, Lichtenstein GR. GI manifestations of Ehlers-Danlos syndrome. Am J Gastroenterol 1996;91(11):2282–2288.
61. Dwivedi M, Misra SP. Blue rubber bleb nevus syndrome causing upper GI hemorrhage: a novel management approach and review. Gastrointest Endosc 2002;55(7):943–6.
62. Walter C, Mbebe T, Caragounis E, Thirsk I. Blue rubber bleb naevus syndrome: a rare cause of gastrointestinal bleeding in an African child. Afr J Paediatr Surg 2010;7 (3):206–8.
63. van Tuyl SA, Letteboer TG, Rogge-Wolf C, Kuipers EJ, Snijder RJ, Westermann CJ, et al. Assessment of intestinal vascular malformations in patients with hereditary hemorrhagic teleangiectasia and anemia. Eur J Gastroenterol Hepatol 2007; 19(2):153–8.
64. Kjeldsen AD, Kjeldsen J. Gastrointestinal bleeding in patients with hereditary hemorrhagic telangiectasia. Am J Gastroenterol 2000;95(2):415–18
65. Sharathkumar AA, Shapiro A. Hereditary haemorrhagic telangiectasia. Haemophilia 2008;14(6):1269–1280.
66. Laube S, Moss C. Pseudoxanthoma elasticum. Arch Dis Child 2005 Jul; 90(7):754–6.
67. Fishman SJ, Smithers CJ, Folkman J, Lund DP, Burrows PE, Mulliken JB, et al. Blue rubber bleb nevus syndrome: surgical eradication of gastrointestinal bleeding. Ann Surg 2005;241(3):523–8.
68. Pore G. GI lesions in Henoch-Schonlein purpura. Gastrointest Endosc 2002; 55(2):283–6.
69. Chae EJ, Do KH, Seo JB, Park SH, Kang JW, Jang YM, et al. Radiologic and clinical findings of Behcet disease: comprehensive review of multisystemic involvement. Radiographics 2008;28(5):e31.

70. Perez RA, Silver D, Banerjee B. Polyarteritis nodosa presenting as massive upper gastrointestinal hemorrhage. Surg Endosc 2000;14(1):87.

71. Pagnoux C, Mahr A, Cohen P, Guillevin L. Presentation and outcome of gastrointestinal involvement in systemic necrotizing vasculitides: analysis of 62 patients with polyarteritis nodosa, microscopic polyangiitis, Wegener granulomatosis, Churg-Strauss syndrome, or rheumatoid arthritis-associated vasculitis. Medicine (Baltimore) 2005; 84(2):115–28.

72. Kuipers EJ, van Leeuwen MA, Nikkels PG, Jager J, van Rijswijk MH. Hemobilia due to vasculitis of the gall bladder in a patient with mixed connective tissue disease. J Rheumatol 1991;18(4):617–18.

73. Steen S, Lamont J, Petrey L. Acute gastric dilation and ischemia secondary to small bowel obstruction. Proc (Bayl Univ Med Cent) 2008;21(1):15–17.

74. Lewis S, Holbrook A, Hersch P. An unusual case of massive gastric distension with catastrophic sequelae. Acta Anaesthesiol Scand 2005;49(1):95–7.

75. Mensink PB, Moons LM, Kuipers EJ. Chronic gastrointestinal ischaemia: shifting paradigms. Gut 2010;60: 722–37.

76. Fiddian-Green RG, Stanley JC, Nostrant T, Phillips D. Chronic gastric ischemia. A cause of abdominal pain or bleeding identified from the presence of gastric mucosal acidosis. J Cardiovasc Surg (Torino) 1989;30(5):852–9.

77. Sharlow JW, Cone JB, Schaefer RF. Acute gastric necrosis in the postoperative period. South Med J 1989;82(4):529–30.

78. Arora M, Goldberg EM. Kaposi sarcoma involving the gastrointestinal tract. Gastroenterol Hepatol (N Y) 2010 Jul; 6(7):459–62.

79. Al-Haddad M, Ward EM, Bouras EP, Raimondo M. Hyperplastic polyps of the gastric antrum in patients with gastrointestinal blood loss. Dig Dis Sci 2007; 52(1):105–9.

80. Chen ZM, Scudiere JR, Abraham SC, Montgomery E. Pyloric gland adenoma: an entity distinct from gastric foveolar type adenoma. Am J Surg Pathol 2009; 33(2):186–93.

81. Vasen HF, Moslein G, Alonso A, Aretz S, Bernstein I, Bertario L, et al. Guidelines for the clinical management of familial adenomatous polyposis (FAP). Gut 2008; 57(5):704–13.

82. Aretz S. The differential diagnosis and surveillance of hereditary gastrointestinal polyposis syndromes. Dtsch Arztebl Int 2010;107(10):163–73.

83. Ramsoekh D, van Leerdam ME, Dekker E, Ouwendijk RT, van Dekken H, Kuipers EJ. Sporadic duodenal adenoma and the association with colorectal neoplasia: a case-control study. Am J Gastroenterol 2008;103(6):1505–1509.

84. Ferlay J, Shin HR, Bray F, Forman D, Mathers C, Parkin DM. Estimates of worldwide burden of cancer in 2008: GLOBOCAN 2008. Int J Cancer 2010;127: 2893–2917.

85. Vial M, Grande L, Pera M. Epidemiology of adenocarcinoma of the esophagus, gastric cardia, and upper gastric third. Recent Results Cancer Res 2010;182: 1–17.

86. Enzinger PC, Mayer RJ. Esophageal cancer. N Engl J Med 2003;349(23):2241–2252.

87. Savides TJ, Jensen DM, Cohen J, Randall GM, Kovacs TO, Pelayo E, et al. Severe upper gastrointestinal tumor bleeding: endoscopic findings, treatment, and outcome. Endoscopy 1996;28(2):244–8.

88. Hyatt BJ, Paull PE, Wassef W. Gastric oncology: an update. Curr Opin Gastroenterol 2009;25(6):570–8.

89. Asakura H, Hashimoto T, Harada H, Mizumoto M, Furutani K, Hasuike N, et al. Palliative radiotherapy for bleeding from advanced gastric cancer: is a schedule of 30 Gy in 10 fractions adequate? J Cancer Res Clin Oncol 2010;137:125–30.

90. Lee HJ, Shin JH, Yoon HK, Ko GY, Gwon DI, Song HY, et al. Transcatheter arterial embolization in gastric cancer patients with acute bleeding. Eur Radiol 2009;19 (4):960–5.

91. Zullo A, Hassan C, Cristofari F, Andriani A, De Francesco V, Ierardi E, et al. Effects of Helicobacter pylori eradication on early stage gastric mucosa-associated lymphoid tissue lymphoma. Clin Gastroenterol Hepatol 2010;8(2):105–10.

92. Capelle LG, de Vries AC, Looman CW, Casparie MK, Boot H, Meijer GA, et al. Gastric MALT lymphoma: epidemiology and high adenocarcinoma risk in a nation-wide study. Eur J Cancer 2008;44(16):2470–2476.

93. Radic-Kristo D, Planinc-Peraica A, Ostojic S, Vrhovac R, Kardum-Skelin I, Jaksic B. Primary gastrointestinal non-Hodgkin lymphoma in adults: clinicopathologic and survival characteristics. Coll Antropol 2010;34(2):413–17.

94. Chen WL, Tsai WC, Chao TY, Sheu LF, Chou JM, Kao WY, et al. The clinicopathological analysis of 303 cases with malignant lymphoma classified according to the World Health Organization classification system in a single institute of Taiwan. Ann Hematol 2010;89(6):553–62.

95. Kim JH, Lee JH, Lee J, Oh SO, Chang DK, Rhee PL, et al. Primary NK-/T-cell lymphoma of the gastrointestinal tract: clinical characteristics and endoscopic findings. Endoscopy 2007;39(2):156–60.

96. Lee HH, Hur H, Jung H, Jeon HM, Park CH, Song KY. Analysis of 151 consecutive gastric submucosal tumors according to tumor location. J Surg Oncol 2010;104: 72–5.

97. Fletcher CD, Berman JJ, Corless C, Gorstein F, Lasota J, Longley BJ, et al. Diagnosis of gastrointestinal stromal tumors: A consensus approach. Hum Pathol 2002; 33(5):459–65.

98. Miettinen M, Lasota J. Gastrointestinal stromal tumors: review on morphology, molecular pathology, prognosis, and differential diagnosis. Arch Pathol Lab Med 2006;130(10):1466–1478.

99. Miettinen M, Sarlomo-Rikala M, Sobin LH, Lasota J. Esophageal stromal tumors: a clinicopathologic, immunohistochemical, and molecular genetic study of 17 cases and comparison with esophageal leiomyomas and leiomyosarcomas. Am J Surg Pathol 2000;24(2):211–22.

100. Rijcken E, Kersting CM, Senninger N, Bruewer M. Esophageal resection for giant leiomyoma: report of two cases and a review of the literature. Langenbecks Arch Surg 2009;394(4):623–9.

101. Chang CW, Chu CH, Shih SC, Chen MJ, Yang TL, Chang WH. Duodenal polypoid lipoma with bleeding. Am J Surg 2010;200(4):e49–50.

102. Sadio A, Peixoto P, Castanheira A, Cancela E, Ministro P, Casimiro C, et al. Gastric lipoma – an unusual cause of upper gastrointestinal bleeding. Rev Esp Enferm Dig 2010;102(6):398–400.

103. Czekajska-Chehab E, Tomaszewska M, Drop A, Dabrowski A, Skomra D, Orlowski T, et al. Liposarcoma of the esophagus: case report and literature review. Med Sci Monit 2009;15(7):CS123–7.

104. Lin CH, Hsu CW, Chiang YJ, Ng KF, Chiu CT. Esophageal and gastric Kaposi's sarcomas presenting as upper gastrointestinal bleeding. Chang Gung Med J 2002;25 (5):329–33.

105. Schuchter LM, Green R, Fraker D. Primary and metastatic diseases in malignant melanoma of the gastrointestinal tract. Curr Opin Oncol 2000;12(2):181–5.

106. Chehab BM, Dakhil SR, Nassif, II. Melanoma metastatic to the duodenum presenting as upper GI bleed: 2 cases and a review of the literature. Gastrointest Endosc 2008; 67(6):998–1000.

107. Kotteas EA, Adamopoulos A, Drogitis PD, Zalonis A, Giannopoulos KV, Karapana-giotou EM, et al. Gastrointestinal bleeding as initial presentation of melanoma of unknown primary origin: report of a case and review of the literature. In Vivo 2009;23(3):487–9.

108. Modlin IM, Oberg K, Chung DC, Jensen RT, de Herder WW, Thakker RV, et al. Gastroenteropancreatic neuroendocrine tumours. Lancet Oncol 2008;9(1): 61–72.

109. Ellis L, Shale MJ, Coleman MP. Carcinoid Tumors of the Gastrointestinal Tract: Trends in Incidence in England Since 1971. Am J Gastroenterol 2010;105: 2563–2569.

110. Sawalakhe NR, Nistala S, Sasidharan M, Narendran RT, Amrapurkar AD, Joshi RM, et al. Solitary type III gastric carcinoid causing upper gastrointestinal bleeding and severe anaemia. Trop Gastroenterol 2010;31(1):43–4.

111. Green LK. Hematogenous metastases to the stomach. A review of 67 cases. Cancer 1990;65(7):1596–1600.

112. Oda, Kondo H, Yamao T, Saito D, Ono H, Gotoda T, et al. Metastatic tumors to the stomach: analysis of 54 patients diagnosed at endoscopy and 347 autopsy cases. Endoscopy 2001;33(6):507–10.

113. Mallory GK, Weiss SW. Hemorrhages from lacerations of the cardiac orifice of the stomach due to vomiting. Am J Med Sci 1929;178: 506–12.

114. Kim JW, Kim HS, Byun JW, Won CS, Jee MG, Park YS, et al. Predictive factors of recurrent bleeding in Mallory-Weiss syndrome. Korean J Gastroenterol 2005;46 (6):447–54.

115. Younes Z, Johnson DA. The spectrum of spontaneous and iatrogenic esophageal injury: perforations, Mallory-Weiss tears, and hematomas. J Clin Gastroenterol 1999;29(4):306–17.

116. Eisen GM, Baron TH, Dominitz JA, Faigel DO, Goldstein JL, Johanson JF, et al. Complications of upper GI endoscopy. Gastrointest Endosc 2002;55(7):784–93.

117. Kortas DY, Haas LS, Simpson WG, Nickl NJ, 3rd, Gates LK, Jr. Mallory-Weiss tear: predisposing factors and predictors of a complicated course. Am J Gastroenterol 2001;96(10):2863–2865.

118. Llach J, Elizalde JI, Guevara MC, Pellise M, Castellot A, Gines A, et al. Endoscopic injection therapy in bleeding Mallory-Weiss syndrome: a randomized controlled trial. Gastrointest Endosc 2001;54(6):679–81.

119. Cho YS, Chae HS, Kim HK, Kim JS, Kim BW, Kim SS, et al. Endoscopic band ligation and endoscopic hemoclip placement for patients with Mallory-Weiss syndrome and active bleeding. World J Gastroenterol 2008;14(13):2080–2084.

120. Huang SP, Wang HP, Lee YC, Lin CC, Yang CS, Wu MS, et al. Endoscopic hemoclip placement and epinephrine injection for Mallory-Weiss syndrome with active bleeding. Gastrointest Endosc 2002;55(7):842–6.

121. Lecleire S, Antonietti M, Iwanicki-Caron I, Duclos A, Ramirez S, Ben-Soussan E, et al. Endoscopic band ligation could decrease recurrent bleeding in Mallory-Weiss syn-drome as compared to haemostasis by hemoclips plus epinephrine. Aliment Phar-macol Ther 2009;30(4):399–405.

122. Park CH, Min SW, Sohn YH, Lee WS, Joo YE, Kim HS, et al. A prospective, randomized trial of endoscopic band ligation vs. epinephrine injection for actively bleeding Mallory-Weiss syndrome. Gastrointest Endosc 2004;60(1):22–7.

123. Yen HH, Soon MS, Chen YY. Esophageal intramural hematoma: an unusual com-plication of endoscopic biopsy. Gastrointest Endosc 2005;62(1):161–3.

124. Cheung J, Muller N, Weiss A. Spontaneous intramural esophageal hematoma: case report and review. Can J Gastroenterol 2006;20(4):285–6.

125. van Heel NC, Haringsma J, Spaander MC, Bruno MJ, Kuipers EJ. Short-term esophageal stenting in the management of benign perforations. Am J Gastroenterol 2010;105(7):1515–1520.

126. Poley JW, Steyerberg EW, Kuipers EJ, Dees J, Hartmans R, Tilanus HW, et al. Ingestion of acid and alkaline agents: outcome and prognostic value of early upper endoscopy. Gastrointest Endosc 2004;60(3):372–7.

127. Kay M, Wyllie R. Caustic ingestions in children. Curr Opin Pediatr 2009;21(5):651–4.

128. Lee M. Caustic ingestion and upper digestive tract injury. Dig Dis Sci 2010; 55(6):1547–1549.

129. Sahin C, Alver D, Gulcin N, Kurt G, Celayir AC. A rare cause of intestinal perforation: ingestion of magnet. World J Pediatr 2010;6(4):369–71.

130. Syrakos T, Zacharakis E, Antonitsis P, Spanos C, Georgantis G, Kiskinis D. Surgical intervention for gastrointestinal foreign bodies in adults: a case series. Med Princ Pract 2008;17(4):276–9.

131. Huiping Y, Jian Z, Shixi L. Esophageal foreign body as a cause of upper gastrointestinal hemorrhage: case report and review of the literature. Eur Arch Otorhinolaryngol 2008;265(2):247–9.

132. Kim YJ, Park JC, Kim JH, Shin SK, Lee SK, Lee YC, et al. Histologic diagnosis based on forceps biopsy is not adequate for determining endoscopic treatment of gastric adenomatous lesions. Endoscopy 2010;42(8):620–6.

133. Kato M, Nishida T, Tsutsui S, Komori M, Michida T, Yamamoto K, et al. Endoscopic submucosal dissection as a treatment for gastric noninvasive neoplasia: a multicenter study by Osaka University ESD Study Group. J Gastroenterol 2010;46: 325–31.

134. Ghazi A, Ferstenberg H, Shinya H. Endoscopic gastroduodenal polypectomy. Ann Surg 1984;200(2):175–80.

135. Reed WP, Kilkenny JW, Dias CE, Wexner SD, Group SEOS. A prospective analysis of 3525 esophagogastroduodenoscopies performed by surgeons. Surg Endosc 2004; 18(1):11–21.

136. Alderliesten J, Conchillo JM, Leeuwenburgh I, Steyerberg EW, Kuipers EJ. Predictors for outcome of failure of balloon dilatation in patients with achalasia. Gut 2010;60: 10–16.

137. Hordijk ML, van Hooft JE, Hansen BE, Fockens P, Kuipers EJ. A randomized comparison of electrocautery incision with Savary bougienage for relief of anastomotic gastroesophageal strictures. Gastrointest Endosc 2009;70(5):849–55.

138. Jamil LH, Krause KR, Chengelis DL, Jury RP, Jackson CM, Cannon ME, et al. Endoscopic management of early upper gastrointestinal hemorrhage following laparoscopic Roux-en-Y gastric bypass. Am J Gastroenterol 2008;103(1): 86–91.

139. Monkhouse SJ, Morgan JD, Norton SA. Complications of bariatric surgery: presentation and emergency management – a review. Ann R Coll Surg Engl 2009; 91(4):280–6.

140. Prata Martins F, Bonilha DR, Correia LP, Paulo Ferrari A. Obstructive jaundice caused by hemobilia after liver biopsy. Endoscopy 2008;40Suppl 2: E265–6.

141. Lee YT, Lin H, Chen KY, Wu HS, Hwang MH, Yan SL. Life-threatening hemobilia caused by hepatic pseudoaneurysm after T-tube choledostomy; report of a case. BMC Gastroenterol 2010;10: 81.

142. Sandblom P. *Hemobilia (Biliary Tract Hemorrhage). History, Pathology, Diagnosis, Treatment*. Springfield, Illinois: Charles C Thomas 1972.

143. Green MH, Duell RM, Johnson CD, Jamieson NV. Haemobilia. Br J Surg. 2001; 88(6):773–86.

144. Hommes M, Kazemier G, van Dijk LC, Kuipers EJ, van Ijsseldijk A, Vogels LM, et al. Complex liver trauma with bilhemia treated with perihepatic packing and endovascular stent in the vena cava. J Trauma 2009;67(2):E51–3.

145. Sandblom P. Gastrointestinal hemorrhage through the pancreatic duct. Ann Surg 1970;171(1):61–6.

146. Etienne S, Pessaux P, Tuech JJ, Lada P, Lermite E, Brehant O, et al. Hemosuccus pancreaticus: a rare cause of gastrointestinal bleeding. Gastroenterol Clin Biol 2005 Mar; 29(3):237–42.

147. Vimalraj V, Kannan DG, Sukumar R, Rajendran S, Jeswanth S, Jyotibasu D, et al. Haemosuccus pancreaticus: diagnostic and therapeutic challenges. HPB (Oxford) 2009 Jun; 11(4):345–50.

148. Kuganeswaran E, Smith OJ, Goldman ML, Clarkston WK. Hemosuccus pancreaticus: rare complication of chronic pancreatitis. Gastrointest Endosc 2000;51(4 Pt 1): 464–5.

149. Shinzeki M, Hori Y, Fujino Y, Matsumoto I, Toyama H, Tsujimura T, et al. Mucinous cystic neoplasm of the pancreas presenting with hemosuccus pancreaticus: report of a case. Surg Today 2010;40(5):470–3.

150. Massani M, Bridda A, Caratozzolo E, Bonariol L, Antoniutti M, Bassi N. Hemosuccus pancreaticus due to primary splenic artery aneurysm: a diagnostic and therapeutic challenge. JOP 2009;10(1):48–52.

151. Seicean A, Stan-Iuga R, Munteanu D. An unusual cause of hemosuccus pancreaticus diagnosed by endoscopic ultrasonography: splenic arterial fistula due to a pancreatic stent (with video). Endoscopy 2010;42 (Suppl 2): E239–40.

152. Hutchison SM, Finlayson ND. Epistaxis as a cause of hematemesis and melena. J Clin Gastroenterol 1987;9(3):283–5.

CHAPTER 9

Lower GI Bleeding: Endoscopic, Radiological and Surgical Diagnosis and Management

Ana Ignjatovic[1], John T. Jenkins[2] & Brian P. Saunders[1]
[1]Wolfson Unit for Endoscopy, Imperial College London, London, UK
[2]Department of Colorectal Surgery, St Mark's Hospital, Imperial College London, London, UK

Introduction

Definition

Lower gastrointestinal bleeding (LGIB) refers to bleeding originating distal to the ligament of Treitz and therefore covers both small bowel and colonic sources. Patients can present with visible bleeding (overt LGIB) or with iron-deficiency anemia or positive fecal occult blood test (FOBT) on screening (occult LGIB). LGIB can be classed as acute or chronic depending on the duration of symptoms, with acute bleeding arbitrarily defined as lasting <3 days. Acute LGIB may be massive and associated with hemodynamic instability, requiring urgent investigations and management. Chronic LGIB can either present with episodic bright red rectal bleeding (haematochezia) or insidiously, with iron-deficiency anemia or a positive FOBT.

Incidence

Rectal bleeding is a common symptom with estimated prevalence of 20% in general population (1) although only about 7 per 1000 patients per year seek medical opinion (2). The LGI tract is the source of bleeding in approximately 20% of patients hospitalized for GI hemorrhage (3). The annual incidence of LGIB requiring hospitalization was estimated by one epidemiological study to be 21/100,000 adults in the USA (4). A recent study demonstrated a trend toward an increasing incidence of LGIB over the last 10 years (from 20/100,000 to 33/100,000) in contrast to a decreasing incidence of UGIB (from 87/100,000 to 47/100,000) (5). Patients who present with LGIB are typically elderly, reflecting the higher incidence of conditions that tend to occur with aging (diverticulosis, angiodysplasia, neoplasms, ischemic colitis). The

Gastrointestinal Bleeding, Second Edition. Edited by Joseph J.Y. Sung, Ernst J. Kuipers and Alan N. Barkun. © 2012 Blackwell Publishing Ltd.
Published 2012 by Blackwell Publishing Ltd.

annual incidence of LGIB increases with age, from 1/100,000 for patients in their twenties to more than 200/100,000 in patients in the ninth decade of life (4). In a number of studies, LGIB was found to be commoner in men than women.

Etiology

It is often difficult to determine the exact source of LGIB, especially if it is intermittent in nature, and in up to 42% of patients no definite source of bleeding is identified after endoscopic and radiological investigations (6). In one study of 80 patients with severe hematochezia and negative nasogastric (NG) aspirate, proctoscopy and rigid sigmoidoscopy, only 74% of bleeding lesions were colonic in origin. Upper GI tract lesions were thought to be a cause in 11% and small bowel lesions in the remaining 9% (7). More than one potential bleeding source may be identified in up to 40% of patients (8, 9), but a definite bleeding site (active bleeding, visible vessels and adherent clots) is identified less frequently, in 21–43% of cases (10, 11). The commonest colonic causes of LGIB are listed in Boxes 9.1 and 9.2. Conditions in italics are the ones most likely to cause acute massive hemorrhage.

Outcomes

LGIB tends to be less severe in presentation than UGIB. Patients with LGIB are likely to have a significantly higher hemoglobin (Hb) level, require fewer blood transfusions and are less hemodynamically unstable than patients with UGIB (16) and 80–85% of bleeding episodes in the LGI tract will stop spontaneously. Reported mortality rates for LGIB are 3–5%, although the patients who develop bleeding whilst hospitalized have higher mortality

---

Box 9.1 Colorectal causes of LGIB

Commonest colorectal causes of LGIB	Frequency (%)[*]
Diverticular disease	5.2-42
Angiodysplasia	1.2-4
Neoplasms (including polyps)	2.9-19
Inflammatory bowel disease	2.3-3.9
Ischemic colitis	7-18
Infectious colitis	2.6
Radiation proctitis	9-13
Anorectal causes (fissures, hemorrhoids)	20
Post-polypectomy hemorrhage	0-12.8
Post-anastomotic bleed	

[*] Sources: Longstreth (4); Green, Rockey, Portwood, et al. (12); Angtuaco, Reddy, Drapkin, et al. (14); and Ohyama, Sakurai, Ito, et al. (15)

Box 9.2 Non-colonic causes of LGIB

Small bowel source (≈10%)
AV malformations
Meckel's diverticulum
IBD
Neoplasia
Vasculitis

UGI source (≈10%)
Ulcer
Neoplasia

---

rates (23%) compared to those who have rectal bleeding before hospital admission (3%) (4). A large cross sectional study of 227,022 hospitalized patients with a diagnosis of LGIB, identified that increasing age, comorbidity, intestinal ischemia, coagulation defects, development of bleeding whilst hospitalized for another condition, hypovolemia, transfusion of packed red blood cells and male gender were all independent predictors of in-hospital mortality (17). Comay et al. assessed economic impact of LGIB and found that the average cost for a hospitalized patient with LGIB in Ontario was $3000, with an average hospital stay of 7.5 days (18).

Unlike with UGIB, there are no commonly accepted criteria used to predict the outcome in patients with LGIB. The "BLEED" classification was devised to stratify patients with both upper and lower GI hemorrhage and predict their risk of adverse events whilst hospitalized. Patients with ongoing bleeding, systolic blood pressure <100 mmHg, prothrombin time >1.2, altered mental state and significant comorbidity were more likely to develop multi-organ failure, require more units of blood and have longer hospital stays (19). Strate and colleagues identified predictors of severe LGIB defined as transfusion of ≥2 units of blood, a decrease in hematocrit of 20% or recurrent rectal bleeding (accompanied by a drop in hematocrit or a need for blood transfusion) within one week (20). Patients could be stratified into low, moderate or high-risk groups using simple clinical parameters:

- heart rate ≥100/min
- systolic blood pressure ≤115 mmHg
- syncope
- non-tender abdominal exam
- rectal bleeding in the first four hours of evaluation
- aspirin use
- presence of >two comorbidities.

The prognostic model was externally validated on 275 patients and it successfully stratified patients into risk groups – patients with three or more of the parameters were at a high risk of severe bleeding ($\approx$80%), those at 1–3 parameters at moderate risk ($\approx$45%) and those with no risk factors at low risk (<10%) (21). Therefore high-risk patients can be identified early and triaged to urgent investigations and management. Artificial neural networks have been used in the prediction of outcome with LGIB and may improve clinical performance and patient outcome (22).

Clinical evaluation

History

Patients with LGIB may present with bright red rectal bleeding, passage of clots and altered blood, or rarely, melena. Presence of symptoms such as dyspnoea, tachypnea, fatigue, chest pain, syncope and postural symptoms suggests potential hemodynamic compromise. Adequate history and examination should take place concurrently with resuscitation. Careful current and past medical history may help determine the etiology of LGIB. Typically melena or dark blood, indicate an upper GI source of bleeding, although proximal colonic lesions may present similarly. Although bright red bleeding is likely to result from the left colon or anorectum, proximal lesions may be found on colonoscopy. There is a degree of subjectivity and lack of consistency when describing the colour of blood, devaluing its predictive value as to the location of the bleeding source (23). A previous history of bloody diarrhea and abdominal pain in younger patients would suggest inflammatory bowel disease whereas in older population, especially those with hypertension or cardiovascular disease, ischemic colitis should be considered. Painless bleeding in patients older than 70 is typical of diverticulosis and angiodysplasia, with the latter thought to be more common in patients with chronic renal failure and valvular heart disease. Ulceration throughout the GI tract and diverticular bleeding are common in patients who regularly use aspirin or other NSAIDs (24). Previous medical interventions may help determine the etiology of bleeding, such as recent colonoscopy and polypectomy (polypectomy bleed), resection of the bowel with formation of anastomosis (anastomotic bleed), previous pelvic radiotherapy (radiation proctopathy) and vascular surgery (aorto-eneteric fistula).

Examination

Presence of hemodynamic compromise is an important factor in risk stratification of the patient. Even in the absence of obvious tachycardia or hypotension, postural blood pressure should be measured and a drop in systolic

BP of more than 15 mmHg from lying to standing indicates a significant compromise. Thorough cardiac, pulmonary, and abdominal examination should be performed. Presence of abdominal tenderness may indicate an inflammatory etiology but is not specific as blood from any source when present in the colonic lumen can cause colicky pain. Digital rectal examination should be performed in all patients presenting with LGIB (25) and in one study 40% of rectal carcinoma were palpable on rectal examination (26).

Initial management

Initial management depends on the severity of bleeding. Patients presenting with minimal intermittent bleeding with no hemodynamic compromise or a drop in Hb can be managed as outpatients. Patients with severe bleeding and hemodynamic compromise need urgent resuscitation, using crystalloids, colloids and blood as required, via large bore cannula, whilst a further management plan is determined. Blood samples for full blood count, electrolytes, liver function test, clotting and cross match should be sent urgently. Thrombocytopenia (platelets $<50 \times 10^9$/L) should be corrected with platelet transfusion and coagulopathy (PT > 15 sec) with fresh frozen plasma. Patients taking NSAIDs and anticoagulants should have those withdrawn, and for the latter group, if bleeding is severe, anticoagulation should be reversed with vitamin K and fresh frozen plasma. Further management depends on severity and cause of hemorrhage.

Acute severe hemorrhage

Diverticulosis (Fig. 9.1) is the commonest cause of acute LGIB, accounting for about 40% of cases (27). The other, less common causes are listed in Box 9.3.

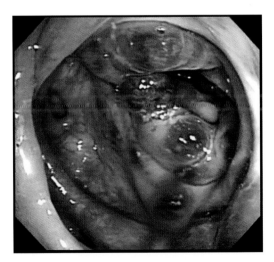

Figure 9.1 Bleeding diverticula

Box 9.3 Common causes of acute severe LGIB

Diverticulosis
Angodysplasia
Ischemic colitis
Inflammatory bowel disease
Ulcers (Ischemic, radiotherapy-induced, infective, Dieulafoy's)
Aorto-enteric fistula
Ruptured splenic artery aneurysm
Erosion of pancreatic pseudocyst
Post–operative/anastomotic hemorrhage
Post-polypectomy
Colonic/rectal/stomal varices

Although bloody diarrhea is common in ulcerative colitis, massive hemorrhage is rare. In a series of 1,526 patients with Crohn's disease, acute bleeding occurred in 1.9% of patients with Crohn's colitis and 0.7% with Crohn's ileitis (28). Although 48% of patients were managed medically without surgery, bleeding recurred in 30% of patients. Conditions such as aorto-enteric fistula, ruptured splenic artery aneurysm and erosion of pancreatic pseudocyst in the colon are relatively rare (29, 30), but may present with torrential bleeding. Colonic and rectal varices (Fig. 9.2) are uncommon in patients with portal hypertension – in one study, the most common finding in patients with portal hypertension and LGIB was angiodysplasia (14/20 patients) (31).

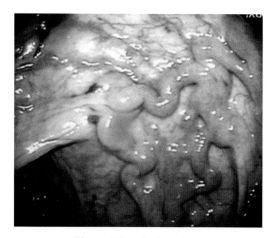

Figure 9.2 Colonic varices

Acute severe hemorrhage will stop spontaneously in 70–90% of patients (32, 33), but patients who are hemodynamically unstable and/or need more than 4 units of blood need urgent investigation and treatment.

Endoscopic investigations

Esophagogastroduodenoscopy

All patients presenting with acute LGIB with hemodynamic compromise should undergo esophagogastroduodenoscopy (OGD) to exclude an UGI source of bleeding which may be found in 10–15% of patients (7). To minimize the potential complications associated with endoscopy, patients should be well resuscitated before the procedure. Complications, such as aspiration pneumonia and myocardial infarction are commoner in the elderly and are usually associated with excessive sedation (34). Therefore careful titration of sedation in patients over 75 is of paramount importance. Heart rate and oxygen saturations should be routinely monitored. Intranasal oxygen prevents de-saturation associated with endoscopy (35) and has been shown to reduce cardiac rhythm disturbances and ischemic changes in patients with pre-existing cardiovascular disease (36). If an UGI source of bleeding is identified, endoscopic treatment is warranted for lesions with recent stigmata of bleeding (frank blood, fresh clot or visible vessel – see Chapter 8).

Colonoscopy – diagnosis

There has been some controversy about the role of colonoscopy in the evaluation of patients with acute LGIB. Although colonoscopy for acute LGIB has been performed since the 1970s, it has not been widely accepted in the acute setting, partly due to fears about poor visibility in the unprepared colon and the potential for an increased risk of complications (37). However, with the improvement in colonoscopic technology, including thinner and more flexible colonoscopes, a number of studies have demonstrated that colonoscopy is safe and effective in the diagnosis of LGIB (7, 12, 13, 15). Maximum dexterity is required when performing colonoscopy in patients with acute LGIB, both to negotiate the scope past residual blood and clots and to navigate a potentially difficult diverticular segment in patients with diverticulosis. As blood is an effective cathartic, there is usually little residual stool in the colon to impede progress; however, views may be impeded by blood and clots. Ideally, large suction channel instruments (3.6 mm or larger) should be used and the colonoscope rotated so that the suction channel is at correct orientation (e.g. 5 o'clock on Olympus colonoscopes) to maximize suction. Ideally an irrigation pump should be available to assist in washing the mucosal surface and to improve visualization. If not available, 50 ml syringes of water flushed down the biopsy channel are a

Table 9.1 Diagnostic yield of colonoscopy.

Study	Year	No. of patients	Diagnosis (%)
Caos (9)	1986	35	77
Jensen (7)	1988	80	74
Chaudhry (32)	1998	85	97
Jensen (11)	2000	121	96
Ohyama (15)	2000	345	89
Angtuaco (13)	2001	39	74
Al Quahtini (38)	2002	152	45
Strate (10)	2003	144	89
Schumlewitz (14)	2003	415	89
Green (12)	2005	50	96

reasonable alternative. The addition of simethicone to water clears the bubbles caused by water irrigation and air insufflation. Position change of the patients is invaluable when performing colonoscopy in patients with LGIB, by redistributing blood and air gravitationally. The left colon, from mid-sigmoid to the distal transverse, is often visualized best in the supine or right lateral position, whereas the rectum, distal sigmoid and right colon in left lateral position.

Diagnostic yield of colonoscopy ranges from 45 to 97% (Table 9.1 summarizes some of the studies).

However, when diagnosis defined by either active bleeding during colonoscopy or stigmata of recent bleeding (visible vessel or a blood clot), the diagnostic yield of colonoscopy is significantly lower. In one study, where colonoscopy was performed within 24 hours of admission, a definite source of bleeding was seen in only 8% compared to a possible source in 67% of patients (19). However, in the only randomized controlled trial on the use of urgent colonoscopy for evaluation of acute LGIB, 42% of patients had a definite diagnosis made when colonoscopy was performed within eight hours of admission (12). There is no consensus regarding the timing of urgent colonoscopy, which is often determined by local resource availability. In the literature colonoscopy within eight hours, 12 hours and 24 hours are all reported as urgent colonoscopies. There is evidence that a definite source of bleeding is identified more often with early colonoscopy (42% vs 22% for standard medical care without colonoscopy (12)). However it is unclear if that has any effect on the outcome. Green et al. (12) showed no difference in mortality, hospital stay, mean transfusion requirements, early or late rebleeding or surgery when comparing urgent colonoscopy (within eight hours) to standard medical care (without colonoscopy but which included angiography). However, two other retrospective studies found that earlier colonoscopy (within 24 hours) was associated with shorter hospital stay (10, 14). In addition, Strate et al. (10) found that earlier colonoscopy resulted in significantly more therapeutic interventions.

Although urgent colonoscopy has been performed without bowel preparation with reasonable diagnostic yield (32), rapid (2–7 hours) oral purge (or via nasogastric tube, for patients unable to tolerate oral) using a balanced electrolyte solution (PEG-based purge, e.g. Kleenprep, GoLytely) ensures better visualization. Zuckerman et al. (25) reviewed 13 studies of colonoscopy in acute LGIB and found overall complication rate of just 1.3%, but a third of those were related to bowel preparation (all heart failure).

Colonoscopy – therapy

There are the following therapeutic options:
- injection of adrenaline 1:10,000
- bipolar electrocoagulation
- argon plasma coagulation (APC)
- endoclips
- banding

Adrenaline

Techniques used for the treatment of UGIB have been adapted for the use in the colon. Like in the UGI tract, immediate hemostasis is best achieved by injection of adrenaline 1:10,000, at 1–2 ml aliquots quadrantically around the bleeding point. The advantage of injection is that precise localization is often not necessary and several injections can be placed around the bleeding vessel. Adrenaline results in hemostasis by a combination of tamponade and vasoconstriction of the bleeding vessel.

Bipolar/Multipolar electrocoagulation

This encompasses use of Goldprobe (Fig. 9.3); Microvasive; BICAP; and ACM endoscopy. The advantage of bipolar coagulation is that the current is delivered to a small area between the two acting electrodes at the tip of the probe, making it safe to use as long as the power settings are low (10–20 W) and the pulses used are of short duration (about 1 second). In addition to delivering thermal therapy, the physical pressure of the probe tip provides a tamponade effect. A disadvantage, however, of any contact probe is that it can at times stick to the underlying tissue and attempts to remove it may precipitate further bleeding. Great care is required when using any thermal modality, particularly in a thin-walled diverticulum or the right colon. Generally, electrocoagulation should only be used when a visible vessel or bleeding point is seen. A new device, Coagrasper (Olympus, Tokyo), combines the mechanical effect of forceps and coagulation and is passed down

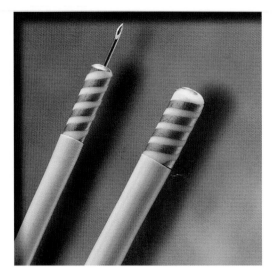

Figure 9.3 Gold probe

the biopsy channel. A bleeding vessel can be grasped, pulled away slightly from the normal mucosa and soft coagulation current applied (60–80 W), cauterizing the bleeding point.

Argon plasma coagulation (APC)(Erbe)

APC is a monopolar, non-contact technique with the current conducted through ionized argon gas flow onto the tissue. As the depth of penetration is limited, it is safe, although like with other thermal techniques, extra care is needed in the proximal, thin walled colon. An advantage of APC is the availability of both forward and side firing catheters allowing access to awkwardly positioned lesions. It is most commonly used for the treatment of radiation-induced proctopathy and angiodysplasia. APC has largely replaced Nd:YAG lasers due to its superior safety and lower cost.

Endoclips (QuickClip2, Olympus; Resolution Clips, Boston Scientific; TriClip, Wilson-Cook Medical)

Clips are particularly useful when an obvious bleeding vessel is seen (Fig. 9.4). They are made from stainless steel and are passed down the biopsy channel via an introducer. A bleeding lesion can be approached either tangentially or en face. Tangential approach allows more surrounding tissue to be grasped within the clip. The "QuickClip" (Olympus) has the advantage of being rotatable, however once it is closed it cannot be re-opened again. The "Resolution®" clip (Boston Scientific) can be opened and closed allowing re-positioning. It is not, however, rotatable but can be moved by rotating the shaft of the colonoscope. "TriClips" (Wilson-Cook

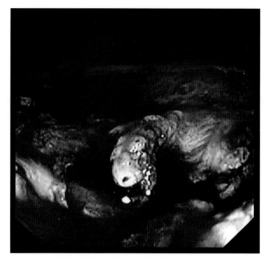

Figure 9.4 Vissible vessel on a post EMR site

Medical) can only be used *en face* and their fine wire prongs may not grasp sufficient tissue to occlude a bleeding vessel. If there is active bleeding, adrenaline can be injected first to enable visualization of a vessel. Small vessels and mucosal defects are ideal for clipping, often with two or three clips applied next to each other (Fig. 9.5). The lesions should ideally be approached tangentially and suction applied as the clip is deployed to draw in a maximum amount of tissue into the clip (39). Once the clip is fired, the introducer can be removed and further clips applied as necessary.

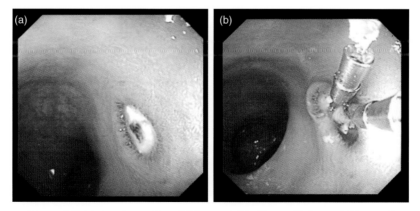

Figure 9.5 (a) An ulcer with a visible vessel.(b) Clips applied to a visible vessel

Banding

One pilot study, *ex-* and *in-vivo* assessed the use of endoscopic band ligation in treatment of bleeding colonic diverticula. In the *ex-vivo* study 11 diverticula were successfully everted and banded in surgical specimens, and no everted diverticula contained muscularis propria or serosal involvement. In the *in-vivo* study, active diverticular bleeding was completely controlled by endoscopic band ligation. No patients rebled or required surgery with a 12 months' follow-up period. Despite these encouraging pilot results, the risk of perforation still precludes the acceptance of banding for treatment of diverticular hemorrhage.

Analogous to bleeding lesions in the UGI tract, recent stigmata of hemorrhage predict likelihood of rebleeding, and endoscopic treatment of bleeding vessel prevents recurrent bleeding (11). In one study, 53% of patients with stigmata of recent hemorrhage who did not have endoscopic therapy had persistent or recurrent bleeding (11). Although there is no evidence specific to the LGI tract with regard to number of modalities used, most colonoscopists infer the findings related to UGI tract bleeding, and apply a combination of two therapies if possible (with adrenaline being one of the modalities) to reduce the likelihood of rebleeding.

Radiological investigations

There are two options:
- Multi-detector row computed tomography (MDCT)
- Mesenteric angiography

MDCT

CT is only recently establishing itself in the algorithm of treatment of patients with acute LGIB. The introduction of multi-slice CT has allowed rapid, non-invasive and quick diagnosis for patients suspected of GI bleeding. Active bleeding is defined if contrast extravasation with a focal area of high attenuation can be found within the bowel lumen (40) on the arterial phase of the scan. Patients are not given any oral contrast or water as extravasation of intravenous contrast may be obscured. Intravenous iodinated contrast material is routinely used, but the image acquisition parameters tend to be locally determined. Patients are frequently pre-hydrated with crystalloids to try and avoid contrast- induced nephropathy. There is a debate whether unenhanced scans should be routinely performed as well. Although, those scans allow identification of hyperdense material in the bowel (drugs, hemostatic clips) that may otherwise be seen as false positives, they expose the patients to higher radiation dose which may not be justified. Portal phase scans are performed as they help detect venous hemorrhage, often associated with tumors. If active contrast exavasation is identified, attenuation values in Hounsfield units should be measured to differentiate active bleeding and clotted blood (41).

There is a paucity of evidence from the use of MDCT in the evaluation of patients with acute LGIB. Tew et al. (42) evaluated 13 patients with acute LBIB and MDCT identified bleeding points in 7/13, five of whom underwent mesenteric angiography and two were treated surgically. Of the six patients who had negative scans, none required further treatment of their LGIB. In the first prospective study, Yoon et al. (43) evaluated accuracy of MDCT in 26 patients with acute LGIB. The sensitivity and specificity of MDCT for detection of GI bleeding were 90.9% and 99% respectively, and the overall patient-based accuracy was 88.5%. Scheffel et al. (44) prospectively evaluated the ability of MDCT to localize LGIB. Although, MDCT demonstrated a potential source of bleeding in 83% of cases, an active extravasation of contrast reflecting a definite, active source of bleeding was found in only 67% of patients. In a study by Frattaroli et al. (45), 18 hemodynamically stable patients with acute severe LGIB (Hb<9 or transfusion of > 4 units of blood) underwent colonoscopy followed by unenhanced and triphasic (arterial, portal venous and late phase) 16-MDCT. The diagnosis was considered correct when the two investigations were concordant, or when it was confirmed at angiography, surgery or at post-mortem examination. Colonoscopy revealed the source of bleeding in 50% of patients, which were all confirmed by MDCT. In only one patient with angiodysplasia, despite being able to determine the location of bleeding, MDCT could not identify the exact source. In the remaining nine patients with negative colonoscopy, MDCT could determine the aetiology in seven – two with colonic lesions (caecal diverticulum and right colon cancer) and five with small bowel lesions (two jejunal and one ileal tumour, one ischemic ileal loop and one caecal varices). In one further patient MDCT was able to localize the bleeding to the right colon, contributing to 100% sensitivity of MDCT for localization of bleeding and 88.2% for determining the exact etiology of acute LGIB.

Although just emerging as the diagnostic option in the management of patients with acute LGIB, the advantage of arterial phase MDCT is that it can localize the source of bleeding rapidly and non-invasively and therefore guide further therapy including endoscopy, mesenteric angiography or surgery.

Mesenteric angiography

Mesenteric angiography can provide accurate localization of bleeding and allow therapy, now most commonly in the form of embolization. The examination is not definite unless extravasation of contrast into the lumen is demonstrated and for this to occur it is estimated that the arterial bleeding rate needs to be 1 ml/min (46). Hemostasis can be achieved either by intra-arterial infusion of vasopressin or embolization of a bleeding vessel. Initially, hemostasis was achieved using a systemic intra-arterial infusion of vasopressin. Although the use of vasopressin led to successful hemostasis in up to 91% of patients (47), it was very resource intensive as it required patients to be managed in intensive care units and was also associated with a 10–20% complication rate in the form of arrhythmias, hypertension and pulmonary edema as a result of systemic vasoconstriction. Further-more, rebleeding occurs in up to 50% (47) of patients after the cessation of infusion.

Intra-arterial embolization as a form of treatment for acute LGIB was first described by Bookstein et al. in 1974 (48), but the initial enthusiasm was dampened by the early reports of significant ischemic colonic complications (up to 33% (49)). Early studies used large 7F catheters that could only achieve embolization of the relatively large, proximal vessels. However, modern hydrophilic 4 and 5-F catheters allow subselective catheterization and can be used in combination with co-axial microcatheters to achieve distal embolization. The aim is to achieve embolization as close as possible to the bleeding source and this is often at the level of the vasa recta. Particular care is needed around watershed areas (caecum, splenic flexure and recto-sigmoid junction). Various embolization agents are used, including micro-coils (2–3 mm diameter), gelfoam and polyvinyl alcohol particles.

Zuckerman et al. reviewed 14 studies in 1998 and found diagnostic yield of angiography to be 61–72% if it is performed in patients who are actively bleeding (25). Much lower diagnostic yield is achieved in patients with a slower rate or intermittent bleeding. Recently Maleux et al. (50) retrospec-tively evaluated the outcome of subselective embolization in 122 patients who presented with acute LGIB and had a failed colonoscopic therapy. Only 35% of patients had angiographic signs of contrast exavasation and there-fore a definitely positive angiogram. Diverticular disease and angiodysplasia are the most common findings when angiography is positive, with the latter being characterized by slow emptying veins and vascular tufts (Fig. 9.6). Exact localization of the bleeding source allows an attempt at embolization and if unsuccessful, surgical management.

Technical success rate of superselective embolization in recent series is 73–100% (51–53). The commonest causes of technical failure are vaso-spasm, vascular distortion and prior surgery. A recent meta-analysis iden-tified 25 studies published from 1997 to 2002 that investigated the use of embolization in the treatment of acute LGIB (54). The clinical success rate, defined as immediate hemostasis, was 36–100% and the median rebleeding rate for LGIB at 30 days post-embolization was 14% (range 0–75%). The most commonly observed complications were ischaemia (range 0–33%) and the need for surgery (0–50%). The average number of days to

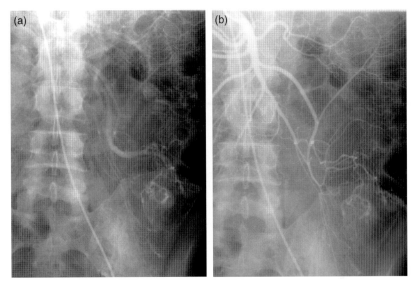

Figure 9.6 A & B: Mesenteric angiogram: angiodysplasia

rebleeding was $4.0 +/-6.1$, with three quarters of rebleeding occurring within 3.5 days of successful localization and embolization. Using random effects model, authors estimated that patients were more likely to rebleed if the cause of bleeding was arterio-venous malformation rather than diverticular disease.

Studies since 2000 have reported even higher success rates of subselective embolization (Table 9.2 lists the most recent ones). In one study in 2002 (55), immediate hemostasis was achieved with superselective embolization in 27/27 patients, five of whom were hemodynamically unstable with systolic BP <80 mmHg. Six patients rebled (22%) in the short term and five/six were treated surgically and one had repeat embolization.

Table 9.2 Outcome following embolization.

Author	Total no. of patients	No. of patients embolized	Hemostasis (%)	Rebleed (early) (%)	Surgery (%)	Ischemic complications needing surgery (%)	Mortality (%)
Koh et al. (108)	68	68	100	18 (9)	15	1.5	0
Tan et al. (109)	265	32	97	34 (22)	28	3	9
Ahmed et al. (53)	20	20	80	27	30	0	25
Maleux (50)	122	39	100	20 (6)	18	10	15

Two patients (7.2%) had post-embolization ischemia – one was treated surgically and one conservatively. Two out of 10 patients available for follow-up rebled – one at 12 and one at 18 months post initial embolization.

Superselective mesenteric angiography remains at the cornerstone of management of patients with acute LGIB, but it is an invasive and time-consuming procedure. In addition, due to its low sensitivity for slower and intermittent bleeding the majority of radiologists now advise the use of a MDCT scan in the arterial phase to demonstrate contrast exavasation and therefore localize the source of bleeding in an attempt to improve the diagnostic yield of mesenteric angiography.

Surgery in acute severe LGIB

Most patients with severe and even prolonged LGIB will not require surgery. Surgery, however, should be considered in patients where the bleeding source has been identified and other interventions have failed or in an unstable patient with unrelenting hemorrhage. Surgical intervention must be timely; must accurately resect the bleeding segment of bowel; must have acceptable mortality; must achieve acceptable morbidity with a low risk of rebleeding; and provide acceptable post-operative bowel function.

Current evidence for best practice in the surgical management of acute severe LGIB is based upon small cohort studies and case-control studies and any recommendation should be regarded as opinion-based rather than strongly evidence-based.

Patients requiring surgery will frequently have failed to respond to endoscopic and/or radiological therapeutic measures. This group will usually have the site of hemorrhage confirmed pre-operatively and the surgical approach will be dictated by the information prior to emergency surgery. However, in patients with acute severe unrelenting LGIB failing to respond to resuscitation, time will be wasted with attempts at endoscopic and radiological control when surgical arrest of hemorrhage is required. Extensive pre-operative work-up, especially when negative may unnecessarily delay surgical therapy in the actively hemorrhaging patient and adversely affect a patient's outcome.

Several surgical options are available; the extent of resection depending upon the extent of the underlying disease process or whether bleeding has been accurately identified prior to surgery. These include; emergency limited segmental resection for an identified bleeding source (directed segmental resection); emergency segmental resection for an unknown source (blind segmental resection); and emergency total colectomy for an unknown colonic bleeding source with or without ileo-rectal anastomosis. Where surgery is required, mortality of up to 40% has historically been recorded. Where a blood loss of greater than 10 units is recorded, mortality rises significantly [7% < 10 units vs 45% > 10 units] (56). Clinicians treating patients with acute continuing LGIB should consider emergency surgical intervention before a patient reaches this transfusion requirement and should seek emergency surgical intervention with > 6 units blood transfusion and continuing hemorrhage. It is crucial to operate before a patient reaches this large transfusion requirement, as delay is likely to adversely affect outcome.

The gold standard for surgical treatment of acute severe LGIB should be directed segmental colectomy based upon aggressive pre-operative identification of the bleeding site and patient stability. In practice, however, this is often difficult to achieve, with many patients undergoing emergency or urgent resection without the bleeding site being localized or patient instability negating the usefulness of endoscopic or radiological assessment. Renzulli et al. (57) successfully localized the site of bleeding in only 14% of patients overall with diverticular bleeding requiring surgery; precise colonoscopic localization was recorded in 5% and 29% of patients undergoing selective mesenteric angiography as a second line investigation. Evidence suggests that 18–25% of patients who require blood transfusion for LGIB will ultimately require surgical intervention (58). In patients with acute severe LGIB, we would advocate surgical intervention when hemodynamic instability persists despite aggressive resuscitation, blood transfusion requirements are > 6 units, severe recurrent bleeding occurs or localized bleeding fails to respond to endoscopic or radiological attempts at endostasis. These criteria are rather arbitrary and deciding upon whether a patient requires surgery in the absence of ongoing severe LGIB will be affected by the individual clinical situation and other factors such as associated comorbidities and patient age. It is clear that accurate localization in patients requiring surgical resection by modalities such as angiography has significantly lower morbidity than in historic controls without angiographic localization [8.6% vs 37%]. Rebleeding rates of 14% after directed segmental resection exist compared with 42% in patients undergoing "blind" or "best-guess" segmental resection with a negative angiographic result (59). Segmental resection based solely upon radionuclide scanning is fraught with significant rebleeding rates and increased morbidity. Blind segmental resections were previously advocated on the basis of the likely bleeding source and diagnosis. Left-sided diverticulosis was once thought to be the source of most lower GI bleeding prompting left-sided colonic resection before right-sided diverticula and right-sided angiodysplasia were recognized as additional significant sources. Such an approach resulted in high rebleeding rates [30%] and high mortality [10–40%]. Rebleeding rates of 0% have been reported after subtotal colectomy.

Subtotal colectomy was first performed for LGIB by Cate in 1953 (60). Historically, the use of subtotal colectomy [STC], in the absence of adequate pre-operative localization, lead to high mortality from rebleeding from missed lesions and fell into disrepute for the treatment of LGIB owing to the assumption that it carried a higher mortality and a perception that disabling post-operative stool frequency and incontinence in the elderly would result. Even recent reviews on the topic of LGIB management report that subtotal colectomy should be used as a "last resort" (61). However, it has been suggested that the reason that STC has historically poor outcomes is owing to its use as "the last resort" where earlier and expeditious use in the setting of unlocalized uncontrolled hemorrhage has similar mortality to "best-guess" segmental resection with significantly reduced rebleeding rates [18% vs 4%] (62) and maintains acceptable bowel function post-operatively (57, 63), particularly if 10 cm of intra-abdominal rectum is retained above the peritoneal reflection (64, 65). The decision to perform an anastomosis will be dictated by the condition of the patient but in the study by Bender et al. (56) where > 10 units of blood were transfused the ileo-rectal anastomotic leak rate and intra-abdominal abscess formation was significantly elevated and in this situation avoiding an anastomosis and fashioning an end ileostomy would be regarded as prudent. Delayed re-anastomosis can be considered after the patient recovers.

Operative technique

Full midline laparotomy is required. There is no role currently for a laparoscopic resection in an unstable patient with LGIB.

At laparotomy, even in the presence of a pre-operatively confirmed source of blood loss, full assessment of the viscera is required. The stomach, duodenum, small intestine then colon are inspected. The areas of the GI tract filled with blood are confirmed and may guide assessment of the origin of bleeding. If only the colon is found to be filled with blood, this narrows the extent of assessment.

Once the abdomen has been assessed then directed segmental resection can be performed if the likely bleeding source is known. Where the small intestine is filled with blood then intra-operative enteroscopy will need to be employed if no obvious source is found at laparotomy. This can be performed via the transoral route or if necessary via a gastrotomy or enterotomy. Intra-operative colonoscopy has also been used with good effect and has been employed after intra-operative colonic lavage (66, 67). Intra-operative clamping of the bowel has a theoretical basis in identifying the location of bleeding but has generally been found to be ineffective in aiding localization.

If no source is identifiable and the bleeding appears to arise from the colon then subtotal colectomy should be performed. If a patient is stable without excessive blood loss [> 10 units] then ileo-rectal or ileo-sigmoid anastomosis may be fashioned; however, if the blood loss is excessive then end ileostomy should be favored.

Acute self-limiting/intermittent hemorrhage

Any of the causes of LGIB can present as self-terminating events.

There is little evidence on the management of acute, severe, self-limiting hemorrhage and at best it can be inferred from the literature concerning acute severe LGIB. In the presence of documented melena and history of NSAIDs use, OGD should be performed first to exclude an upper GI source. Proctoscopy to assess for anorectal cause of bleeding should be performed prior to elective colonoscopy, followed by full bowel preparation. If OGD, proctoscopy and colonoscopy do not reveal the source of bleeding, investigation of the small bowel should be undertaken. MDCT will reveal obvious blood clot or neoplasia as well as the overall morphology of the bowel. Unless there is active arterial bleeding at a rate 0.5–1.0 ml/min mesenteric angiography is unlikely to determine the location of the bleed and provocation angiography with vasodilators, anticoagulants or thrombolytics should be considered (see Chapter 11). An alternative approach is to arrange for an immediate access for endoscopic examination (enteroscopy or colonoscopy) should bleeding recur.

Chronic/Intermittent bleeding

Occult
Patients with occult GI bleeding present with a positive fecal occult blood test FOBT) or iron deficiency anemia. Rockey et al. (68) performed OGD and colonoscopy in 248 FOBT positive patients with mean age 61 (range 40–89) (patients with active bleeding and iron deficiency anemia were excluded). Lesions likely to have been responsible for bleeding were detected in 119 patients (48%) – in 45% of those they were colonic in origin. The most common colonic lesions were adenomas >1 cm (29%), cancer (13%), colitis (5%) and angiodysplasia (5%). In 100 patients with iron-deficiency anemia, OGD and colonoscopy reveled a potential bleeding source in 62%, with lesions located in colon in 25%, nearly half of which were cancers (69). However, addition of positive FOBT and lower GI symptoms lead to a positive predictive value of 86% for detecting lesions in the LGI tract. Therefore, patients with iron deficiency anemia and change in bowel habit or positive FOBT should have a colonoscopy first, followed by an OGD as 1% of patients had bleeding lesions in both upper and lower GI tract. Patients in whom a cause for bleeding is not found following an OGD, colonoscopy and some form of small bowel imaging (MDCT/small bowel enteroclysis/capsule endoscopy and enteroscopy), are deemed to have obscure GI bleeding. The investigation and management of those patients is covered in Chapter 11.

Overt

Anorectal causes are the commonest causes of chronic, intermittent, bright red rectal bleeding. These include:
- hemorrhoids
- anal fissures
- IBD (predominantly UC)
- radiation proctopathy
- solitary rectal ulcer syndrome
- neoplasia (adenomas/cancers)

Proctoscopy and flexible sigmoidoscopy should be performed in younger patients; in those >50 years or with alarm symptoms (weight loss, change in bowel habit) a full colonoscopy should be performed to exclude proximal colonic lesions.

Specific conditions

Diverticulosis

The most common cause of life-threatening LGI hemorrhage is a diverticular bleed.

Forty percent of LGIB is diverticular in origin, yet bleeding complicates less than 5% of all cases of diverticulosis (70). Diverticulosis is common in the developed world and increases with age – the prevalence of diverticulosis is < 10% in adults under 40 and increases in up to 60% in those aged 80. Despite the fact that 90% of diverticula are in the left colon, at least 60% of bleeding colonic diverticula documented at angiography are proximal to splenic flexure (71). The exact etiology of diverticular bleeding is not clear. Although it is thought to be a result of an acute rupture of the vasa recta close to the neck of a diverticulum, it is unclear what precipitates the rupture. In a case-control study of 44 patients with diverticular bleed and 88 controls, multivariate analysis showed that NSAIDs (OR 15.6, 95% CI 1.1–214), hypertension (OR 6.6, 95% CI 2.1–20.5) and aspirin ± another anticoagulant (OR 3, 95% CI 1.04–8.6) were significant risk factors for diverticular bleeding (72). In a prospective cohort study by Strate et al., body mass index, waist circumference and waist-to-hip ratio were found to significantly increase the risk of diverticular bleeding (73). In a study of 78 patients who were admitted 106 times for LGIB (74), bleeding stopped spontaneously in 75% of episodes and 99% of patients required < 4 units of blood transfusion per day. On the other hand, 60% of patients who required more than 4 units of blood per day came to emergency surgery. Thirty-eight percent of patients who were discharged from hospital without surgical intervention had recurrence of bleeding. Longstreth et al. (4) observed similar recurrence rates in 88 patients who had no definite therapy for the initial bleed (9% at one year, 10% at two years, 90% at three years and 25% at four years). Endoscopic treatment of diverticular bleeding aims to achieve hemostasis and therefore reduce blood transfusion requirements, reduce rebleeding and avoid surgery.

There are a number of studies supporting the role of urgent (within 12–24 hrs) colonoscopy for diverticular bleed. Although diverticulosis is thought to account for 40% of LGIB, when the definite stigmata of recent bleeding are used for a definitive diagnosis, that figure drops to 15–20% (11, 75). Jensen et al. (11) prospectively studied acute LGIB and compared patients with definite stigmata of bleeding who were treated endoscopically by a combination of adrenaline injection and bipolar coagulation (n = 10) with historical controls who were not treated endoscopically (n = 17). None of the endoscopically treated patients had recurrent bleeding or needed surgery after 30 months compared to controls, 52% of whom rebled and 35% required surgery. Bloomfeld et al. (76) used similar methods of endoscopic hemostasis, with a combination of adrenaline and thermal therapy, in 13 patients with stigmata of recent diverticular bleed and although there were no immediate complications of endoscopic therapy, 38% of patients had early rebleeding (within 30 days) and 80% of those required surgical management. A further 23% of patients were admitted for late rebleeding. In a recent study, 58% of patients with active bleeding and stigmata had endoscopic therapy, which was found to be safe and effective. This study also assessed the timing of colonoscopy and found no association between the timing of colonoscopy and definite diagnosis of diverticular bleeding. In contrast, another study (12) showed that urgent colonoscopy identified a definite source of bleeding more often than angiography and expectant colonoscopy, but had no significant effect on patient outcomes, including mortality, hospital stay, rate of rebleeding or requirement for surgery.

Endoscopic treatment modalities include adrenaline injection, thermal therapy and more recently clips. A quantity of 1–2 ml of adrenaline 1:10,000 should be injected quadrantically or close to the mouth of the diverticulum to achieve tamponade (11). If a clot is present, adrenaline should again be injected in 4 quadrants before attempting to remove the clot, either by copious washes or using a cold snare. If a vessel is exposed it should be coagulated (bipolar coagulation) or clipped. Using bipolar coagulation (Gold probe, Microvasive) with 10–15 W of power, short 1–2 s pulses and gentle pressure, should be safe and effective. The evidence for the use of Endoclips in the treatment of diverticular bleeding comes from a few case reports (77–79) and small case series (80). Eleven patients with acute diverticular hemorrhage and active bleeding or non-bleeding visible vessel were treated with endoclips and followed up for median 15 months (range 1–22 months). In all cases, hemostasis was achieved at endoscopy and no patients had recurrent bleeding within three days or necessitated further blood transfusion or surgery. Late bleeding occurred in two patients (18%) at five and six months respectively. An important practical point is to tattoo the site of diverticulum bleeding, even if it has been successfully stopped. This allows recognition at laparotomy should torrential bleeding occur.

In the event of acute severe hemorrhage that cannot be controlled endoscopically, MDCT is performed to attempt to localize the site of hemorrhage before proceeding to mesenteric angiography or surgery. Recently a case report described successful embolization for the treatment of a bleeding diverticulum, using newly available equipment that allows CT and angiography simultaneously (81). A meta-analysis of six published studies demonstrated that embolization for diverticular bleeding is more effective than for other pathologies (54).

Angiodysplasia (vascular ectasia)

Angiodysplasia is defined by the presence of ectasia of normal pre-existing intestinal submucosal veins and overlying mucosal capillaries. They are an acquired condition that is associated with aging, although exact aetiology is not known. They are common in the right colon, but have been described in the whole GI tract and can present with acute, chronic or occult bleeding. Colonoscopy studies have identified angiodysplasia in 0.9–6.2% of patients having the procedure performed for various indications, with detection rates of 0.2–2.9% in asymptomatic patients (82–84) and 2.6–6.2% of patients evaluated for anemia, FOBT or LGIB. Although, angiodysplasias were thought to account for up to 30% of acute LGIB, they may not be the source of bleeding in some patients. When colonoscopy was performed for other indications, the proportion of bleeding angiodysplasias ranged from 20% to 90% (82, 83, 85). Foutch et al. (86) followed eight patients who were found to have an incidental finding of angiodysplasia at colonoscopy over a period of three years. Mean size of lesions was 4 mm and 62% were located in proximal colon. All patients maintained their hemoglobin and none bled during follow up. Similarly Richter et al. (87) reported on 101 patients with colonic angiodysplasias. Fifteen asymptomatic patients were followed for a mean 23 months (up to 68) and none experienced a bleeding episode. However, 31 patients with anemia or overt bleeding and managed by blood transfusions alone had a rebleeding rate of 26% at one year and 46% at three years. One study (88) assessed bleeding rates in five patients with colonic and small bowel angiodysplasia treated conservatively. Over the period of time, there was 91% decrease in transfused units of blood per month, suggesting bleeding from angiodysplasia may diminish spontaneously over time. Angiodysplasia is associated with chronic renal failure, von

Willebrands' disease, aortic stenosis, cirrhosis and pulmonary disease, although the strength of association has been questioned (89). Colonoscopy is probably the most sensitive test for detection of angiodysplasia although comparative sensitivities are not known (90). At colonoscopy, they appear as flat, small 4–10 mm lesions with a central feeding vessel or surrounding pale mucosal halo (86) but may be masked in patients who are severely anaemic or volume depleted or given opiate analgesia, which all lead to a reduction in mucosal blood flow. Administration of an opiate antagonist was reported to increase both the number and size of angiodysplasias visualized at colonoscopy (91). CT angiography has been reported as relatively sensitive and specific tool for diagnosis of angiodysplasias. In 28 patients who presented with LGIB, 18 were found to have angiodysplasia using colonoscopy and angiography and 14 using CT angiogram. This resulted in 70% sensitivity and 100% specificity of the CT angiogram for detection of angiodysplasias (92). Mesenteric angiography with embolization should be the next step if extravasation of contrast is demonstrated on CT although as the bleeding from angiodysplasia is typically intermittent, this may not be seen and provocation angiography should be considered. At angiography, angiodysplasia is characterized by abnormal cluster of small arteries seen during arterial phase of the scan, early opacification and delayed emptying of the veins (93). If bleeding angiodysplasias are seen at colonoscopy, they should be treated with APC, with extra care taken in the right colon. Out of 15 patients who presented with LGIB secondary to angiodysplasia, 13 were treated successfully by fulguration, with no incidence of rebleeding over 1–7 year follow-up (94).

Colitis (IBD/ischemic)

Although IBD, especially UC, often present with bloody diarrhea, acute massive LGIB is rare. In one study, massive hemorrhage accounted for only 0.1% of admissions for UC and 1.2% for Crohn's disease. Most of the patients were managed medically, but 39% came to surgery for ongoing or recurrent bleeding (95). Belaiche et al. (96) analysed 34 patients with Crohn's disease who presented with acute LGIB and required at least 2 units of blood in 24 hours and found that colonic disease was more likely to present with acute hemorrhage than isolated small bowel disease and that the bleeding lesion was most frequently an ulcer in the left colon. Only 21% of patients needed surgical treatment (one third had a colectomy) and bleeding recurred in just over a third of patients during follow up (mean 3 years, range 4 days to 8 years). Acute GI bleeding in IBD should be investigated and managed in the same way as any other cause of acute GI bleeding.

If risk factors for ischemic colitis are present and it is confirmed at colonoscopy then resection is only considered in the presence of increasing tenderness or patient deterioration. Most cases will settle with active observation.

Anorectal conditions

Hemorrhoids

Hemorrhoids are a cause of minor to moderate chronic rectal bleeding. Rarely is emergency surgery required for bleeding hemorrhoids. The exact incidence of this common condition is difficult to estimate as many people are reluctant to seek medical advice for various personal, cultural, and socioeconomic reasons, but epidemiological studies report a prevalence varying from 4.4% in adults in the United States to over 30% in general practice in London (97, 98). Though rare, significant hemorrhage has been reported and therefore it is mandatory to exclude an obvious source by anoscopy prior to further investigation.

Treatment is dependent upon the severity of symptoms and the whether there is hemorrhoidal prolapse. Options include observation, rubber band ligation, injection sclerotherapy, infrared coagulation, hemorrhoidal ligation, hemorrhoidectomy and stapled anopexy.

Rubber band ligation is the best outpatient treatment for hemorrhoids with up to 80% of patients being satisfied with the short-term outcome. Surgery is considered in patients with large symptomatic hemorrhoids that do not respond to outpatient treatment. These aspects of hemorrhoidal disease are beyond the scope of this chapter.

Anal fissure

Anal fissures will usually cause minimal bleeding and patients will mainly complain of significant proctalgia on defecation. They may develop a fear of defecation owing to the pain. It is diagnosed clinically with evidence of the fissure edge present at the distal anal canal. Digital rectal examination is unlikely to add more information once a fissure is identified and is likely to cause significant discomfort. Proctoscopy will cause unnecessary discomfort.

Anal fissures may be acute or chronic [> 6 weeks duration + / − features of chronicity]. The location of the fissure provides an indication to their likely etiology. Anterior and posterior fissures are predominantly classical high- pressure fissures. Anterior fissures have been identified in the immediate postpartum period and have been supposed to have a low-pressure etiology, generated by shear stress upon the anal canal during delivery. A greater number of anterior fissures have underlying sphincter injuries and surgical treatment such as sphincterotomy should be more cautious in this group (99). Lateral fissures are more concerning and can be associated with Crohn's disease, UC, HIV, malignancy, syphilis, and tuberculosis.

Acute fissures will usually respond to conservative measures with fiber supplements. The modern options for treatment of chronic fissure include lateral internal sphincterotomy [open or closed], "chemical sphincterotomy" with agents such as topical glyceryl trinitrate [GTN], diltiazem and Botox injections.

Radiation proctopathy

Radiation proctopathy or proctitis can cause chronic LGIB and is seen frequently at endoscopy in patients who have undergone radiation therapy to the pelvic organs in the treatment of pelvic malignancies (Fig. 9.7). Pelvic irradiation, either alone or in combination with other treatment modalities such as surgery, chemotherapy and hormonal therapy, is commonly used in the curative management of gynaecological and urological malignant diseases. Over 75% of patients receiving pelvic radiotherapy develop acute anorectal symptoms, and up to 20% will develop persistent radiation-induced proctopathy and this is likely to be an underestimate. Anorectal sequelae predominate in the increasing numbers of patients now being treated by external beam radiotherapy for prostate cancer. Five years after radiotherapy for early prostate carcinoma, 48%, 23% and 25% of the patients reported urgency of defaecation, mucous incontinence and rectal bleeding, respectively. Prospective, longitudinal data based on quantitative endoscopic and anorectal manometric evaluation indicate that abnormalities are observed in up to 68% of patients 2–5 years after radiotherapy for prostate cancer.

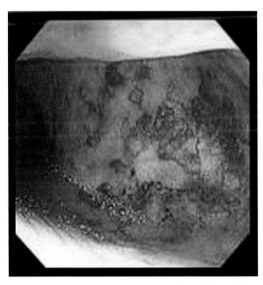

Figure 9.7 Radiation proctopathy

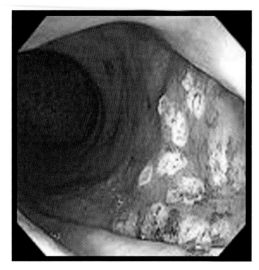

Figure 9.8 Radiation proctopathy after application of APC

A variety of therapeutic options have been investigated including pharmacotherapy (oral and rectal 5-ASA products, steroids, sucralfate), hyperbaric oxygen, endoscopic therapy for rectal bleeding, and surgery.

Endoscopic therapy with argon plasma coagulation therapy (100) is generally accepted as the most suitable treatment (Fig. 9.8) with the local application of formalin in the event of failure. Should this fail, topical formalin therapy has been found to be effective (101). The technique reduces rectal bleeding in 80–90% of cases. Topical formalin therapy depends on direct application of a 4% concentration of the chemical soaked in gauze to the haemorrhagic areas under direct vision using a rigid sigmoidoscope under general anaesthesia. Outpatient 2% retention enemas and 10% direct application with cotton tip applicator have also been used though these studies have been small with shorter follow-up than the 4% formalin preparation though the approach avoids general anesthesia and bowel preparation. Thrombosis of the neovasculature and coagulation necrosis of the superficial mucosa ensues, with a complete response rate of 78%. While topical formalin appears to be slightly less effective than argon plasma coagulation therapy, formalin application alone or a combination of the two treatments has been advocated for severe cases of hemorrhagic radiation proctitis. Low-dose thalidomide has been employed with some success in the treatment of haemorrhagic radiation proctitis as it inhibits angiogenesis.

Hyperbaric oxygen has been used on the basis that it may attend to the microvascular changes that occur in the bowel wall following radiotherapy.

Hyperbaric oxygen treatment has been submitted to randomised study identifying a success rate of 53% (102).

Anastomotic bleeding

Rectal bleeding following stapled colorectal anastomosis is common but usually self-limited. Continuous hemorrhage is rare, and when it occurs, often requires further treatment. It is a rare event for severe LGIB from the staple line of an intestinal anastomosis to require intervention either endoscopic or surgical. Endostasis should the first line of therapy in the event of staple-line LGIB (103). Endoclips, adrenalin injection and cautery have been used effectively. Other options include: rectal packing, angiographic identification of the bleeding site with vasopressin infusion or embolization, and endoscopic eletrocoagulation.

Malik et al. (104) identified six patients from a prospective series of 777 patients (0.8%) that had a stapled anastomosis that suffered a staple-line hemorrhage that necessitated intervention with 50% controlled by endostasis with good patient outcomes thereafter. Linn et al. (105) identified a 4% staple-line hemorrhage rate and noted the rate to be increased if the inferior mesenteric artery was preserved. All patients in this group responded to endostasis.

Post-polypectomy bleeding

Bleeding is the commonest serious colonoscopic complication. Generally, simple cold biopsy with standard pinch biopsy forceps is safe even in patients on anticoagulation with rates of 0–0.04% reported. As expected rates of bleeding after polypectomy are higher (0–4% in studies performed in the last decade). Patients undergoing polypectomy or dilatation should have anticoagulation withdrawn prior to colonoscopy to reduce the risk of bleeding. ASGE recommends that aspirin does not need to be stopped prior to routine polypectomy. Patients on clopidogrel are particularly at

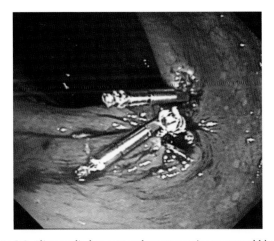

Figure 9.9 Clips applied to post-polypectomy site to control bleeding

risk of bleeding and ideally this drug should be stopped for 10 days prior to therapeutic intervention bearing in mind the risk of in-stent thrombosis in patients with recent insertion of drug-eluting coronary stents.

Bleeding after therapy can be immediate or delayed for up to 3 weeks after colonoscopy. One study found that old age, cardiovascular and chronic renal disease, anticoagulant use, polyp size >1 cm, pedunculated or laterally spreading tumours, use of cutting rather than blended or coagulation current and poor bowel preparation were all risk factors for immediate post-polypectomy bleeding (106).

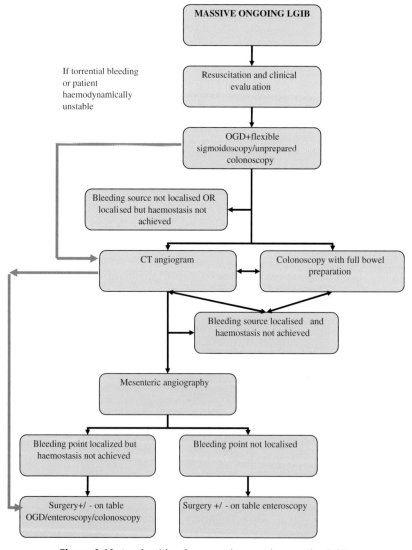

Figure 9.10 An algorithm for managing massive ongoing LGIB

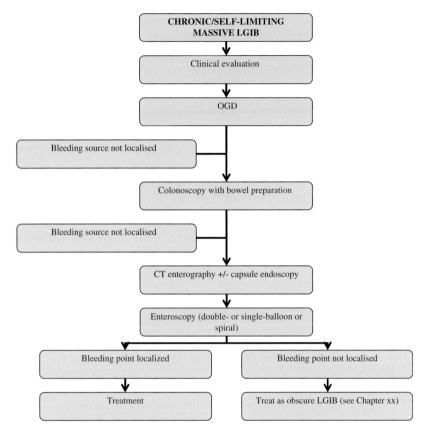

Figure 9.11 An algorithm for managing chronic/intermittent LGIB

Delayed bleeding presents with hemotochesia, decrease in hemoglobin and subsequent hemodynamic instability. Risk factors associated with delayed bleeding include increasing polyp size and resumption of anticoagulation following polypectomy (107). The majority of patients stop bleeding spontaneously with conservative management, which includes correction of any clotting abnormality and blood transfusion. Repeat colonoscopy may be necessary to identify the bleeding point and apply therapy. Endoclips (Fig. 9.9), endo-loops, adrenaline injection and thermal modalities have all been used successfully either as single modalities or in combination. If endoscopic therapy fails angiography and segmental embolization may be attempted prior to segmental colonic resection.

Conclusion

Although minor rectal bleeding is common, severe bleeding associated with hemodynamic compromise is rare. Majority of acute LGIB episodes will stop spontaneously and for those patients in whom bleeding is severe there are a number of endoscopic and radiological techniques that could be used to attempt to achieve hemostasis. Surgery is reserved for patients in whom those techniques have failed to control the bleeding or who present with unrelenting torrential hemorrhage (Fig. 9.10 and Fig. 9.11).

References

1. Jones R, Lydeard S. Irritable bowel syndrome in the general population. BMJ 1992; 304(6819):87–90.
2. Fijten GH, Muris JW, Starmans R, Knottnerus JA, Blijham GH, Krebber TF. The incidence and outcome of rectal bleeding in general practice. Fam Pract 1993; 10(3):283–7.
3. Gostout CJ, Wang KK, Ahlquist DA, Clain JE, Hughes RW, Larson MV, et al. Acute gastrointestinal bleeding. Experience of a specialized management team. J Clin Gastroenterol 1992;14(3):260–7.
4. Longstreth GF. Epidemiology and outcome of patients hospitalized with acute lower gastrointestinal hemorrhage: a population-based study. Am J Gastroenterol 1997; 92(3):419–24.
5. Lanas A, Garcia-Rodriguez LA, Polo-Tomas M, Ponce M, Alonso-Abreu I, Perez-Aisa MA, et al. Time trends and impact of upper and lower gastrointestinal bleeding and perforation in clinical practice. Am J Gastroenterol 2009;104(7):1633–41.
6. Brackman MR, Gushchin VV, Smith L, Demory M, Kirkpatrick JR, Stahl T. Acute lower gastroenteric bleeding retrospective analysis (the ALGEBRA study): an analysis of the triage, management and outcomes of patients with acute lower gastrointestinal bleeding. Am Surg 2003;69(2):145–9.
7. Jensen DM, Machiado GA. Diagnosis and treatment os severe haematochezia. The role of urgent colonoscopy after purge. Gastroenterology 1988;95: 1569–74.
8. Cairns S, Scholefield JH. Guidelines for colorectal cancer screening in high risk groups. Gut 2002;51 Suppl 5:V1–2.
9. Caos A, Benner KG, Manier J, McCarthy DM, Blessing LD, Katon RM, et al. Colonoscopy after Golytely preparation in acute rectal bleeding. J Clin Gastroenterol 1986;8(1):46–9.
10. Strate LL, Syngal S. Timing of colonoscopy: impact on length of hospital stay in patients with acute lower intestinal bleeding. Am J Gastroenterol 2003;98 (2):317–22.
11. Jensen DM, Machicado GA, Jutabha R, Kovacs TO. Urgent colonoscopy for the diagnosis and treatment of severe diverticular hemorrhage. N Engl J Med 2000 Jan 13; 342(2):78–82.
12. Green BT, Rockey DC, Portwood G, Tarnasky PR, Guarisco S, Branch MS, et al. Urgent colonoscopy for evaluation and management of acute lower gastrointestinal hemorrhage: a randomized controlled trial. Am J Gastroenterol 2005;100 (11):2395–2402.
13. Angtuaco TL, Reddy SK, Drapkin S, Harrell LE, Howden CW. The utility of urgent colonoscopy in the evaluation of acute lower gastrointestinal tract bleeding: a 2-year experience from a single center. Am J Gastroenterol 2001;96(6):1782–1785.
14. Schmulewitz N, Fisher DA, Rockey DC. Early colonoscopy for acute lower GI bleeding predicts shorter hospital stay: a retrospective study of experience in a single center. Gastrointest Endosc 2003;58(6):841–6.

15. Ohyama T, Sakurai Y, Ito M, Daito K, Sezai S, Sato Y. Analysis of urgent colonoscopy for lower gastrointestinal tract bleeding. Digestion 2000;61(3):189–92.

16. Peura DA, Lanza FL, Gostout CJ, Foutch PG. The American College of Gastroenterology Bleeding Registry: preliminary findings. Am J Gastroenterol 1997; 92(6):924–8.

17. Strate LL, Ayanian JZ, Kotler G, Syngal S. Risk factors for mortality in lower intestinal bleeding. Clin Gastroenterol Hepatol 2008;6(9).

18. Comay D, Marshall JK. Resource utilization for acute lower gastrointestinal hemorrhage: the Ontario GI bleed study. Can J Gastroenterol 2002;16(10):677–82.

19. Kollef MH, O'Brien JD, Zuckerman GR, Shannon W. BLEED: a classification tool to predict outcomes in patients with acute upper and lower gastrointestinal hemorrhage. Crit Care Med 1997l;25(7):1125–1132.

20. Strate LL, Orav EJ, Syngal S. Early predictors of severity in acute lower intestinal tract bleeding. Arch Intern Med 2003;163(7):838–43.

21. Strate LL, Saltzman JR, Ookubo R, Mutinga ML, Syngal S. Validation of a clinical prediction rule for severe acute lower intestinal bleeding. Am J Gastroenterol 2005;100(8):1821–1827.

22. Das A, Ben-Menachem T, Cooper GS, Chak A, Sivak MV, Jr., Gonet JA, et al. Prediction of outcome in acute lower-gastrointestinal haemorrhage based on an artificial neural network: internal and external validation of a predictive model. Lancet 2003;362(9392):1261–1266.

23. Zuckerman GR, Trellis DR, Sherman TM, Clouse RE. An objective measure of stool colour for differentiation upper from lower gastrintestinal bleeding. Dig Dis Sci 1995; 40.

24. Chan FK, Lanas A, Scheiman J, Berger MF, Nguyen H, Goldstein JL. Celecoxib versus omeprazole and diclofenac in patients with osteoarthritis and rheumatoid arthritis (CONDOR): a randomised trial. Lancet. [Randomized Controlled Trial Research Support, Non-U.S. Gov't]. 2010;376(9736):173–9.

25. Zuckerman GR, Prakash C. Acute lower intestinal bleeding: part I: clinical presentation and diagnosis. Gastrointest Endosc 1998;48(6):606–17.

26. Cheung PS, Wong SK, Boey J, Lai CK. Frank rectal bleeding: a prospective study of causes in patients over the age of 40. Postgrad Med J 1988;64.

27. Davila RE, Rajan E, Adler DG, Egan J, Hirota WK, Leighton JA, et al. ASGE Guideline: the role of endoscopy in the patient with lower-GI bleeding. Gastrointest Endosc 2005;62(5):656–60.

28. Robert JR, Sachar DB, Greenstein AJ. Severe gastrointestinal hemorrhage in Crohn's disease. Ann Surg 1991;213(3):207–11.

29. Hong GS, Wong CY, Nambiar R. Massive lower gastrointestinal haemorrhage from a splenic artery pseudoaneurysm. Br J Surg 1992;79(2):174.

30. Santos JC, Jr., Feres O, Rocha JJ, Aracava MM. Massive lower gastrointestinal hemorrhage caused by pseudocyst of the pancreas ruptured into the colon. Report of two cases. Dis Colon Rectum 1992;35(1):75–7.

31. Pickens CA, Tedesco FJ. Colonic varices. Unusual cause of rectal bleeding. Am J Gastroenterol 1980;73(1):73–4.

32. Chaudhry V, Hyser MJ, Gracias VH, Gau FC. Colonoscopy: the initial test for acute lower gastrointestinal bleeding. Am Surg 1998 Aug; 64(8):723–8.

33. Billingham RP. The conundrum of lower gastrointestinal bleeding. Surg Clin North Am 1997;77

34. Lipper B, Simon D, Cerrone F. Pulmonary aspiration during emergency endoscopy in patients with upper gastrointestinal haemorhage. Crit Care Med 1991;19: 330–3.

35. Griffin SM, Chung SC, Leung JW, Li AC. Effect of intranasal oxygen on hypoxia and tachycardia during endoscopic cholangiopancreaography. BMJ 1990;300: 83–4.

36. Bell GD, Bown s, Morden A, et al. Prevention of hypoxaemia during upper gastro-intestinal endoscopy by means of oxygen via nasal cannulae. Lancet 1987;1: 1022–1024.

37. Steer ML, Silen W. Diagnostic procedures in gastrointestinal hemorrhage. N Engl J Med 1983;309(11):646–50.

38. Al Qahtani AR, Satin R, Stern J, Gordon PH. Investigative modalities for massive lower gastrointestinal bleeding. World J Surg 2002 May; 26(5):620–5.

39. Anastassiades CP, Baron TH, Wong Kee Song LM. Endoscopic clipping for the management of gastrointestinal bleeding. Nat Clin Pract Gastroenterol Hepatol 2008;5(10):559–68.

40. Yoon W, Jeong YY, Kim JK. Acute gastrointestinal bleeding: contrast-enhanced MDCT. Abdom Imaging 2006;31(1):1–8.

41. Willmann JK, Roos JE, Platz A, Pfammatter T, Hilfiker PR, Marincek B, et al. Multidetector CT: detection of active hemorrhage in patients with blunt abdominal trauma. AJR Am J Roentgenol 2002;179(2):437–44.

42. Tew K, Davies RP, Jadun CK, Kew J. MDCT of acute lower gastrointestinal bleeding. AJR Am J Roentgenol 2004;182(2):427–30.

43. Yoon W, Jeong YY, Shin SS, Lim HS, Song SG, Jang NG, et al. Acute massive gastrointestinal bleeding: detection and localization with arterial phase multi-detector row helical CT. Radiology 2006;239(1):160–7.

44. Scheffel H, Pfammatter T, Wildi S, Bauerfeind P, Marincek B, Alkadhi H. Acute gastrointestinal bleeding: detection of source and etiology with multi-detector-row CT. Eur Radiol 2007;17(6):1555–1565.

45. Frattaroli FM, Casciani E, Spoletini D, Polettini E, Nunziale A, Bertini L, et al. Prospective Study Comparing Multi-Detector Row CT and Endoscopy in Acute Gastrointestinal Bleeding. World J Surg 2009 Aug. 5

46. Zuckerman DA, Bocchini TP, Birnbaum EH. Massive hemorrhage in the lower gastrointestinal tract in adults: diagnostic imaging and intervention. AJR Am J Roentgenol 1993;161(4):703–11.

47. Browder W, Cerise EJ, Litwin MS. Impact of emergency angiography in massive lower gastrointestinal bleeding. Ann Surg 1986 Nov; 204(5):530–6.

48. Bookstein JJ, Chlosta EM, Foley D, Walter JF. Transcatheter hemostasis of gastro-intestinal bleeding using modified autogenous clot. Radiology 1974;113(2):277–85.

49. Guy GE, Shetty PC, Sharma RP, Burke MW, Burke TH. Acute lower gastrointestinal hemorrhage: treatment by superselective embolization with polyvinyl alcohol par-ticles. AJR Am J Roentgenol 1992;159(3):521–6.

50. Maleux G, Roeflaer F, Heye S, Vandersmissen J, Vliegen AS, Demedts I, et al. Long-term outcome of transcatheter embolotherapy for acute lower gastrointestinal hemorrhage. Am J Gastroenterol 2009;104(8):2042–2046.

51. Bandi R, Shetty PC, Sharma RP, Burke TH, Burke MW, Kastan D. Superselective arterial embolization for the treatment of lower gastrointestinal hemorrhage. J Vasc Interv Radiol 2001;12(12):1399–405.

52. Funaki B, Kostelic JK, Lorenz J, Ha TV, Yip DL, Rosenblum JD, et al. Superselective microcoil embolization of colonic hemorrhage. AJR Am J Roentgenol 2001;177(4): 829–36.

53. Ahmed TM, Cowley JB, Robinson G, Hartley JE, Nicholson AA, Lim M, et al. Long term follow up of transcatheter coil embolotherapy for major colonic haemorrhage. Colorectal Dis 2010;12(10):1013–1037.

54. Khanna A, Ognibene SJ, Koniaris LG. Embolization as first-line therapy for diverticulosis-related massive lower gastrointestinal bleeding: evidence from a meta-analysis. J Gastrointest Surg 2005;9(3):343–52.

55. DeBarros J, Rosas L, Cohen J, Vignati P, Sardella W, Hallisey M. The changing paradigm for the treatment of colonic hemorrhage: superselective angiographic embolization. Dis Colon Rectum 2002;45(6):802–8.

56. Bender JS, Wiencek RG, Bouwman DL. Morbidity and mortality following total abdominal colectomy for massive lower gastrointestinal bleeding. Am Surg 1991; 57(8):536–40; discussion 40.

57. Renzulli P, Maurer CA, Netzer P, Dinkel HP, Buchler MW. Subtotal colectomy with primary ileorectostomy is effective for unlocalized, diverticular hemorrhage. Langenbecks Arch Surg 2002;387(2):67–71.

58. Farrell JJ, Friedman LS. Review article: the management of lower gastrointestinal bleeding. Aliment Pharmacol Ther 2005;21(11):1281–1298.

59. Parkes BM, Obeid FN, Sorensen VJ, Horst HM, Fath JJ. The management of massive lower gastrointestinal bleeding. Am Surg 1993;59(10):676–8.

60. Cate WR, Jr., Colectomy in the treatment of massive melena secondary to diverticulosis. Ann Surg 1953;137(4):558–60.

61. Rockey DC. Lower gastrointestinal bleeding. Gastroenterology 2006 Jan; 130 (1):165–71.

62. Farner R, Lichliter W, Kuhn J, Fisher T. Total colectomy versus limited colonic resection for acute lower gastrointestinal bleeding. Am J Surg 1999;178(6):587–91.

63. Baker R, Senagore A. Abdominal colectomy offers safe management for massive lower GI bleed. Am Surg 1994;60(8):578–81; discussion 82.

64. Aranha GV, Walsh RM, Jacobs HK, Freeark RJ, Harford FJ, Keshavarzian A, et al. Factors influencing bowel function following total abdominal colectomy. Dis Colon Rectum 1996 Dec; 39(12):1418–1422.

65. Papa MZ, Karni T, Koller M, Klein E, Scott D, Bersuk D, et al. Avoiding diarrhea after subtotal colectomy with primary anastomosis in the treatment of colon cancer. J Am Coll Surg 1997;184(3):269–72.

66. Campbell WB, Rhodes M, Kettlewell MG. Colonoscopy following intraoperative lavage in the management of severe colonic bleeding. Ann R Coll Surg Engl 1985; 67(5):290–2.

67. Batch AJ, Pickard RG, De Lacey G. Peroperative colonoscopy in massive rectal bleeding. Br J Surg 1981;68(1):64.

68. Rockey DC, Koch J, Cello JP, Sanders LL, McQuaid K. Relative frequency of upper gastrointestinal and colonic lesions in patients with positive fecal occult-blood tests. N Engl J Med 1998;339(3):153–9.

69. Rockey DC, Cello JP. Evaluation of the gastrointestinal tract in patients with iron-deficiency anemia. N Engl J Med 1993 Dec 2; 329(23):1691–1695.

70. Tudor RG, Farmakis N, Keighley MR. National audit of complicated diverticular disease: analysis of index cases. Br J Surg 1994 May; 81(5):730–2.

71. Lewis M. Bleeding colonic diverticula. J Clin Gastroenterol 2008;42(10):1156–1158.

72. Yamada A, Sugimoto T, Kondo S, Ohta M, Watabe H, Maeda S, et al. Assessment of the risk factors for colonic diverticular hemorrhage. Dis Colon Rectum 2008;51(1):116–20.

73. Strate LL, Liu YL, Aldoori WH, Syngal S, Giovannucci EL. Obesity increases the risks of diverticulitis and diverticular bleeding. Gastroenterology. [Research Support, N.I.H., Extramural Research Support, U.S. Gov't, P.H.S.]. 2009;136(1):115–22 e1.

74. McGuire HH, Jr., Bleeding colonic diverticula. A reappraisal of natural history and management. Ann Surg. 1994;220(5):653–6.

75. Smoot RL, Gostout CJ, Rajan E, Pardi DS, Schleck CD, Harmsen WS, et al. Is early colonoscopy after admission for acute diverticular bleeding needed? Am J Gastroenterol 2003;98(9):1996–1999.

76. Bloomfeld RS, Rockey DC, Shetzline MA. Endoscopic therapy of acute diverticular hemorrhage. Am J Gastroenterol 2001 Aug; 96(8):2367–2372.

77. Hokama A, Uehara T, Nakayoshi T, Uezu Y, Tokuyama K, Kinjo F, et al. Utility of endoscopic hemoclipping for colonic diverticular bleeding. Am J Gastroenterol 1997;92(3):543–6.

78. Rino Y, Imada T, Iwasaki H, Tanabe H, Toyoda H, Kato N, et al. Hemostasis of colonic diverticular bleeding with hemoclips under endoscopic control: report of a case. Hepatogastroenterology 1999;46(27):1733–1735.

79. Simpson PW, Nguyen MH, Lim JK, Soetikno RM. Use of endoclips in the treatment of massive colonic diverticular bleeding. Gastrointest Endosc 2004;59(3):433–7.

80. Yen EF, Ladabaum U, Muthusamy VR, Cello JP, McQuaid KR, Shah JN. Colonoscopic treatment of acute diverticular hemorrhage using endoclips. Dig Dis Sci 2008; 53(9):2480–2485.

81. Hizawa K, Miura N, Matsumoto T, Iida M. Colonic diverticular bleeding: precise localization and successful management by a combination of CT angiography and interventional radiology. Abdom Imaging 2008 Oct 24.

82. Heer M, Sulser H, Hany A. Angiodysplasia of the colon: an expression of occlusive vascular disease. Hepatogastroenterology 1987;34(3):127–31.

83. Danesh BJ, Spiliadis C, Williams CB, Zambartas CM. Angiodysplasia – an uncommon cause of colonic bleeding: colonoscopic evaluation of 1,050 patients with rectal bleeding and anaemia. Int J Colorectal Dis 1987;2(4):218–22.

84. Richter JM, Hedberg SE, Athanasoulis CA, Schapiro RH. Angiodysplasia. Clinical presentation and colonoscopic diagnosis. Dig Dis Sci 1984;29(6):481–5.

85. Hochter W, Weingart J, Kuhner W, Frimberger E, Ottenjann R. Angiodysplasia in the colon and rectum. Endoscopic morphology, localisation and frequency. Endoscopy 1985;17(5):182–5.

86. Foutch PG, Rex DK, Lieberman DA. Prevalence and natural history of colonic angiodysplasia among healthy asymptomatic people. Am J Gastroenterol 1995;90 (4):564–7.

87. Richter JM, Christensen MR, Colditz GA, Nishioka NS. Angiodysplasia. Natural history and efficacy of therapeutic interventions. Dig Dis Sci 1989;34(10):1542–1546.

88. Hutcheon DF, Kabelin J, Bulkley GB, Smith GW. Effect of therapy on bleeding rates in gastrointestinal angiodysplasia. Am Surg 1987 Jan; 53(1):6–9.

89. Imperiale TF, Ransohoff DF. Aortic stenosis, idiopathic gastrointestinal bleeding, and angiodysplasia: is there an association? A methodologic critique of the literature. Gastroenterology 1988;95(6):1670–1676.

90. Foutch PG. Angiodysplasia of the gastrointestinal tract. Am J Gastroenterol 1993;88 (6):807–18.

91. Brandt LJ, Spinnell MK. Ability of naloxone to enhance the colonoscopic appearance of normal colon vasculature and colon vascular ectasias. Gastrointest Endosc 1999; 49(1):79–83.

92. Junquera F, Quiroga S, Saperas E, Perez-Lafuente M, Videla S, Alvarez-Castells A, et al. Accuracy of helical computed tomographic angiography for the diagnosis of colonic angiodysplasia. Gastroenterology 2000;119(2):293–9.

93. Baum S, Athanasoulis CA, Waltman AC, Galdabini J, Schapiro RH, Warshaw AL, et al. Angiodysplasia of the right colon: a cause of gastrointestinal bleeding. AJR Am J Roentgenol 1977;129(5):789–94.

94. Santos JC, Jr., Aprilli F, Guimaraes AS, Rocha JJ. Angiodysplasia of the colon: endoscopic diagnosis and treatment. Br J Surg 1988;75(3):256–8.

95. Pardi DS, Loftus EV, Jr., Tremaine WJ, Sandborn WJ, Alexander GL, Balm RK, et al. Acute major gastrointestinal hemorrhage in inflammatory bowel disease. Gastrointest Endosc 1999;49(2):153–7.

96. Belaiche J, Louis E, D'Haens G, Cabooter M, Naegels S, De Vos M, et al. Acute lower gastrointestinal bleeding in Crohn's disease: characteristics of a unique series of 34 patients. Belgian IBD Research Group. Am J Gastroenterol 1999;94(8):2177–2181.

97. Johanson JF, Sonnenberg A. The prevalence of hemorrhoids and chronic constipation. An epidemiologic study. Gastroenterology 1990;98(2):380–6.

98. Gazet JC, Redding W, Rickett JW. The prevalence of haemorrhoids. A preliminary survey. Proc R Soc Med 1970;63Suppl: 78–80.

99. Jenkins JT, Urie A, Molloy RG. Anterior anal fissures are associated with occult sphincter injury and abnormal sphincter function. Colorectal Dis 2008;10(3):280–5.

100. Postgate A, Saunders B, Tjandra J, Vargo J. Argon plasma coagulation in chronic radiation proctitis. Endoscopy 2007;39(4):361–5.

101. Haas EM, Bailey HR, Farragher I. Application of 10 percent formalin for the treatment of radiation-induced hemorrhagic proctitis. Dis Colon Rectum 2007;50(2):213–7.

102. Marshall GT, Thirlby RC, Bredfeldt JE, Hampson NB. Treatment of gastrointestinal radiation injury with hyperbaric oxygen. Undersea Hyperb Med 2007;34(1):35–42.

103. Perez RO, Sousa A, Jr., Bresciani C, Proscurshim I, Coser R, Kiss D, et al. Endoscopic management of postoperative stapled colorectal anastomosis hemorrhage. Tech Coloproctol 2007;11(1):64–6.

104. Malik AH, East JE, Buchanan GN, Kennedy RH. Endoscopic haemostasis of staple-line haemorrhage following colorectal resection. Colorectal Dis 2008;10(6):616–18.

105. Linn TY, Moran BJ, Cecil TD. Staple line haemorrhage following laparoscopic left-sided colorectal resections may be more common when the inferior mesenteric artery is preserved. Tech Coloproctol 2008;12(4):289–93.

106. Kim HS, Kim TI, Kim WH, Kim YH, Kim HJ, Yang SK, et al. Risk factors for immediate postpolypectomy bleeding of the colon: a multicenter study. Am J Gastroenterol 2006;101(6):1333–1341.

107. Sawhney MS, Salfiti N, Nelson DB, Lederle FA, Bond JH. Risk factors for severe delayed postpolypectomy bleeding. Endoscopy 2008;40(2):115–19.

108. Koh DC, Luchtefeld MA, Kim DG, Knox MF, Fedeson BC, Vanerp JS, Mustert BR. Efficacy of transarterial embolization as definitive treatment in lower gastrointestinal bleeding. Colorectal Dis 2009;11(1):53–9 Epub 2008 Apr. 28.

109. Tan KK, Wong D, Sim R. Superselective embolization for lower gastrointestinal hemorrhage: an institutional review over 7 years. World J Surg 2008;32(12): 2707–2715.

CHAPTER 10

Small Bowel Bleeding

Daniela E. Serban[1] & Ernest G. Seidman[2]

[1]Pediatric Clinic II, Emergency Hospital for Children, University of Medicine and Pharmacy "Iuliu Haţieganu", Cluj-Napoca, Romania

[2]McGill Center for IBD Research, Montreal General Hospital, Montreal, Canada

Epidemiology and terminology

Obscure gastrointestinal bleeding (OGIB) is defined as bleeding from the GI tract that persists or recurs without an obvious etiology after esophagogastroduodenoscopy, colonoscopy, and radiologic evaluation of the small bowel. OGIB could be categorized into obscure overt and obscure occult bleeding, based on the presence or absence of clinically evident bleeding. OGIB may account for ~ 5% of all GI bleedings (1). Most OGIB lesions are located in the small bowel. Small bowel bleeding (SBB) is defined as bleeding between the ampulla of Vater and the terminal ileum (2).

Etiology

A comprehensive list of the various causes of SBB is presented in Box 10.1 (3–13). The most common include vascular lesions (accounting for 50–70% of cases), especially in people over age 60, tumors (4–15%) and ulcers/erosions (3–16%). Etiologies of SBB by age are summarized in Box 10.2.

Diagnosis

The SB is the most challenging bowel segment to examine, because of its extensive length, contractility, overlapping loops, and free intraperitoneal location (1). Localization of the bleeding site cannot be identified by the clinical history. Consequently, patients with SBB generally undergo

---

Gastrointestinal Bleeding, Second Edition. Edited by Joseph J.Y. Sung, Ernst J. Kuipers and Alan N. Barkun. © 2012 Blackwell Publishing Ltd.
Published 2012 by Blackwell Publishing Ltd.

Box 10.1 Etiology of Small Bowel Bleeding

Vascular lesions (congenital or acquired)
Angioectasia (angiodysplasia), Dieulafoy's lesion, varices (3); multiple phlebectasia,
  telangiectasia (Osler-Rendu-Weber disease; or associated with Turner Syndrome,
  systemic sclerosis or mixed connective tissue disease), hemangioma (± as part of a
  syndrome – Blue Rubber-bleb Naevus Syndrome, Klippel-Trenaunnay-Webber
  Syndrome), disorders of connective tissue (Ehlers-Danlos Syndrome, pseudo-xanthoma
  elasticum) (4)
Tumors
Primary:
– Benign: giant ileal lymphoid hyperplasia, (5) lipoma, inflammatory polyp, lymphangioma,
  leiomyoma, polyps/polyposis (adenomas/familial adenomatous polyposis, hamartomas –
  Peutz Jeghers Syndrome) (5, 6)
– Malignant: lymphomas, carcinoid tumors, adenocarcinoma, GI stromal tumor (6)
Metastatic: melanoma, breast cancer, renal-cell carcinoma (6)
Ulcers/Erosions
Inflammatory diseases: Crohn's disease, celiac disease, vasculitides (6), ischemic
  enteritis, (7) radiation enteritis (3), infectious enteritis [tuberculosis, (7) hookworms],
  eosinophilic or allergic enteritis (8)
Medication induced: nonsteroidal anti-inflammatory drugs (NSAIDs) (3),
  chemotherapy
Meckel diverticulum (3)
Diverticula (3)
Aorto-enteric fistulas, after abdominal aortic aneurysm repair (3)
Non-specific ulcer(s) (3)
Duplication of the intestine (9)
Ectopic pancreas (10)
Miscellaneous
Lymphangiectasia (11), amyloidosis (12), intestinal intussusception (13);

---

numerous diagnostic procedures, require more blood transfusions, have longer hospitalizations, and have higher health care expenditures than patients who have upper or lower GI bleeding (15).

Radiological studies

Radiological imaging has been the principal method of evaluating the SB for nearly a century (16). Techniques include *barium studies*, such as SB follow-through (SBFT) and enteroclysis (1); *angiography* (1); *cross-sectional imaging* (computed tomography (CT) and magnetic resonance (MR) imaging with enteroclysis or enterography (17, 18), CT angiography (1), and *radio-isotope scans* (1)).

Since most of these expose patients to radiation, they are contraindicated in pregnancy.

Box 10.2 Common causes of Small Bowel Bleeding According to Age

Children and adolescents [+]
Angioectasia
Celiac disease (ulcerative jejunitis)
Congenital vascular disorders
Crohn's disease
Eosinophilic gastroenteropathy
Henoch-Schonlein purpura (14)
Infectious enteritis
Meckel's diverticulum
NSAID-enteropathy
Polyps/polyposis
Varices
Young Adults < 40 years [++]
Angioectasia
Celiac disease (ulcerative jejunitis)
Crohn's disease
Dieulafoy's lesions
Meckel's diverticulum
Tumors
Older Adults > 40 years [++]
Angioectasia
Celiac disease (ulcerative jejunitis)
NSAID-enteropathy
Tumors

[+] Modified from Seidman et al. (8)
[++] Modified from Raju et al. (1)

SBFT and enteroclysis

SBFT

This is a series of abdominal x-rays taken at different times after the ingestion of barium sulfate (19).

Double-Contrast enteroclysis

This involves insertion of barium directly into the SB through a catheter fixed in the descending duodenum or at the ligament of Treitz, by means of inflating a balloon. Barium is then slowly injected until the terminal ileum is filled. The SB is then inflated with air (or CO_2), injected through the tube. When sufficient inflation is achieved, scopolamine butylbromide or glucagon can be injected to inhibit peristalsis. The double-contrast agent can be methylcellulose, but air is considered better in terms of showing mucosal details, and is preferred for cases of SBB. Bowel preparation typically includes a low-residue diet, ample fluids, laxative on the day prior to the examination, and nothing by mouth on the day of the examination (20).

- *Advantages*:
  - ○ visualization of the entire SB
- *Disadvantages*:
  - ○ radiation
  - ○ enteroclysis – less pleasant for the patient.
- *Contraindications*:
  - ○ pregnancy
  - ○ complete intestinal obstruction
  - ○ acute GI bleeding (21).
- *Yield of: SBFT and Enteroclysis in OGIB:* very low – 0%–5.6% and 10%–21%, respectively. The tests are able to show sizeable abnormalities (enteritis or tumors), but miss many smaller (flat, vascular or inflammatory) lesions (22).
- *Comparative Studies::* A recent meta-analysis has shown that, compared with SBFT, the diagnostic yield of capsule endoscopy (CE) is significantly higher in detecting SB lesions (67% vs 8%; $p < 0.00001$ and clinically significant findings (42% vs 6%), with a number needed to test of three (23). In another prospective study, the diagnostic potential of SBFT in OGIB was much lower than CE (5% vs 31%, $p < 0.05$) (24). In a retrospective review in 98 patients, enteroclysis changed management in only 10% of patients (25). In another study, none of the patients with a negative CE had findings on push enteroscopy and SBFT (26).
- *Conclusion::* Given the extremely low diagnostic yield of SBFT and enteroclysis, their role in the evaluation of OGIB has waned substantially, since the advent of CE and enteroscopy. Therefore, unless the clinical findings suggest SB obstruction due to malignancy, Crohn's disease (CD), or prior use of NSAIDs, there is no role for either SBFT or enteroclysis in the evaluation of OGIB (1).

Mesenteric angiography

This examines the blood vessels that supply the small and large bowel (celiac axis, superior and inferior mesenteric arteries), usually using the Seldinger technique (27, 28). Although *provocative* angiography can be performed safely (with vasodilators, anticoagulants, or thrombolytic agents), the overall yield of this technique is low (29).

- *Indication::* As a primary imaging test in patients with brisk bleeding or who are hemodynamically unstable due to hemorrhage, especially as a localization technique for embolization, or prior to surgery. (21) It may detect both acute bleeding (extravasation of contrast dye in the bowel lumen) and non-bleeding lesions (particularly angioectasias – which often have characteristic features and tumors) (1, 28). Angiographic criteria of angioectasias are: a densely opacified, slowly emptying, dilated tortuous vein within the intestinal wall; a vascular tuft; and/or an early filling vein (28).

- *Advantages*:
  - ○ lack of need for bowel preparation
  - ○ ability to precisely localize a bleeding source (if identified)
  - ○ potentially therapeutic (30).
- *Disadvantages*:
  - ○ requires a minimal active bleeding rate (>0.5–1 mL/min)
  - ○ often unable to determine a specific cause
  - ○ potential complications (listed below), especially with therapeutic procedures (1)
  - ○ radiation exposure.
- *Angiographic therapy*:: Usually reserved for acutely bleeding lesions detected during diagnostic angiography. Selective intra-arterial vasopressin therapy had been considered the standard therapy, but has been associated with complications and a rebleeding rate of 50% (21). Superselective embolotherapy with microcoils alone or with gelatin sponge pledglets or polyvinyl alcohol embolospheres is becoming increasingly popular (1). After finding a lesion, success at initial hemostasis ranges from 73% to 100%, with rebleeding seen in 1–14% of cases (30). The major advantage of successful embolotherapy is immediate cessation of bleeding, which avoids the risk of prolonged catheter placement and systemic complications of vasopressin (31).

  In mesentic arterial stenosis (which could lead to ischemic enteritis), revascularization of the vessels can be achieved also by endovascular percutaneous transluminal angioplasty, with or without stent placement. This technique is associated with a high primary technical success rate of 90–100%, with symptom relief in 73–99% of patients. However, the relapse rate due to restenosis of the artery or in-stent stenosis is around 28% (range 11–39%), necessitating new endovascular interventions (32).
- *Complications (in 5–15%)*:
  - ○ access site thrombosis or hemorrhage
  - ○ contrast reactions
  - ○ acute renal failure
  - ○ transient cerebral ischemia
  - ○ injury to target vessels (33)
  - ○ related to vasopressin: myocardial ischemia, arrhythmias, bowel infarction, arterial vasospasm, lower extremity ischemia and cerebral edema (21).

- *Yield in*: *OGIB:* Data for OGIB are limited. (1) Its overall yield in detecting a GI bleeding source ranges from 27 to 77% (34). The specificity is 100%, but sensitivity varies with the pattern of bleeding, ranging from 47% with acute – to 30% with recurrent bleeding (35).
- *Comparative studies:*: A study compared CE with various endoscopic and imaging techniques in 56 patients with OGIB. The yield of CE was 68%, compared to only 16% with angiography (36).

Cross-sectional imaging
The multi-detector row helical CT technique
This recent technique combines the advantages of enteral volume challenge to optimize bowel distention, cross-sectional imaging, multiplanar reformatted imaging, and imaging in both arterial and venous phases (13).

CT enteroclysis
This combines standard enteroclysis to distend the SB with helical CT (37). It uses a negative (hypodense) luminal contrast medium (0.5% methylcellulose or pure water), with intravenous (IV) iodinated contrast medium. Bowel preparation is the same as for enteroclysis (21). Images are analysed primarily in the axial plane and then multiplanar reconstruction (MPR) and maximum intensity projection (MIP) images are generated in the coronal and sagittal planes (13).

- *Advantages*:
  - detection of very small lesions (polyps, tumors, vascular malformations) (37), and of Meckel diverticulum (17)
  - hyperdense foci extending into the intestinal wall, as seen on CT images acquired in the arterial or venous phase, are interpreted as vascular lesions (38)
  - assessment of CD activity is best done in the portal venous phase, whereas the arterial phase may detect vascular pathologies, such as arteriovenous malformations (37).
- *Disadvantages*:
  - naso-enteric tube (17)
  - high radiation exposure (39)
  - increased cost
  - requires IV contrast
  - inability to detect mild inflammation (37).
- *Contraindications*:
  - complete bowel obstruction (17)
  - severe allergy to contrast dye (iodine)
  - significant renal insufficiency (40).

- *Complications (rare):*
  - ○ bowel perforation
  - ○ contrast aspiration
  - ○ respiratory depression (sedation) (17).
- *Yield in: OGIB:* In a small prospective study, the detection rate of the bleeding source was 47%: findings were 64% in patients with overt compared to only 14% in those with occult bleeding (13).
- *Comparative Studies::* In a retrospective study in OGIB, CE was superior to CT enteroclysis with neutral enteral contrast, barium-carbon dioxide or barium-methylcellulose enteroclysis in detecting flat mucosal lesions (like vascular lesions) (40). In patients with ongoing overt OGIB, the association of CE and CT enteroclysis had an overall diagnostic yield of 72%. As in the previous study, CE was superior to CT enteroclysis in detecting flat lesions (6).

CT enterography

The invasive nature of CT enteroclysis can be eliminated by ingesting the agent. CT enterography refers to the use of IV contrast material-enhanced abdomino-pelvic CT following ingestion of a large volume of neutral oral contrast agent. This method may be more suitable for the evaluation of OGIB (41), especially when expertise for CT enteroclysis is unavailable (17). Some lesions diagnosed by CT enteroclysis or enterography, in patients assessed for OGIB, are illustrated in Fig. 10.1.

- *Comparative Studies::* In a recent study, CT enterography identified a bleeding source in 45% of 22 OGIB cases. Eight of 10 positive findings were later confirmed. CT enterography correctly identified three lesions undetected at CE, whereas a lesion was detected by CE in only 1 of 4 patients with negative CT enterography (41).
- *Conclusion::* CT enteroclysis or enterography may play a complementary role to CE in evaluating OGIB (17, 41). Others have suggested that these CT techniques should precede CE in order to exclude strictures and to detect tumors that could be missed by CE (6).

Magnetic resonance studies

These can be performed with *enteroclysis* or *enterography*. Enterography is generally the routine technique for both CT and MR imaging, reserving enteroclysis for selected indications such as low-grade small bowel obstruction (18).

- *Advantages over CT imaging:*
  - ○ excellent soft tissue contrast resolution
  - ○ lack of ionizing radiation (40)

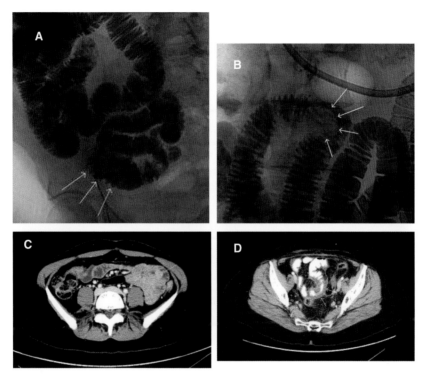

Figure 10.1 Representative images of small bowel lesions causing bleeding diagnosed by CT enteroclysis or enterography: (A) radiation ileitis; (B) Peutz-Jeghers polyp; (C) ileal carcinoid; (D) Ileal lymphoma. (Courtesy of Dr. Laurence A. Stein, Royal Victoria Hospital, McGill University Health Center, Montreal.)

- o ability to perform real-time and functional imaging
  - o safety profile of gadolinium IV contrast agents (18).
- *Disadvantages*:
  - o spatial resolution of MR imaging – inferior to CT (small bowel mucosa cannot be analyzed in as much detail)
  - o longer overall examination time
  - o high cost (18).
- *Comparative Studies*:: In a prospective comparison between MR enteroclysis and CT enteroclysis, the latter had higher sensitivity and inter-observer agreement (42).

CT angiography (CTA)
This involves helical CT angiography before and after intra-arterial injections of contrast medium (1, 43). The site of hemorrhage is recognized as a hyperdense area due to the extravasation of contrast into the lumen. Angiography can be realized also with MR.

- *Yield in OGIB::* Helical CTA revealed the site of hemorrhage in 72% of patients (43).
- *Comparative studies::* In 28 patients with OGIB, CE detected a source in 72% of patients – compared to 24% by CTA or 56% by standard mesenteric angiography. CE identified a source in 100% of patients diagnosed by CTA and in 86% by standard angiography. Moreover, CE was positive in 63% of negative cases using CTA and in 55% with negative standard angiography. Agreement between CE and the other two techniques was 52% (p = 0.03). Therapeutic intervention was undertaken in 47% patients as a result of the CE findings (44).

    CTA or MR arteriography, abdominal duplex ultrasound and the new functional tests for assessment of mucosal perfusion (*GI tonometry* and *visible-light spectroscopy for detection of mucosal hypoxaemia*) are good diagnostic tools in chronic GI ischemia. CTA is the 'gold standard' for diagnosing and staging of gastrointestinal arterial stenosis (32).

Scintigraphy (nuclear scans, radioisotope scans)

Tests can be performed with technetium (^{99m}Tc)-labeled red blood cells (half-life 24 h) or ^{99m}Tc sulfur colloid (half-life 3 min) (45). ^{99m}Tc-pertechnate is used to detect a Meckel diverticulum (46). Using erythrocytes for the detection of extravasated blood, 1–3 mL of the patient's blood are withdrawn, labeled with ^{99m}Tc, and then re-injected (21). Early scanning (30 min to 4 h) is recommended (47); although images can be obtained for up to 24 h, localization accuracy decreases over time (1). The ^{99m}Tc sulfur colloid has the advantage of no preparation time delay. However, given its very short half-life, it is helpful only in immediate, ongoing bleeding. Furthermore, uptake into the liver and spleen restricts the image area.

- *Indication::* active bleeding in hemodynamically stable patients.
- *Advantages*:
  - noninvasive;
  - relatively easy to perform
  - no preparation needed (47).
- *Disadvantages*:
  - minimum bleeding rate (>0.1 mL/min) required
  - inaccurate localization (45)
  - inability to determine a specific cause
  - high false negative rate
  - radiation.

  Erythrocyte scan results should be verified by a second method (angiography, endoscopy, CE), before surgery is performed (45).
- *Yield::* In acute lower GI bleeding, the accuracy is highly variable, averaging 78% (range 41–97%); early scanning (2 h) is most sensitive (34).

Giving its disadvantages, studies are limited in OGIB. A retrospective series of 92 patients reported a positive result in 73%, with only 4% false positive. (47) The sensitivity for GI bleeding due to a Meckel's diverticulum is approximately 75%. A positive result indicates the presence of ectopic gastric mucosa, but is not proof of causality. Moreover, a negative result does not exclude a Meckel's diverticulum (46).

- *Comparative studies::* A positive scintigram increased the diagnostic yield of subsequent angiography in acute lower GI bleeding (22% to 53%) (48). However, these results were not confirmed in another study (49).
- *Conclusion::* The role of nuclear scans (in particular, using red blood cells) is limited in patients with OGIB (1).

Videocapsule endoscopy

CE has revolutionized the exploration of SB diseases (50–52). It enabled, for the first time, the visualization of the entire SB in a noninvasive manner and has become the gold standard to identify a bleeding source in OGIB (8, 53). CE transmits images to a digital recorder worn on a belt, which are subsequently downloaded to a PC workstation with dedicated software (54). The need for a bowel preparation or a prokinetic is controversial (55). Three SB capsules are now marketed in North America, with a 7–10 hour lifespan (54). PillCam models SB1 and SB2 (11 mm × 26 mm, with a complementary metal oxide semiconductor, manufactured by Given Imaging, Yoqneam, Israel) were the first introduced and are most widely used. Endocapsule (same dimensions, with a charge-coupled device, Olympus Medical Systems Corporation, Tokyo, Japan) is also available. Recently, the MiRo capsule has been introduced (Intro Medic Ltd, Seoul, Korea). Another capsule, not yet FDA approved, is the OMOM device (Chongqing Jinshan Science & Technology Group Co., Ltd, Chongqing, China).

One study comparing CE devices in OGIB found a statistically nonsignificant trend for the EndoCapsule in detecting more bleeding sources than did the PillCam SB. However, the authors speculated that the longer recording times might have provided more data (56). In our experience, the software and image quality of the Given Imaging system are superior to that of the Olympus capsule.

- *Indication::* as an initial step in the assessment of OGIB (1), especially if the patient does not have massive bleeding and is hemodynamically stable (no therapeutic immediate measures required) (1, 44, 57).
- *Advantages*:
  o ability to image the entire SB noninvasively
  o no radiation or sedation (51, 54)

- o readily performed
- o ability to review and share images
- o patient preference; outpatient procedure (54)
- o safety profile.
- The description of lesions uses the classic endoscopic terminology (58). For vascular lesions, the Yano-Yamamoto classification has been proposed (as detailed below in the double-balloon endoscopy section). According to the risk of bleeding, intestinal lesions can be classified as follows (59):
  - o P0 (low relevance):: lesions with no potential for bleeding, including visible submucosal veins, diverticula without the presence of blood, or nodules without mucosal alterations
  - o P1 (uncertain relevance):: lesions with uncertain hemorrhagic potential, such as red spots on the intestinal mucosa, or small or isolated erosions
  - o P2 (high relevance):: lesions with high potential for bleeding, such as typical angiodysplasia, large ulcerations, tumors, or varices.

    In Fig. 10.2, we illustrate some lesions diagnosed by CE, in patients presenting with OGIB.
- *Disadvantages* : (13, 16)
  - o inability to perform biopsies or therapeutic procedures
  - o risk of capsule retention
  - o over-estimation of trivial lesions (the clinical significance of small lesions such as petechiae or focal erythematous spots remains questionable)
  - o poor localization of lesions
  - o cessation of battery power prior to reaching the cecum (in 15–20% of cases) (54)
  - o high cost
  - o time required for interpretation of the images
  - o inability to provide information on the intestinal wall and mesentery
  - o impossibility to distinguish between an extra-mucosal SB wall tumor and an extra-intestinal lesion
  - o inadequate cleansing of the SB, not permitting full visualization (up to 50% of procedures) (54)
  - o inability to evaluate a lesion in a to-and-fro manner (60)
  - o need for second investigation in positives as well as negatives with persistent bleeding.
- *Contraindications – recently reviewed* : (54, 61)
  - o absolute::
    - ❖ evidence of SB obstruction
    - ❖ very small children [although CE use in this age group has been reported (8, 62) and recently reviewed (63)].

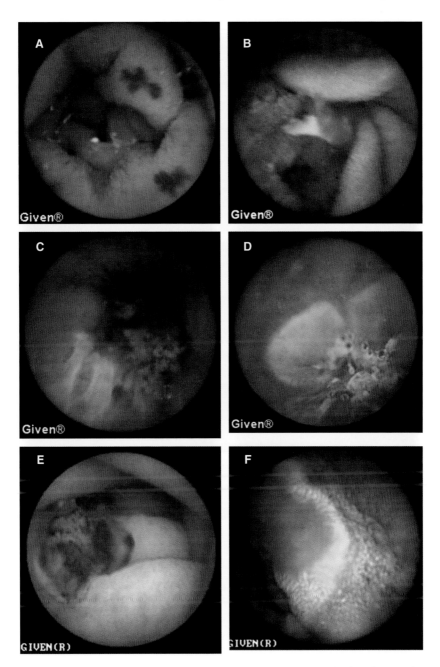

Figure 10.2 Representative images of small bowel lesions causing bleeding diagnosed by capsule endoscopy: (A) angioectasias; (B) jejunal ulcer due to Crohn's disease; (C) ulcerated ileal stricture due to Crohn's disease; (D) ulcerated ileal stricture due to chronic NSAID use; (E) ulcerative jejunitis due to celiac disease; (F) denuded jejunal mucosa due to eosinophilic gastroenteritis; (G) jejunal hamartomatous polyp in Peutz-Jeghers Syndrome; (H) adenocarcinomas; (I) metastatic melanoma; (J) distal duodenal gastrointestinal stromal tumor; (K) carcinoid; (L) lymphoma; (M) varix due to portal hypertension; (N) hemangioma.

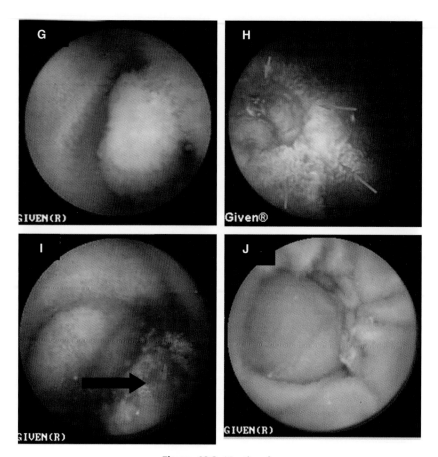

Figure 10.2 (*Continued*)

○ relative:
  ❖ cardiac pacemakers or other implanted electromedical devices (however, we have reported on the safe use of CE in such patients using the Given Pillcam) (64)
  ❖ dysphagia or other swallowing problems such as in young children (16) can be overcome by delivering the capsule endoscopically directly into the duodenum (8).
• *Complications::* Capsule retention is defined as failure of the capsule to be excreted after more than two weeks without surgical, endoscopic, or medical interventions (65). The risk in OGIB is low (0.1%). However, retention has been reported in up to 5% of high risk cases (54). Risk factors include Crohn's disease (with undetected strictures), chronic NSAID use, history of intestinal surgery, suspected tumor, history of abdominal radiotherapy, and suspected mesenteric ischemia (60). When a stricture is suspected, a patency capsule can be used first to reduce retention risk (Agile®, Given Imaging Ltd, Yoqneam, Israel) (66).

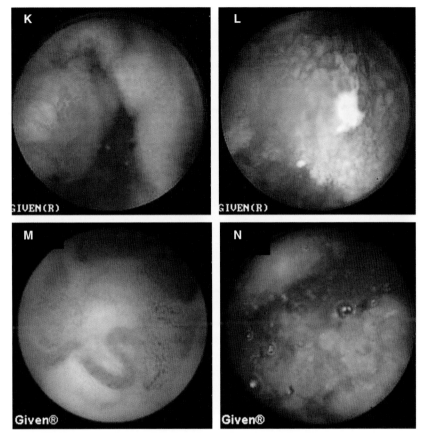

Figure 10.2 (*Continued*)

- *Yield in*: *OGIB:* The diagnostic yield of CE has been reported to vary between 31% (24) and 76% (67), with most studies showing yields of 60–70% [reviewed in (1, 63)]. The sensitivity, specificity, positive and negative predictive values are 89%, 95%, 97% and 83% (68) and 95%, 75%, 95% and 86% (69), respectively, in two studies. Conditions that increase the diagnostic yield of CE are: a. the indication (68–70) and b. the timing (71–73).
  a. Carey et al. (70) analysed 15 studies that were performed in patients with *ongoing* GI bleeding and found that the yield in this group was significantly higher than that in patients with *prior overt* OGIB (87% vs 56%, p = 0.02). Yields are lower in patients with *occult* OGIB (68–70). A very recent study confirmed that the diagnostic yield for *ongoing overt* bleeding (88%) was significantly higher than that of *previous overt* and *occult bleeding* (48%) (74).

b. The diagnostic yield was 92% if CE was performed within 48 hours of a bleeding episode (73). The yield for CE was also higher (91% vs 34%) if performed within 2 weeks of a bleeding episode (72). After a negative initial CE in OGIB, a repeat CE identified findings in 75% (75).

The positive findings of CE impacted on management in 37%–66% of cases [studies reviewed in (1)], with resolution of bleeding observed in about 65% (68). During a median follow-up of 13 months, diagnoses of specific diseases by CE led to a favorable outcome in 64% of cases, whereas negative CE cases were associated with no further bleeding in 80% (35).

Published data in the pediatric population are limited. Case reports documented the feasibility of CE in patients with OGIB, later confirmed by larger series (7, 8, 14, 62), recently reviewed (63). The youngest reported case thus far has been 18 months (5).

- *Comparative studies:*: The superior yield of CE over other imaging techniques has been reviewed above (6, 11, 23, 24, 26, 36, 40, 44). The American Society for Gastrointestinal Endoscopy Technology Assessment Committee concluded that CE using the PillCam SB (Given Imaging) provided a superior yield compared with both radiographic contrast studies and push enteroscopy (76). Two meta-analyses have shown the superiority of the CE in OGIB. The first, published in 2005 (23), included 14 studies. The yield for CE was 63% vs 28% for push enteroscopy (PE) (for any finding), with an incremental yield of 35% ($p < 0.00001$) and 56% vs 26%, respectively (for clinically significant findings) (incremental yield of 30%, $p < 0.00001$) (23). The second (77) included 17 studies. The absolute pooled difference in the rate of positive findings between CE and alternative modalities (PE, SBFT or enteroclysis) for SB diseases was 41% and for occult GI bleeding – 37%. Compared with PE, CE significantly increased the probability of a positive finding (OR 4.3, 95% CI 3.1–6.0, $P < 0.001$) (77). Studies comparing CE and DBE are presented below.
- *Conclusion:*: CE should be part of the initial investigation in patients with OGIB. CE is helpful in achieving effective decision-making concerning subsequent investigations and treatments (51, 77). CE should be performed early after a bleeding episode (71).

Cable endoscopic techniques

These include sonde enteroscopy, push enteroscopy, single- and double-balloon enteroscopy, spiral enteroscopy and intraoperative enteroscopy.

Sonde enteroscopy

This involves peroral placement of a long (3 m) enteroscope with a distal balloon into the proximal small intestine that is propelled by peristaltic activity into the ileum. Because of prolonged examination (7 hours), patient discomfort, and the inability to carry out therapeutic interventions, this technique is now rarely used (1, 78).

Push enteroscopy

Although it uses an enteroscope with a working length of > 220 cm, looping generally limits visualization to only the proximal 50–150 cm of SB (1, 57). Use of an overtube can prevent looping and improve the depth of insertion. However, this has not been shown to impact on diagnostic yield (1) and is associated with increased complications. Therefore, PE has been replaced in many practices in favor of CE and/or balloon enteroscopy (57).

- *Advantages*:
  - provides diagnostic and therapeutic capabilities during a single procedure
  - can be performed in an outpatient setting
  - no need for a pump control system
  - shorter procedure time vs balloon-assisted enteroscopy (79).
- *Disadvantages*:
  - limited SB examination
  - patient discomfort (1)
  - invasiveness.
- *Complications* (infrequent, < 1%, mostly related to overtube use):
  - pharyngeal or Mallory–Weiss tear
  - esophageal perforation
  - pancreatitis
  - gastric mucosal stripping.
- *Yield in*: *OGIB:* The diagnostic yield of PE ranges between 19% (80) and 78% (81), all studies being reviewed in (1, 63). In a recent AGA review on OGIB, endoscopic therapy was reported in 12.5%–100% of cases. In patients with angioectasia who underwent endoscopic therapy, bleeding cessation ranged from 27% to 85% per year (1).
- *Comparative Studies::* The two meta-analyses comparing CE and PE are detailed in the CE section above. The studies comparing PE with DBE are presented in the balloon enteroscopy section below.
- *Contraindications::* Analogous to upper gastrointestinal endoscopy and colonoscopy. Although adhesions are not a contraindication, they may limit the procedure, as a fixed SB limits the insertion depth and often causes considerable patient discomfort (57).

Double-balloon enteroscopy (push-and-pull enteroscopy)

Double-balloon endoscopy (DBE), devised in 2001 by Yamamoto et al., may allow the visualization of the entire SB mucosa (82). The principle of DBE is

based on alternating "push-and-pull" maneuvers, with inflation and deflation of the balloons and telescoping of the intestine onto the overtube
(82, 83). DBE can be carried out via both oral and anal routes.

The choice of the initial route depends on the suspected location of the
pathology. CE can assist in this decision: if the ratio of time to reach the lesion
to the time to reach the cecum is < 0.75, the oral route should be considered
first (84). When performing balloon enteroscopy, a tattoo and/or marking-
clip is placed at the deepest insertion point to assist in confirming total
enteroscopy during the subsequent procedure from the opposite direction (57). No specific preparation is required for the oral route, whereas
bowel cleansing is required for the retrograde approach. Although many
centers use general anesthesia, DBE can be safely performed under conscious sedation (1, 57). Preliminary data suggest that DBE in pediatric
patients is safe, and that diagnostic yield, insertion depth, and procedure
duration appear to be similar to that in adults (57, 85).

- *Advantages*:
  - total visualization of the SB
  - compared to CE, DBE affords:
    - improved visualization by: virtue of ability to insufflate air, irrigate
      and suction any obscuring mucus/material and by focusing exam-
      ination on any mucosal abnormality
    - tissue sampling
    - therapeutic intervention (82, 83).

      The diagnostic and therapeutic procedures are the same as with
      other endoscopic techniques: chromoendoscopy; biopsy; selective
      enteroclysis; marking with India ink; hemostasis (injection of various
      agents, thermocoagulation, clip application); polypectomy; endo-
      scopic mucosal resection; dilation; foreign-body extraction; implan-
      tation of self-expanding enteral metal stents (83). The techniques for
      achieving hemostasis are the same as in other digestive segments.

- *Disadvantages*:
  - time-consuming (2–4 h)
  - not widely available (16).

- *Endoscopic Classification of*: *SB Vascular Lesions*: A recent endoscopic classification proposed by Yano–Yamamoto is shown in Fig. 10.3 (86).
  - Types 1a and 1b lesions are derived from a normal vein in the submu-
    cosal layer and dilation of capillary blood vessels in the lamina propria.
    The clinical condition is a tortuous abnormal blood vessel with path-
    ologic venous characteristics corresponding to angioectasia (7).
    Angioectasia appears usually as a 1–10-mm flat or slightly raised, bright
    red spot, with uniform or irregular margins (28). Sedation for endos-
    copy, especially using meperidine, may, however, make these lesions
    disappear (87).

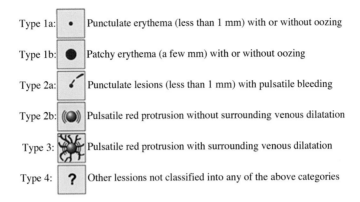

Type 1a: •   Punctulate erythema (less than 1 mm) with or without oozing

Type 1b: ●   Patchy erythema (a few mm) with or without oozing

Type 2a: Punctulate lesions (less than 1 mm) with pulsatile bleeding

Type 2b: ((○)) Pulsatile red protrusion without surrounding venous dilatation

Type 3:   Pulsatile red protrusion with surrounding venous dilatation

Type 4:   ?   Other lessions not classified into any of the above categories

Figure 10.3 Endoscopic classification of small-intestinal vascular lesions (Reproduced from Yano et al. (86) with permission from Elsevier.)

- ○ Types 2a and 2b correspond to Dieulafoy's lesion (4), which can cause major hemorrhage because of an abnormally thick artery meandering in the submucosa contiguous with the surface mucosa, causing an erosion to form by mechanical pressure.
- ○ Type 3 is a lesion within an anastomosis or in the transitional part between comparatively large arteries and veins. Such lesions are comparatively large, arteriovenous malformations (AVM), reaching the serosal surface and not limited to the submucosa.

  This classification is also practical for selection of treatment methods. Coagulation of lesion types 1a and 1b with a high-frequency current such as argon plasma coagulation (APC), hemostasis of types 2a and 2b with clip placement, and, for type 3, placement of a clip to block the inflow blood vessel or surgical removal are recommended. (7) Endoscopic mucosal biopsies of vascular lesions generally are not recommended because of the low diagnostic yield and risk of provoking hemorrhage (87). In Fig. 10.4, we show some lesions in patients presenting with OGIB, diagnosed by DBE.

- • *Complications* : (88)
  - ○ low rate for diagnostic procedures (0.8%); pancreatitis may result from the antegrade approach
  - ○ much higher rate in therapeutic DBE (4.3% – perforation, bleeding).
- • *Yield in*: OGIB: A systematic review from 2007 analysed 13 studies involving 906 patients. The diagnostic yield of DBE was 66% (95% CI 63–69). Subsequent management (medical, surgical or endoscopic) was influenced by DBE findings in 44% of patients, including endoscopic treatment in 26.6% of patients (95% CI 23.4–30) (89). Restricting our review to analysing the diagnostic yield of DBE in OGIB (9, 12, 46, 74, 90–122), yielded data for 2908 patients. The diagnostic yield ranged from 25% (94)

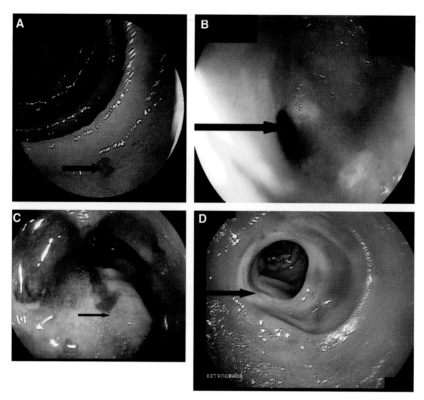

Figure 10.4 Representative lesions causing small bowel bleeding observed by double-balloon endoscopy: (A) angioectasia; (B) stricture due to Crohn's disease; (C) adenocarcinoma; (D) diaphragm disease associated with chronic use of non-steroidal anti-inflammatory drugs. (Courtesy of Dr. Jonathan A. Leighton, Mayo Clinic, Scottsdale.)

to 92% (102), with a median of 73% and a mean of 67.7% (95% CI 62.9–72.6). Use of enteroscopic therapy was noted for patients with OGIB in 31 of the 37 above mentioned studies and ranged from 10% (99) to 78.4% (113) of patients investigated by DBE, with a median of 34.4% and a mean of 37.6% (95% CI 30–45.3). In very recent studies, DBE has had an influence on patient management (including medical measures, endoscopic and surgical procedures) in 51% (109)–73% (110). The sensitivity, specificity, and positive and negative predictive values of DBE in the diagnosis of SB lesions in patients with OGIB were 92.7%, 96.4%, 98.1%, and 87.1%, with a 94.0% overall accuracy (111).

The *diagnostic yield* of DBE depends on a combination of factors, including indication, performance of a pre-DBE CE, timing of DBE, and quality and completeness of pre-DBE endoscopic investigations. Higher yields have generally been achieved when the indication was *overt-ongoing* OGIB as compared to *overt-previous* or to *occult* OGIB (60). In three very recent series, the diagnostic yields were as follows: 100% for *overt-ongoing*, 48% for *overt-previous*, and 42% for *occult* bleeding (111), respectively; 77% for *overt-ongoing* bleeding, 58% for *overt-previous bleeding of sporadic type*, 47% for *overt-previous bleeding of first attack only*, 71% for *occult bleeding with continuous positive fecal occult blood test*, and 60% for *occult bleeding with 1 positive fecal occult blood test with iron deficiency anemia* (12); and 87% for *ongoing-overt* vs 52% for *previous-overt* and *occult bleeding* (74). Generally, studies with the highest yield include numerous patients with a previous CE (60). CE followed by DBE also has a positive influence on management in 91% of cases (84).

A Japanese study examined clinical outcome after DBE-induced therapy for OGIB (101). Ninety-one percent of the patients treated endoscopically or surgically did not experience further bleeding after 8.5±0.6 months. In a recent survey, up to 60% of patients with OGIB reported no further bleeding at 30 months after DBE. Patients with AVM or normal examinations to the depth of insertion were most likely to report recurrent hemorrhage (123). Another series reported that the rate of rebleeding in patients who had undergone interventions (20%) was similar to that in patients who had not (18%) (124). Moreover, the rate of bleeding recurrence in patients with negative DBE findings (9.8%) was not significantly different from that in patients with positive DBE findings (7.7%) (111).

- *Comparative studies*:
  a. *DBE vs PE*. DBE was more effective than PE in two prospective comparative studies (79, 99). It was superior in depth of SB exploration and diagnostic yield (79). In the other study involving OGIB, the overall diagnostic yield with DBE (73%) was also superior to PE (44%). DBE identified additional lesions in deeper parts of the small bowel in PE-positive patients in 78% of cases (9).

  b. *DBE vs CE*. One comparative study in OGIB favored CE (diagnostic yield 80% vs 60% for DBE), (97) while another reported DBE to be superior (87.5% vs 25% for CE). (125) DBE has been reported to diagnose lesions (especially tumors) missed by CE (126, 127). However, a recent meta-analysis of 11 studies (2003–2006) concluded that diagnostic yields for CE and DBE are similar in SB diseases (60% vs 57%), including OGIB (128). Two very recent papers (not included in the meta-analysis) confirmed these results – the overall diagnostic yield between DBE (64% and 65.6%, respectively) and CE (54% and 71.9%, respectively) was similar (74, 114). The latter study concluded that whereas CE is superior in detecting abnormal mucosal lesions, DBE affords endoscopic management (114). Another very recent meta-analysis, including 10 studies, concluded that CE and DBE provide similar diagnostic yields in patients with OGIB. The pooled diagnostic yield for CE was 62% (95% CI 47.3–76.1) and for DBE was 56% (95% CI 48.9–62.1), with an odds ratio for CE compared to DBE of 1.39 (95% CI 0.88–2.20; p = 0.16). Subgroup analysis demonstrated the yield for DBE performed after a previously positive CE was 75.0% (95% CI 60.1–90.0), with the odds ratio for successful diagnosis with DBE after a positive CE compared to DBE in all patients of 1.79 (95% CI 1.09–2.96; p = 0.02). In contrast, the yield for DBE after a previously negative CE was only 27.5% (95% CI 16.7–37.8). The results have thus proved that the diagnostic yield of DBE is significantly higher when performed in patients with a positive CE (129).

In a US multicenter trial, calculated miss rates were 28% for DBE and 20% for CE (91). In another OGIB study, agreement between CE and DBE was observed in 92% of cases; however, the yield in patients with polyposis was 67% for DBE compared with only 33% for CE (127).

In OGIB, angioectasias are the most common finding in European and North/South American series, whereas in series from Far Eastern countries ulcers and erosions are reported most often (60). This could be perhaps be explained by ethnic factors or differences inherent in the DBE and CE modalities (7, 111). For example, CE studies tend to report non-specific red spots as vascular lesions, which may account for higher diagnostic yields. Insufflation of air during DBE may obscure small vascular lesions and explain the comparatively lower diagnostic rates for those lesions (111).

• *Conclusion::* Even if DBE does not allow visualization of the entire SB in one examination compared with CE, it is associated with an equivalent detection rate, has the capability to detect lesions missed by CE, and offers the advantages of therapeutic treatment (1). The disadvantages, as noted above, are availability and invasiveness compared to CE.

Single-balloon enteroscopy (SBE)

SBE is performed with a high-resolution videoendoscope (Olympus XSIF-Q260Y). The single silicon balloon is firmly attached to the tip of an overtube, and is inflated/deflated with air from a pressure-controlled pump system (pressure-setting range: ±6 mm Hg). With this method, after the endoscope has been inserted maximally, the tip of the endoscope is bent through 180° to its maximum up-angle or down-angle. Using this hook shape of the scope in SBE instead of an inflated balloon on the tip as in DBE, the endoscope can hold the SB in the same position, and the overtube can be inserted further without stretching the intestine. When the distal tip of the overtube reaches just before the bent region of the endoscope, the overtube balloon is inflated to grip the intestine. After returning the tip of the endoscope to the neutral position, both the endoscope and the overtube are gently withdrawn in order to shorten the intestine. Repeats of these maneuvers enable the endoscope and overtube to be inserted further into the intestine. As with DBE, both the oral and anal approaches can be used (theoretically allowing total enteroscopy), under conscious sedation or anesthesia (130).

- *Advantages over*: DBE
  - may be easier to perform and less time consuming (130)
- *Possible limits compared to*: DBE: Fewer full papers employing SBE have been published to date (130, 131). Larger studies are required to confirm the ability to insert the scope as far into the SB as the DBE system without additional risk of perforation due to angulation of the tip of the scope. (132)
- *Contraindications*:: as for PE (57).
- *Complications*:: no serious complications have been reported yet (57, 130–133).
- *Yield in OGIB*:: range from 33.3% (130) to 77% (133).
- *A unifying terminology for DBE and SBE has been proposed as "balloon-enteroscopy" or "balloon-assisted enteroscopy"*(134).

Spiral enteroscopy

Another new technique for deep SB intubation has recently been described (135) using a special overtube (Discovery Small Bowel, DSB, Spirus Medical Inc., Soughton, MA, USA) to pleat the SB onto the entero-scope, while advancing through it. The overtube can be used with "slim" enteroscopes (Fujinon EN-450T5 or Olympus SIF-Q180) or a pediatric colonoscope. The DSB has raised helices at the distal end and clockwise rotation of the DSB pleats the SB onto the overtube (Fig. 10.5).

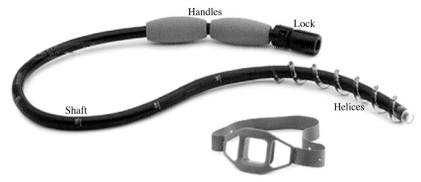

Figure 10.5 Endo-Ease Discovery SB overtube (Reproduced from Akerman et al. (135) with permission from Springer.)

- *Advantages*:
  - ○ depth of insertion comparable with other deep enteroscopy techniques
  - ○ much less time consuming (135, 136).
- *Complications:*: generally minor (minimal mucosal trauma and sore throat) (135, 136).
- *Yield in*: *OGIB*: In a study involving 27 patients the diagnostic yield was 33% (135). Future studies comparing the Discovery SB with balloon enteroscopy are needed.

Intraoperative enteroscopy

Generally performed as procedure last resort in OGIB, after all other techniques failed, or when DBE is either unavailable or cannot be successfully performed (due to the presence of abdominal adhesions or other technical factors) (1).

The endoscope can be inserted via the oral or anal routes, or through an operative enterotomy, while a surgeon telescopes the bowel over the tip of the endoscope by laparotomy or laparoscopy (1, 137).

- *Advantages:*: Using the oral and/or anal approaches, the terminal ileum can be reached in more than 90% of patients (1).
- *Pitfall:*: Trauma induced by insertion of the endoscope and bowel manipulation can be confused with angioectasias while the enteroscope is withdrawn (1).
- *Disadvantages:*: invasive, with high complication rates.
- *Complications:*: significant morbidity (including ileus, bacteremia) and high mortality (up to 17%). (1)
- *Yield in*: *OGIB*: Diagnostic yield is between 58%–88%. However, after therapy, bleeding has been reported to recur in 12.5%–60% (1).
- *Comparative Studies:*: In a prospective study, the sensitivity of CE (compared by IOE as a standard) was 95%, and the positive and negative predictive values – 95% and 86%, respectively. (69) Therefore, CE should be performed prior to consideration of intraoperative enteroscopy.

Guidelines, algorithms and integrative approach to small bowel bleeding

The European Society of Gastrointestinal Endoscopy (ESGE) has recently published a set of guidelines on the use of flexible enteroscopy for diagnosis and treatment of SB diseases (57). The recommendations pertinent to SBB are summarized in Table 10.1. The levels of evidence shown are based on the Oxford Centre for Evidence Based Medicine (138).

Table 10.1 Summary of ESGE guidelines for flexible endoscopy (pertinent to SBB), including category of evidence and grading of recommendations.

ESGE guidelines for flexible enteroscopy	Category of evidence	Grading of recommendation
Diagnostic efficacy of DBE for mid-gastrointestinal bleeding is superior to PE (79, 99)	1b	A
Diagnostic efficacy of DBE for mid-gastrointestinal bleeding is similar to CE (96, 97, 127)	1b	A
Patients with bleeding sites identified on CE should subsequently undergo flexible enteroscopy for endoscopic treatment (82, 90–92, 98, 100, 107, 130)	2b	B
Flexible enteroscopy is the preferred primary approach in patients with active ongoing mid-gastrointestinal bleeding with high probability of therapeutic interventions	2b	B
Intraoperative endoscopy should be reserved for patients with persistent significant mid-gastrointestinal bleeding in whom the bleeding source remains undiagnosed by flexible enteroscopy	5	B
The choice of either anal or oral route for the primary procedure depends on the suspected location of pathology within the small bowel (e.g. pathological findings detected by CE or other imaging modalities) (84)	2b	B
Resection of polyps within the small bowel can be performed with a complication risk similar to that of polyps in the right colon (88)	4	C

DBE, double-balloon enteroscopy; PE, push-enteroscopy; CE, video capsule endoscopy.
Adapted from Pohl et al. [57] with permission from Springer.

Two recent cost-benefit analyses examined the optimal management strategy for OGIB. One (33) compared no therapy (reference arm) to 5 competing modalities for a 50-year-old patient with *overt* OGIB:

1 PE,
2 IOE;
3 angiography;
4 initial anterograde DBE followed by retrograde DBE if the patient had ongoing bleeding; and
5 CE followed by DBE, guided by the CE findings.

It was suggested that DBE might be a more cost-effective modality than CE, especially when AVM were the cause for the bleeding. An initial CE was more costly and less effective. Moreover, the initial DBE arm resulted in an 86% bleeding cessation rate compared to 76% for the CE arm and 59% for the no-therapy arm. However, CE-directed DBE may be associated with better long-term outcomes because of the potential for fewer complications and decreased utilization of endoscopic resources (33). The second analysis (139)

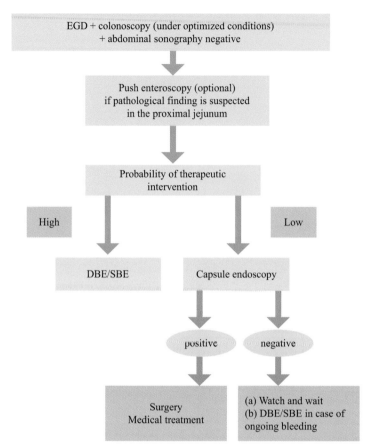

Figure 10.6 Algorithmic approach to mid-gastrointestinal bleeding. DBE, double-balloon enteroscopy; EGD, esophagogastroduodenoscopy; SBE, single-balloon enteroscopy. (Reproduced from Pohl et al. (57) with permission from Springer.)

compared five strategies: initial SBFT, enteroclysis, PE, CE, or DBE. The authors concluded that an initial DBE may be the least expensive strategy when treatment or definitive diagnosis is necessary and initial CE may be preferred when visual identification is sufficient. In settings where DBE is not available as an initial test, initial CE may be the preferred strategy (139).

Proposed algorithms for the investigation of mid-GI bleeding are based on patient clinical presentation, as well as on feasibility and technical considerations (57, 59). The recent ESGE algorithm (Fig. 10.6) recommended that *CE should be the initial diagnostic test* because of its noninvasive quality, tolerance, and ability to view the entire SB, as well as for *determining the initial route of flexible enteroscopy* (57). Flexible enteroscopy was advocated as a *follow-up procedure* in patients with a *positive finding on CE* requiring a biopsy or therapeutic intervention or if suspicion for a SB lesion is *high despite a negative CE* (57) *(i.e. in patients with overt-ongoing mid-GI bleeding)* (60).

Conversely, *flexible enteroscopy should be the first-line exploration* in patients with *active ongoing bleeding*, having a high probability of therapeutic interventions, in patients with *surgically modified anatomy*, especially those with an intestinal afferent loop (that cannot be assessed by CE), and in patients with *suspected stenosis* (clinically or by other imaging modalities). Although balloon-assisted enteroscopy might be considered the first step for most of these cases, PE is an easy-to-apply alternative in cases of suspected bleeding in the proximal jejunum or if DBE/SBE is not readily available (57). Despite the clinical utility of this algorithm, no recommendations are provided for the use of any imaging techniques such as scintigraphy, angiography, CT or MR studies. No algorithm recommendations have yet incorporated the newer spiral enteroscopy technique.

A recent algorithm (60) for cases of *occult* OGIB recommends starting with a CE, and performing DBE only if a potential source is identified. In patients with *overt* OGIB, DBE was proposed as the initial test because of the high likelihood of finding a potentially treatable lesion. The timing of DBE in OGIB has not been defined, but it is commonly considered 'emergent' when performed within the first 48 h of presentation. In their opinion, a true emergent DBE should be performed within 24 h, and preferably 12 h, of patient presentation (60).

The algorithm from the American Gastroenterological Association on obscure OGIB (Fig. 10.7) also recommends angiography for overt massive bleeding, but does not include DBE as a first line investigation in overt bleeding (1).

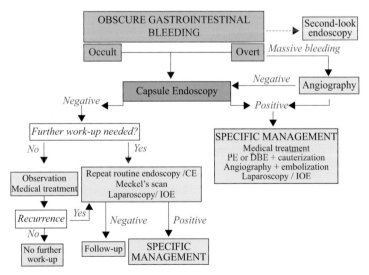

Figure 10.7 Proposed algorithm for the diagnosis and management of obscure GI bleeding. PE, push enteroscopy; IOE, intra-operative enteroscopy; CE, capsule endoscopy. (Reproduced from Raju et al. (1) with permission from Elsevier.)

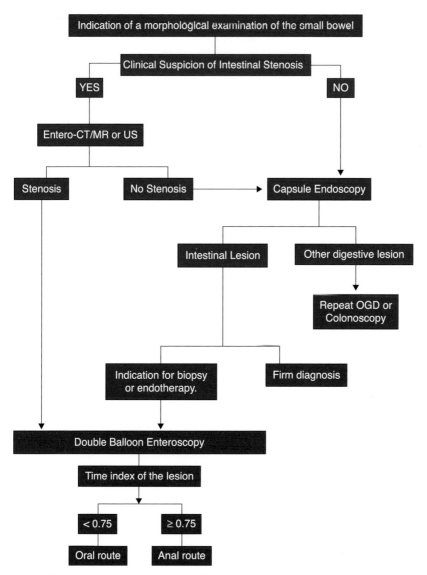

Figure 10.8 Algorithm proposed for the diagnostic work-up of patients with obscure digestive bleeding, integrating a combined approach by capsule endoscopy (CE) followed by push–pull enteroscopy when needed. CT, computed tomography; MR, magnetic resonance; US, ultrasound; OGD, esophagogastroduodenoscopy. (Reproduced from Delvaux et al. (53) with permission from Elsevier.)

The recent algorithm by Delvaux and Gay **(**Fig. 10.8**)** highlights the need to ascertain the absence of a stenosis before proceeding to CE in OGIB (53). In the latter situation, CT or MR studies should be done first. It also adds the concept of the time index of the lesion, using CE findings, to direct the route of DBE.

References

1. Raju GS, Gerson L, Das A, Lewis B, American Gastroenterological Association. AGA Institute technical review on obscure gastrointestinal bleeding. Gastroenterology 2007;133:1697–1717.
2. Ell C, May A. Mid-gastrointestinal bleeding: capsule endoscopy and push-and-pull enteroscopy give rise to a new medical term. Endoscopy 2006;38:73–5.
3. Carey EJ, Fleischer DE. Investigation of the small bowel in gastrointestinal bleeding – enteroscopy and capsule endoscopy. Gastroenterol Clin N Am 2005;34:719–34.
4. Gordon FH, Watkinson A, Hodgson H. Vascular malformations of the gastrointestinal tract. Best Pract Res Clin Gastroenterol 2001;15:41–58.
5. de' Angelis GL, Fornaroli F, de' Angelis N. et al. Wireless capsule endoscopy for pediatric small-bowel diseases. Am J Gastroenterol 2007;102:1749–57.
6. Filippone A, Cianci R, Milano A. et al. Obscure gastrointestinal bleeding and small bowel pathology: comparison between wireless capsule endoscopy and multidetector-row CT enteroclysis. Abdom Imaging 2008;33:398–406.
7. Sunada K, Yamamoto H. Double-balloon endoscopy: past, present, and future. J Gastroenterol 2009;44:1–12.
8. Seidman E, Dirks MH. Capsule endoscopy in the pediatric patient. Curr Treat Options Gastroenterol 2006;9:416–22.
9. Wu CR, Huang LY, Song B. et al. Application of double-balloon enteroscopy in the diagnosis and therapy of small intestinal diseases. Chin Med J 2007;120:2075–80.
10. Chen HL, Li SC, Chang W. et al. Identification of ectopic pancreas in the ileum by capsule endoscopy. J Formos Med Assoc 2007;106:240–3.
11. Stovicek J, Keeil R, Pálová S, Lochmannová J. Intestinal lymphangiectasia: a rare cause of gastrointestinal bleeding? Scand J Gastroenterol 2007;42:418.
12. Ohmiya N, Yano T, Yamamoto H et al. Diagnosis and treatment of obscure GI bleeding at double balloon endoscopy. Gastrointest Endosc 2007;66: S72–7.
13. Jain TP, Gulati MS, Makharia GK et al. CT enteroclysis in the diagnosis of obscure gastrointestinal bleeding: initial results. Clinical Radiology 2007;62:660–7.
14. Preud'homme DL, Michail S, Hodges C. et al. Use of wireless capsule endoscopy in the management of severe Henoch-Schonlein purpura. Pediatrics 2006;118:904–6.
15. Prakash C, Zuckerman GR. Acute small bowel bleeding: a distinct entity with significantly different economic implications compared with GI bleeding from other locations. Gastrointest Endosc 2003;58:330–5.
16. Sandrasegaran K, Maglinte DDT, Jennings SG, Chiorean MV. Capsule endoscopy and imaging tests in the elective investigation of small bowel disease. Clin Radiol 2008;63:712–23.
17. Maglinte DDT, Sandrasegaran K, Lappas JC, Chiorean M. CT Enteroclysis. Radiology 2007;245:661–71.
18. Fidler J. MR imaging of the small bowel. Radiol Clin North Am 2007;45:317–31.
19. Thoeni RF. Radiography of the small bowel and enteroclysis: a perspective. Invest Radiol 1987;22:930–6.
20. Maglinte DDT, Lappas JC, Heitkamp D.E. et al. Technical refinements in enteroclysis. Radiol Clin N Am 2003;41:213–29.
21. Padia SA, Bybel B, Newman JS. Radiologic diagnosis and management of acute lower gastrointestinal bleeding. Cleve Clin J Med 2007;74:417–20.
22. Moch A, Herlinger H, Kochman M.L. et al. Enteroclysis in the evaluation of obscure gastrointestinal bleeding. Am J Roentgenol 1994;163:1381–84.

23. Triester SL, Leighton JA, Leontiadis G.I. et al. A meta-analysis of the yield of capsule endoscopy compared to other diagnostic modalities in patients with obscure gastrointestinal bleeding. Am J Gastroenterol 2005;100;2407–18.

24. Costamagna G, Shah SK, Riccioni M.E. et al. A prospective trial comparing small bowel radiographs and video capsule endoscopy for suspected small bowel disease. Gastroenterology 2002;123:999–1005.

25. Malik A, Lukaszewski K, Caroline D. et al. A retrospective review of enteroclysis in patients with obscure gastrointestinal bleeding and chronic abdominal pain of undetermined etiology. Dig Dis Sci 2005;50:649–55.

26. Leighton JA, Sharma VK, Hentz J.G. et al. Capsule endoscopy versus push enteroscopy for evaluation of obscure gastrointestinal bleeding with 1-year outcomes. Dig Dis Sci 2006;51:891–9.

27. Higgs ZC, Macafee DA, Braithwaite BD, Maxwell-Armstrong CA. The Seldinger technique: 50 years on. Lancet 2005;366:1407–09.

28. Junquera F, Quiroga S, Saperas E. et al. Accuracy of helical computed tomographic angiography for the diagnosis of colonic angiodysplasia. Gastroenterology 2000; 119:293–9.

29. Bloomfeld RS, Smith TP, Schneider AM, Rockey DC. Provocative angiography in patients with gastrointestinal hemorrhage of obscure origin. Am J Gastroenterol 2000;95:2807–12.

30. Miller M, Smith TP. Angiographic diagnosis and endovascular management of non-variceal gastrointestinal hemorrhage. Gastroenterol Clin North Am 2005;34:735–53.

31. Kramer SC, Gorich J, Rilinger N. et al. Embolization for gastrointestinal hemorrhages. Eur Radiol 2000,10:802–5.

32. Mensink PB, Moons LM, Kuipers EJ. Chronic gastrointestinal ischaemia: shifting paradigms. Gut 2011;60:722–37.

33. Gerson L, Kamal A. Cost-effectiveness analysis of management strategies for obscure GI bleeding. Gastrointest Endosc 2008;68:920–36.

34. Zuckerman GR, Prakash C. Acute lower intestinal bleeding: part I: clinical presentation and diagnosis. Gastrointest Endosc 1998;48:606–17.

35. Fiorito JJ, Brandt LJ, Kozicky O. et al. The diagnostic yield of superior mesenteric angiography: correlation with the pattern of gastrointestinal bleeding. Am J Gastroenterol 1989;84:878–81.

36. Neu B, Ell C, May A. et al. Capsule endoscopy versus standard tests in influencing management of obscure digestive bleeding: results from a German multicenter trial. Am J Gastroenterol 2005;100:1736–42.

37. Engin G. Computed tomography enteroclysis in the diagnosis of intestinal diseases. J Comput Assist Tomogr 2008;32:9–16.

38. Miller FH, Hwang CM. An initial experience using helical CT imaging to detect obscure gastrointestinal bleeding. Clin Imaging 2004;28:245–51.

39. Peloquin JB, Pardi DS, Sandborn W.J. et al. Diagnostic ionizing radiation exposure in a population-based cohort of patients with inflammatory bowel disease. Am J Gastroenterol 2008;103:2015–22.

40. Rajesh A, Sandrasegaran K, Jennings S.G. et al. Comparison of capsule endoscopy with enteroclysis in the investigation of small bowel disease. Abdom Imaging 2009;34:459–66.

41. Huprich JE, Fletcher JG, Alexander J. et al. Obscure gastrointestinal bleeding: 64-channel multiphase, multiplanar CT enterography has a role. Radiology 2008;246:562–71.

42. Schmidt S, Lepori D, Meuwly J.Y. et al. Prospective comparison of MR enteroclysis with multidetector spiral-CT enteroclysis: interobserver agreement and sensitivity by means of "sign-by-sign" correlation. Eur Radiol 2003;13:1303–11.

43. Ettorre GC, Francioso G, Garribba A.P. et al. Helical CT angiography in gastrointestinal bleeding of obscure origin. Am J Roentgenol 1997;168:727–31.

44. Saperas E, Dot J, Videla S. et al. Capsule endoscopy versus computed tomographic or standard angiography for the diagnosis of obscure gastrointestinal bleeding. Am J Gastroenterol 2007;102:731–7.

45. Edelman DA, Sugawa C. Lower gastrointestinal bleeding: a review. Surg Endosc 2007;21:514–20.

46. Suzuki T, Matsushima M, Okita I. et al. Clinical utility of double-balloon enteroscopy for small intestinal bleeding. Dig Dis Sci 2007;52:1914–18.

47. Brünnler T, Klebl F, Mundorff S. et al. Significance of scintigraphy for the localization of obscure gastrointestinal bleedings. World J Gastroenterol 2008; 14:5015–19.

48. Gunderman R, Leef J, Ong K, et al. Scintigraphic screening prior to visceral arteriography in acute lower gastrointestinal bleeding. J Nucl Med 1998;39:1081–83.

49. Pennoyer WP, Vignati PV, Cohen JL. Mesenteric angiography for lower gastrointestinal hemorrhage: are there predictors for a positive study? Dis Colon Rectum 1997;40:1014–18.

50. Iddan G, Meron G, Glukhovsky A, Swain P. Wireless capsule endoscopy. Nature 2000;405:17.

51. Pennazio M, Eisen G, Goldfarb N. ICCE consensus for obscure gastrointestinal bleeding. Endoscopy 2005;37:1046–50.

52. ASGE Technology Status Evaluation Report: wireless capsule endoscopy. Gastrointest Endosc 2006;63:539–45.

53. Delvaux M, Gay G. Capsule endoscopy: technique and indications. Best Prac Res Clin Gastroenterol 2008;22:813–37.

54. Waterman M, Eliakim R. Capsule enteroscopy of the small intestine. Abdom Imaging 2009;34:452–8.

55. Rey JF, Ladas S, Alhassani A, Kuznetsov K. European Society of Gastrointestinal Endoscopy (ESGE). Video capsule endoscopy: update to guidelines (May 2006). Endoscopy 2006;38:1047–53.

56. Hartmann D, Eickhoff A, Damian U, Riemann JF. Diagnosis of small-bowel pathology using paired capsule endoscopy with two different devices: a randomized study. Endoscopy 2007;39:1041–45.

57. Pohl J, Delvaux M, Ell C. et al. ESGE Clinical Guidelines Committee. European Society of Gastrointestinal Endoscopy (ESGE) Guidelines: flexible enteroscopy for diagnosis and treatment of small-bowel diseases. Endoscopy 2008;40:609–18.

58. Delvaux M, Friedman S, Keuchel M. et al. Structured terminology for capsule endoscopy: results of retrospective testing and validation in 766 small-bowel investigations. Endoscopy 2005;37:945–50.

59. Saurin JC, Delvaux M, Gaudin J.L. et al. Diagnostic value of endoscopic capsule in patients with obscure digestive bleeding: blinded comparison with push enteroscopy. Endoscopy 2003;35:576–84.

60. Monkemuller K, Bellutti M, Fry CL, Malfertheiner P. Enteroscopy. Best Pract Res Clin Gastroenterol 2008;22:789–811.

61. Ho KK, Joyce AM. Complications of capsule endoscopy. Gastrointest Endosc Clin N Am 2007;17:169–78.

62. Guillion de Araujo Sant'Anna AM, Dubois J, Miron MC, Seidman EG. Wireless capsule endoscopy for obscure small-bowel disorders: final results of the first pediatric controlled trial. Clin Gastroenterol Hepatol 2005;3:264–70.

63. El-Matary W. Wireless capsule endoscopy: indications, limitations, and future challenges. J Pediatr Gastroenterol Nutr 2008;46:4–12.

64. Dirks MH, Costea F, Seidman EG. Successful videocapsule endoscopy in patients with an abdominal cardiac pacemaker. Endoscopy 2008;40:73–5.

65. Cave D, Legnani P, de Franchis R. et al. ICCE consensus for capsule retention. Endoscopy 2005;37:1065–67.

66. Herrerias JM, Leighton JA, Costamagna G. et al. Agile patency system eliminates risk of capsule retention in patients with known intestinal strictures who undergo capsule endoscopy. Gastrointest Endosc 2008;67:902–9.

67. Hartmann D, Schilling D, Bolz G. et al. Capsule endoscopy versus push enteroscopy in patients with occult gastrointestinal bleeding. Z Gastroenterol 2003;41:377–82.

68. Pennazio M, Santucci R, Rondonotti E. et al. Outcome of patients with obscure gastrointestinal bleeding after capsule endoscopy: report of 100 consecutive patients. Gastroenterology 2004;126:643–53.

69. Hartmann D, Schmidt H, Bolz G. et al. A prospective two-center study comparing wireless capsule endoscopy with intraoperative enteroscopy in patients with obscure GI bleeding. Gastrointest Endosc 2005;61:826–32.

70. Carey EJ, Leighton JA, Heigh R.I. et al. A single-center experience of 260 consecutive patients undergoing capsule endoscopy for obscure gastrointestinal bleeding. Am J Gastroenterol 2007;102:89–95.

71. Hindryckx P, Botelberge T, De Vos M, De Looze D. Clinical impact of capsule endoscopy on further strategy and long-term clinical outcome in patients with obscure bleeding. Gastrointest Endosc 2008;68:98–104.

72. Bresci G, Parisi G, Bertoni M et al. The role of video capsule endoscopy for evaluating obscure gastrointestinal bleeding: usefulness of early use. J Gastroenterol 2005;40:256–9.

73. Apostolopoulos P, Liatsos C, Gralnek I.M. et al. Evaluation of capsule endoscopy in active, mild-to-moderate, overt, obscure GI bleeding. Gastrointest Endosc 2007;66:1174–81.

74. Arakawa D, Ohmiya N, Nakamura M. et al. Outcome after enteroscopy for patients with obscure GI bleeding: diagnostic comparison between double-balloon endoscopy and videocapsule endoscopy. Gastrointest Endosc 2009;69:866–74.

75. Jones BH, Fleischer DE, Sharma V.K. et al. Yield of repeat wireless video capsule endoscopy in patients with obscure gastrointestinal bleeding. Am J Gastroenterol 2005;100:1058–64.

76. Mishkin DS, Chuttani R, Croffie J. et al. ASGE Technology Status Evaluation Report: wireless capsule endoscopy. Gastrointest Endosc 2006;63:539–45.

77. Marmo R, Rotondano G, Piscopo R. et al. Meta-analysis: capsule enteroscopy vs. conventional modalities in diagnosis of small bowel diseases. Aliment Pharmacol Ther 2005;22:595–604.

78. Gostout C.J. Sonde enteroscopy. Technique, depth of insertion, and yield of lesions. Gastrointest Endosc Clin North Am 1996;6:777–92.

79. Matsumoto T, Moriyama T, Esaki M. et al. Performance of antegrade double-balloon enteroscopy: comparison with push enteroscopy. Gastrointest Endosc 2006;62:392–8.

80. Mata A, Bordas JM, Feu F. et al. Wireless capsule endoscopy in patients with obscure gastrointestinal bleeding: a comparative study with push enteroscopy. Aliment Pharmacol Ther 2004;20:189–94.

81. Adrain AL, Dabezies MA, Krevsky B. Enteroscopy improves the clinical outcome in patients with obscure gastrointestinal bleeding. J Laparoendosc Adv Surg Tech A 1998;8:279–84.

82. Yamamoto H, Sekine Y, Sato Y. et al. Total enteroscopy with a nonsurgical steerable double-balloon method. Gastrointest Endosc 2001;53:216–20.

83. May A, Ell C. Push-and-pull enteroscopy using the double-balloon technique/ double-balloon enteroscopy. Dig Liv Dis 2006;38:932–8.

84. Gay G, Delvaux M, Fassler I. Outcome of capsule endoscopy in determining indication and route for push-and-pull enteroscopy. Endoscopy 2006;38:49–58.

85. Xu CD, Deng CH, Zhong J, Zhang CL. Application of double-balloon push enteroscopy in diagnosis of small bowel disease in children. Zhonghua Er Ke Za Zhi 2006;44:90–2.

86. Yano T, Yamamoto H, Sunada K. et al. Endoscopic classification of vascular lesions of the small intestine. Gastrointest Endosc 2008;67:169–72.

87. Regula J, Wronska E, Pachlewski J. Vascular lesions of the gastrointestinal tract. Best Pract Res Clin Gastroenterol 2008;22:313–28.

88. Mensink P, Haringsma J, Kucharzik T.F. et al. Complications of double balloon enteroscopy: a multicenter survey. Endoscopy 2007;39:613–15.

89. Pasha SF, Leighton JA, Das A. et al. Diagnostic yield and therapeutic utility of double-balloon enteroscopy (DBE) in patients with obscure gastrointestinal bleeding (OGIB): a systematic review [abstract]. Gastrointest Endosc 2007;65:AB366.

90. Yamamoto H, Kita H, Sunada K. et al. Clinical outcomes of double-balloon endoscopy for the diagnosis and treatment of small-intestinal diseases. Clin Gastroenterol Hepatol 2004;2:1010–16.

91. Mehdizadeh S, Ross A, Gerson L. et al. What is the learning curve associated with double balloon enteroscopy? Technical details and early experience in 6 U.S. tertiary care centers. Gastrointest Endosc 2006;64:740–50.

92. Ell C, May A, Nachbar L. et al. Push-and-pull enteroscopy in the small bowel using the double-balloon technique: results of a prospective European Multicenter Study. Endoscopy 2005;37:613–16.

93. Di Caro S, May A, Heine DG et al. DBE-European Study Group. The European experience with double-balloon enteroscopy, indications, methodology, safety, and clinical impact. Gastrointest Endosc 2005;62:545–50.

94. Akahoshi K, Kubokawa M, Matsumoto M. et al. Double-balloon endoscopy in the diagnosis and management of GI tract diseases: methodology, indications, safety, and clinical impact. World J Gastroenterol 2006;12:7654–59.

95. Mönkemüller K, Weigt J, Treiber G. et al. Diagnostic and therapeutic impact of double-balloon enteroscopy. Endoscopy 2006;38:67–72.

96. Hadithi M, Heine GD, Jacobs M.A. et al. A prospective study comparing video capsule endoscopy with double-balloon enteroscopy in patients with obscure gastrointestinal bleeding. Am J Gastroenterol 2006;101:52–7.

97. Nakamura M, Niwa Y, Ohmiya N. et al. Preliminary comparison of capsule endoscopy and double-balloon enteroscopy in patients with suspected small-bowel bleeding. Endoscopy 2006;38:59–66.

98. Heine GD, Hadithi M, Groenen M.J. et al. Double-balloon enteroscopy: indications, diagnostic yield, and complications in a series of 275 patients with suspected small-bowel disease. Endoscopy 2006;38:42–8.

99. May A, Nachbar L, Schneider M, Ell C. Prospective comparison of push enteroscopy and push-and-pull enteroscopy in patients with suspected small-bowel bleeding. Am J Gastroenterol 2006;101:2016–24.

100. Sun B, Rajan E, Cheng S. et al. Diagnostic yield and therapeutic impact of double-balloon enteroscopy in a large cohort of patients with obscure gastrointestinal bleeding. Am J Gastroenterol 2006;101:2011–15.

101. Manabe N, Tanaka S, Fukumoto A. et al. Double-balloon enteroscopy in patients with GI bleeding of obscure origin. Gastrointest Endosc 2006;64:135–40.

102. Zhi FC, Yue H, Jiang B. et al. Diagnostic value of double balloon enteroscopy for small-intestinal disease: experience from China. Gastrointest Endosc 2007;66: S19–21.

103. Hsu CM, Chiu CT, Su M.Y. et al. The outcome assessment of double-balloon enteroscopy for diagnosing and managing patients with obscure gastrointestinal bleeding. Dig Dis Sci 2007;52:162–6.

104. Safatle-Ribeiro AV, Kuga R, Ishida R. et al. Is double-balloon enteroscopy an accurate method to diagnose small-bowel disorders? Surg Endosc 2007;21:2231–36.

105. Mönkemüller K, Fry LC, Neumann H. et al. Diagnostic and therapeutic utility of double balloon endoscopy: experience with 225 procedures. Acta Gastroenterol Latinoam 2007;37:216–23.

106. Kaffes AJ, Siah C, Koo JH. Clinical outcomes after double-balloon enteroscopy in patients with obscure GI bleeding and a positive capsule endoscopy. Gastrointest Endosc 2007;66:304–9.

107. Zhong J, Ma T, Zhang C. et al. A retrospective study of the application on double-balloon enteroscopy in 378 patients with suspected small-bowel diseases. Endoscopy 2007;39:208–15.

108. Jacobs MA, Mulder CJ. Double-balloon enteroscopy in GI hemorrhage. Gastrointest Endosc 2007;66: S60–2.

109. Byeon JS, Chung JW, Choi K.D. et al. Clinical features predicting the detection of abnormalities by double balloon endoscopy in patients with suspected small bowel bleeding. J Gastroenterol Hepatol 2008;23:1051–55.

110. Hendel JW, Vilmann P, Jensen T. Double-balloon endoscopy: Who needs it? Scand J Gastroenterol 2008;43:363–7.

111. Tanaka S, Mitsui K, Yamada Y. et al. Diagnostic yield of double-balloon endoscopy in patients with obscure GI bleeding. Gastrointest Endosc 2008;68:683–91.

112. Lin TN, Su MY, Hsu C.M. et al. Combined use of capsule endoscopy and double-balloon enteroscopy in patients with obscure gastrointestinal bleeding. Chang Gung Med J 2008;31:450–6.

113. Kamalaporn P, Cho S, Basset N. et al. Double-balloon enteroscopy following capsule endoscopy in the management of obscure gastrointestinal bleeding: outcome of a combined approach. Can J Gastroenterol 2008;22:491–5.

114. Kameda N, Higuchi K, Shiba M. et al. A prospective, single-blind trial comparing wireless capsule endoscopy and double-balloon enteroscopy in patients with obscure gastrointestinal bleeding. J Gastroenterol 2008;43:434–40.

115. Lakatos PL, Fuszek P, Horvath H.C. et al. Double-balloon enteroscopy for the diagnosis and treatment of obscure bleeding, inflammatory bowel diseases and polyposis syndromes: we see more but do we know more? Hepatogastroenterology 2008;55:133–7.

116. Fujimori S, Seo T, Gudis K. et al. Diagnosis and treatment of obscure gastrointestinal bleeding using combined capsule endoscopy and double balloon endoscopy: 1-year follow-up study. Endoscopy 2007;39:1053–58.

117. Nakase H, Matsuura M, Mikami S, Chiba T. Diagnosis and treatment of obscure GI bleeding with double balloon endoscopy. Gastrointest Endosc 2007;66: S78–81.

118. Vilmann P, Jensen T, Hendel J. Double balloon endoscopy in obscure GI bleeding: the Danish experience. Gastrointest Endosc 2007;66: S63–5.

119. Choi H, Choi KY, Eun C.S. et al. Korean experience with double balloon endoscopy: Korean Association for the Study of Intestinal Diseases multi-center study. Gastrointest Endosc 2007;66: S22–5.

120. Li XB, Ge ZZ, Dai J. et al. The role of capsule endoscopy combined with double-balloon enteroscopy in diagnosis of small bowel diseases. Chin Med J (Engl) 2007;120:30–5.

121. Kuga R, Safatle-Ribeiro AV, Ishida R.K. et al. Small bowel endoscopy using the double-balloon technique: four-year results in a tertiary referral hospital in Brazil. Dig Dis 2008;26:318–23.

122. Schäfer C, Rothfuss K, Kreichgauer HP, Stange EF. Efficacy of double-balloon enteroscopy in the evaluation and treatment of bleeding and non-bleeding small bowel disease. Z Gastroenterol 2007;45:237–43.

123. Gerson LB, Batenic MA, Newsom S.L. et al. Long-term outcomes after double-balloon enteroscopy for obscure gastrointestinal bleeding. Clin Gastroenterol Hepatol 2009;7:664–9.

124. Madisch A, Schmolders J, Brückner S. et al. Less favorable clinical outcome after diagnostic and interventional double balloon enteroscopy in patients with suspected small-bowel bleeding? Endoscopy 2008;40:731–4.

125. Zhong J, Zhang CL, Ma T.L. et al. Comparative study of double-balloon enteroscopy and capsule endoscopy in etiological diagnosis of small intestine bleeding. Chin J Dig (Chin) 2004;24:741–4.

126. Ross A, Mehdizadeh S, Tokar J. et al. Double balloon enteroscopy detects small bowel mass lesions missed by capsule endoscopy. Dig Dis Sci 2008;53:2140–43.

127. Matsumoto T, Esaki M, Moriyama T. et al. Comparison of capsule endoscopy and enteroscopy with the double-balloon method in patients with obscure bleeding and polyposis. Endoscopy 2005;37:827–32.

128. Pasha SF, Leighton JA, Das A. et al. Double-balloon enteroscopy and capsule endoscopy have comparable diagnostic yield in small-bowel disease: a meta-analysis. Clin Gastroenterol Hepatol 2008;6:671–6.

129. Teshima CW, Kuipers EJ, Van Zanten SV, Mensink PB. Double balloon enteroscopy and capsule endoscopy for obscure gastrointestinal bleeding: an updated meta-analysis. J Gastroenterol Hepatol 2011;26:796–801.

130. Tsujikawa T, Saitoh Y, Andoh A. et al. Novel single-balloon enteroscopy for diagnosis and treatment of the small intestine: preliminary experiences. Endoscopy 2008;40:11–15.

131. Kawamura T, Yasuda K, Tanaka K. et al. Clinical evaluation of a newly developed single-balloon enteroscope. Gastrointest Endosc 2008;68:1112–16.

132. Hartmann D, Eickhoff A, Tamm R, Riemann JF. Balloon assisted enteroscopy using a single-balloon technique. Endoscopy 2007;39: E276.

133. Ramchandani M, Reddy DN, Rao G.V. et al. Diagnostic yield and therapeutic impact of single balloon enteroscopy; a series of 60 patients with suspected small bowel disease [abstract]. Gastrointest Endosc 2008;67:AB269.

134. Mönkemüller K, Fry LC, Bellutti M, Malfertheiner P. Balloon-assisted enteroscopy: unifying double-balloon and single-balloon enteroscopy. Endoscopy 2008;40: 537–8.

135. Akerman PA, Agrawal D, Cantero D, Pangtay J. Spiral enteroscopy with the new DSB overtube: a novel technique for deep peroral small-bowel intubation. Endoscopy 2008;40:974–8.

136. Akerman PA, Agrawal D, Chen W. et al. Spiral enteroscopy: a novel method of enteroscopy by using the Endo-Ease Discovery SB overtube and a pediatric colonoscope. Gastrointest Endosc 2009;69:327–32.

137. Bowden TA Jr, Hooks VH 3rd, Teeslink C.R. et al. Occult gastrointestinal bleeding: locating the cause. Am Surg 1980;46:80–7.

138. Oxford Centre for Evidence-based Medicine – Levels of, Evidence., [Online]. 2009 March. [Cited 2009 May 22]. Available from: URL: http://www.cebm.net/index. aspx?o=1025

139. Somsouk MA, Gralnek IM, Inadomi JM. Management of obscure occult gastrointestinal bleeding: a cost-minimization analysis. Clin Gastroenterol Hepatol 2008;6:661–70.

CHAPTER 11

Gastrointestinal Bleeding of Unknown Origin

Larry H. Lai, Aric J Hui & James Y.W. Lau
Institute of Digestive Disease, The Chinese University of Hong Kong, Hong Kong, China

Introduction

The diagnosis and management of gastrointestinal bleeding (GIB) have always been a challenge to clinicians. The condition is a common presentation of a wide array of lesions along the gastrointestinal tract. The advent of video capsule endoscopy (VCE) and balloon-assisted endoscopy (BAE) has significantly impacted the management of such patients. The diagnosis of small bowel bleeding is now easier with VCE. Access to small bowel lesions for biopsy and endoscopic therapy is also possible with the use of BAE.

Definitions

The American Gastroenterological Association (AGA) medical position statement defines obscure GIB as 'bleeding from the GI tract that persists or recurs without an obvious etiology after esophagogastroduodenoscopy (EGD), colonoscopy and radiologic evaluation of a small bowel such as small bowel follow-through or enteroclysis' (1). The condition can be further categorized into overt and occult bleeding depending on the presence or absence of visible signs of bleeding. Overt bleeding can be active or inactive at presentation. Occult GIB is often detected by a positive fecal blood test in a patient with iron deficiency anemia.

Traditionally, GIB is classified into bleeding from an upper or lower gastrointestinal source. Bleeding proximal to the ligament of Treitz is defined as upper GIB. With the establishment of the role and reach of EGD and colonoscopy, a new nomenclature has been proposed. Upper GIB is defined as bleeding from a source above the Ampulla of Vater in the second part of the duodenum. This is within reach of EGD. Mid-GIB refers to

Gastrointestinal Bleeding, Second Edition. Edited by Joseph J.Y. Sung, Ernst J. Kuipers and Alan N. Barkun. © 2012 Blackwell Publishing Ltd.
Published 2012 by Blackwell Publishing Ltd.

bleeding from the Ampulla of Vater to ileocecal valve. Colonic and rectal bleeding then defines lower GIB.

Etiology

The epidemiology of obscure GIB is not well defined owing to the diverse nature of these lesions. Patients with obscure gastrointestinal bleeding (Table 11.1) constitute approximately 5% of all cases. They include missed or overlooked lesions from EGD and colonoscopy and true small bowel lesions. Missed lesions include those from the upper tract, such as erosions or ulcers in a hiatus hernia (Cameron lesion), peptic ulcers or Dieulafoy lesions along the lesser curve of the stomach or in the duodenum, angiodysplasia, and antral ectasia. A Dieulafoy lesion is classically described to be found within 6 cm of the cardia. Lower gastrointestinal (GI) tract lesions include angiodysplasia, a cancer in the colon, or a diverticulum.

The differential diagnosis of patients with mid-GIB is somewhat dependent on his/her age. Young patients (those aged less than 40) are more likely to bleed from a Meckel diverticulum, small bowel tumors, Crohn disease, or celiac disease. Older patients tend to bleed from nonsteroidal anti-inflammatory drug (NSAID) enteropathy and angiodysplasia. There are uncommon causes such as hemobilia, hemosuccus pancreaticus, and aortoenteric fistulation in someone with prior abdominal aortic surgery.

Patients with an obscure GIB (OGIB) often require multiple procedures, prolonged and often recurrent admissions before a definite diagnosis is

Table 11.1 Etiology of obscure gastrointestinal bleeding.

Upper GI and lower GI bleeding overlooked	Mid GI bleeding
Upper GI lesions	Younger than 40 years of age
Cameron's erosions	Tumors
Fundic varices	Meckel's diverticulum
Peptic ulcer	Dieulafoy's lesion
Angiectasia	Crohn's disease
Dieulafoy's lesion	Celiac disease
Gastric antral vascular ectasia	Older than 40 years of age
Lower GI lesions	Angiectasia
Angiectasia	NSAID enteropathy
Neoplasms	Celiac disease
	Uncommon
	Hemobilia
	Hemosuccus pancreaticus
	Aortoenteric fistula

Adapted from Raju et al. [1] with permission from Elsevier.

made. The condition can therefore be costly to both the patients and the healthcare system.

Patient's evaluation and assessment

Taking a thorough history and performing a detailed physical examination remain integral to the patient's assessment. They provide useful information to guide diagnosis and subsequent management. Blood loss from gross hematuria and menorrhagia should be excluded. The characteristics of the blood loss provide a clue to the source of the GIB. A definite history of coffee ground or fresh hematemesis would suggest a lesion proximal to the ligament of Treitz, such as a Dieulafoy lesion. A drug history should be sought, including over-the-counter prescriptions. NSAID enteropathy causing small bowel bleeding is not uncommon among elderly patients. A family history may alert us to certain hereditary syndromes.

Certain cutaneous skin signs can enable physicians to deduce the etiology of an obscure GIB (2). Many syndromes associated with skin signs may be complicated with GIB. Commonly described congenital syndromes include Peutz Jeghers syndrome (intestinal hamartomatous polyps and mucocutaneous melanocytic macules), blue rubber bleb nevus syndrome (skin cavernous lesions which are typically bluish in color and compressible, and vascular malformation in the GI tract) and hereditary hemorrhagic telangiectasia (an autosomal dominant condition characterized by mucocutaneous telangiectases and visceral arteriovenous malformations (Figure 11.1). Other uncommon diseases include celiac disease with associated dermatitis herpetiformis in 2% of cases, Plummer-Vinson syndrome (koilonychias, angular cheilitis, glossitis, and post-cricoid web) and acquired immunodeficiency syndrome with Kaposi sarcoma.

Investigations

Repeat EGD and colonoscopy

In a significant proportion of patients with obscure GIB (OGIB), the bleeding source is within reach of conventional upper and lower endoscopy. From case series of patients with OGIB investigated by push enteroscopy, 10–64% of the identified lesions were within reach of EGD or colonoscopy. Zaman and Katon (3) used push enteroscopy to evaluate patients with OGIB. Of 39 lesions found in 95 patients, 25 (64%) were found at or above the major duodenal papilla. These included Cameron ulcers and AVM of stomach and proximal duodenum. Case series on the use of a double balloon enteroscopy (DBE) (4, 5) and video capsule endoscopy (6, 7) also support the benefit of

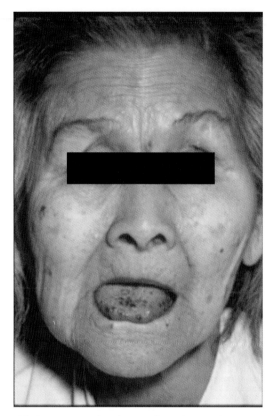

Figure 11.1 An elderly patient with Osler Rendu Weber syndrome. She has multiple mucocutaneous vascular lesions and visceral arteriovenous malformations.

repeating upper and/or lower endoscopy. Fry et al. identified a source of bleeding in 51 of 107 patients (47.6%) with the use of DBE. In 26 patients (24.3%), lesions were outside the small bowel (4). In another series consisting of 179 patients, the yield of DBE for a bleeding lesion was 65.9%. In 44 (24.6%) patients, lesions were not located in the small bowel (5), but were mostly vascular lesions. VCE examinations also found lesions outside the small bowel. In a prospective series of 143 patients with OGIB, 11 of them (3.5%) had a source in either stomach (GAVE and pyloric canal polyp) or colon (cancer and angiodysplasia) (7).

Colon lesions can often be missed. Leapers et al. retrospectively reviewed 286 patients with diagnosed colon cancers; 5.9% of these patients had received a colonoscopy within 6 weeks of diagnosis (8). The reasons for missed cancers were incomplete examination, poor bowel preparation, and misinterpretation of endoscopy findings. In a large community-based cohort study of 32,203 patients, Singh et al. found that 0.5% of those patients with negative colonoscopy had colorectal cancer diagnosed within 6 months of the index endoscopy (9).

Repeating EGD and/or colonoscopy as guided by clinical presentations may be worth while. In patients undergoing VCE or enteroscopy examinations, physicians should be vigilant in looking for a lesion in the upper or lower GI tract.

Small bowel series and enteroclysis

Small bowel series and enteroclysis (Figure 11.2) involve the ingestion or infusion of a radio-opaque contrast, usually barium sulfate through an endoscopically placed duodenal tube. Serial radiographs are then taken to visualize the small bowel as contrast propagates distally with peristalsis. Air or methylcellulose is often administered to distend the small bowel for better visualization. In an early series of OGIB, the diagnostic yield with small bowel enteroclysis was between 10 and 20% (10, 11). Rex et al. found a yield of 10% in 124 consecutive patients. Moch et al. found 27 (21%) lesions in 128 patients who underwent the technique for OGIB (11). The lesions consisted of small bowel tumors (13%) and AVM (2%). The technique is poor in finding mucosal lesions such as angioectasias. Small bowel series and conventional enteroclysis have largely been replaced by modern imaging techniques.

Radionuclide scan

A radionuclide scan using technetium–99m (^{99m}Tc) sulfur colloid or ^{99m}Tc pertechnate-labeled autologous red blood cells is theoretically a sensitive test even for slow bleeding at a rate of 0.1 ml per minute (Figure 11.3).

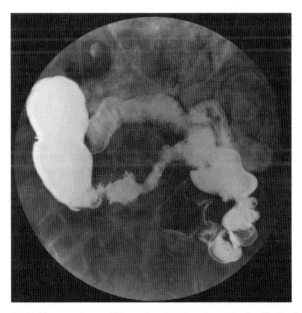

Figure 11.2 Picture of a small bowel series showing a Crohn ileal stricture.

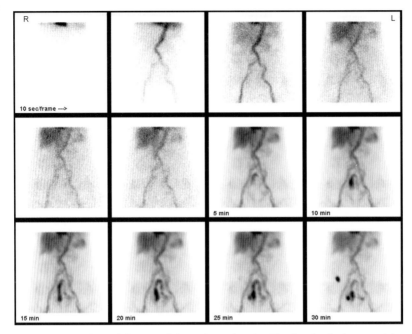

Figure 11.3 A radionuclide scan of the patient, showing bleeding in the bottom right section.

A positive scan can be seen in up to 60% of patients. Localization of the bleeding site is unfortunately poor, especially those in the foregut. A positive scan often fails to direct the definitive treatment. In 103 patients with bleeding, Voeller et al. compared findings from a radionuclide scan to bleeding sites determined at surgery, angiography, or endoscopy. A bleeding site in 85 patients was identified during scanning. In 29 patients with an upper GI bleeding source, sensitivity of the scan was only 8%; 5 positive scans had incorrectly localized the source. The sensitivity for lower GI bleeding was 23%. Surgery was required in 18 patients for bleeding,; 11 of whom had negative scans for bleeding. Half of the patients with negative scans for bleeding had positive localizing arteriograms (12). Of 137 patients who underwent a technetium 99 red cell scan, 70 were positive. The correct site of bleeding was localized in a third as foregut bleeding. The localization of colonic bleeding was higher (15 of 20 cases) (13). In a recent series, Brunnler et al. retrospectively reviewed 92 cases and found positive scintigraphies in 73% of these cases. The bleeding source was reliably localized (37% in the small bowel, 25% in the right colon) (14).

Mesenteric angiogram
Mesenteric angiography has the advantages of an immediate diagnosis, accurate localization of the site of bleeding, and does not require bowel

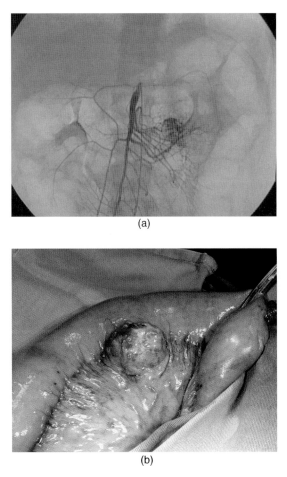

(a)

(b)

Figure 11.4 (a) A mesenteric angiogram of proximal jejunal bleeding. (b) At laparotomy, a bleeding jejunal diverticulum was found.

preparation. It also has a potential for therapeutic intervention (15–18). The examination involves selective cannulation of mesenteric arteries and injection of contrast under fluoroscopy. Active bleeding can be seen as extravasation of contrast (Figures 11.4a and 11.4b). Abnormal vasculature of tumors and angiodysplasia can sometimes be seen. In a Meckel diverticulum, a persistent vitelline artery can be seen. The diagnostic yield of mesenteric angiography is dependent on the speed of bleeding and the expertise of the interventional radiologists. Most of the series reported a high yield on the use of angiography in patients with massive bleeding. Typically, bleeding at a rate of 0.5 ml per minute or more can be readily diagnosed. Mesenteric angiography is therefore particularly useful when active and significant bleeding is suspected. An improved yield has been reported with the use of provocative tests such as an intra-arterial injection of tolazoline. Embolization using a biodegradable gelatin sponge or micro-coils provides a more definitive hemostasis. Embolization is, however, associated with a risk of small bowel infarction. Kramer reported a complication rate of 14% in 35 patients, including 4 fatal deaths from intestinal ischemia (15).

Push enteroscopy

A push enteroscope (PE) is a longer version (2.5 m) of an upper GI endoscope. Often a pediatric or standard colonoscope is used. It is passed per orally with the patient in a left lateral decubitus position similar to an EGD examination. The instrument is advanced as far as possible into the small bowel. The scope is then withdrawn with a clockwise torque in order to straighten the loop. The maneuver is then repeated. Scope advancement can be aided with the use of abdominal pressure, change of patient's position, or the use of an overtube to avoid the formation of the stomach loop. An overtube needs to be back-loaded onto the scope itself. Having reached the second or third part of duodenum, the scope is then straightened. The overtube can then be slid over the scope in the proximal duodenum before further advancement. A PE can often reach beyond the ligament of Treitz for a further distance of 80 cm without the assistance of balloons or overtubes. The procedure can be performed under fluoroscopy. It can, however, examine only a portion of proximal small bowel. The diagnostic yield of PE varied from 24 to 56% in reported series (19–21).

Intra-Operative enteroscopy

Intra-operative enteroscopy can be performed during a laparotomy or laparoscopy in some centers. It is reserved as a method of last resort for patients in whom a source remains elusive despite extensive investigations. The endoscope is commonly introduced per orally or occasionally via an enterostomy. A surgeon then gently telescopes the small bowel over the endoscope. Inspection of the entire length of the small bowel is possible in over 90% of cases (22). Intra-operative enteroscopy was once the gold standard in small bowel examination before the era of balloon-assisted enteroscopy. Intra-operative enteroscopy has been associated with complications of a laparotomy and general anesthesia. In addition, the procedure carries the complications of serosal tear, mesenteric hematoma and prolonged post-operative ileus. Manipulation of the small bowel often causes artifacts to the small bowel mucosa and makes interpretation difficult. The advent of balloon-assisted enteroscopy has helped to avoid a laparotomy in most patients. Intra-operative enteroscopy is used only when a laparotomy becomes necessary because of massive bleeding in patients in whom balloon-assisted enteroscopy hasd failed to reach the target lesion and for confirmatory purposes.

Computer tomography enterocylsis

Computer tomography (CT) enteroclysis combines small bowel enteroclysis with CT helical scanning using multi-detector systems. The combined imaging modality provides better quality images and diagnostic yield when compared to conventional small bowel enteroclysis alone. It has the advantages of detecting extraluminal lesions such as tumors, fluid collections, and fistulations (Figure 11.5). The examination requires the insertion of a duodenal tube with an EGD to allow for infusion of a high volume of methylcellulose. CT enterocylsis has a specific role for imaging suspected Crohn disease in patients with suspected intestinal obstruction in whom VCE is contraindicated or small bowel mass lesions. Series in the literature have reported a diagnostic yield between 36 and 48% (23–25).

With the aid of computerized reformatting, CT angiography is now possible and is comparable to diagnostic mesenteric angiography in its diagnostic yield (Figure 11.6). In an earlier study, Ettorre et al. found bleeding sites in 13 of 18 patients with active bleeding. The sites of bleeding were confirmed either at surgery or percutaneous angiography in all patients (26). In 22 patients with acute massive bleeding, Huprich et al. showed that CT angiography was able to identify the source of bleeding in 10 of them (27). Yoon et al. detected extravasation of contrast in 21 of 26 patients with bleeding (28). In a recent series, CT angiography found active bleeding in 22 of 86 examinations (26%). No further intervention was needed in 59 of 64 patients after a negative examination. A 92% negative

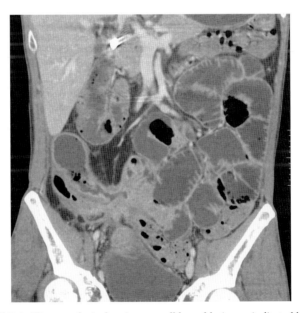

Figure 11.5 A CT enteroclysis showing a small bowel lesion as indicated by arrows.

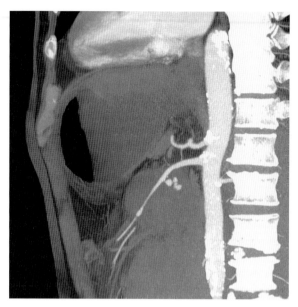

Figure 11.6 A reformatted film of a CT angiography showing active bleeding from jejunal branch of superior mesenteric artery.

predictive value was reported (29). In patients with active bleeding, CT angiography using a multi-detector row appears to be moderately sensitive and highly specific in diagnosing the source of bleeding.

Video capsule endoscopy

VCE systems

Currently four VCE systems are available: PillCam® SB (Given Imaging Ltd., Yoqneam, Israel), EndoCapsule® (Olympus Corp., Tokyo, Japan), MiroCam® (IntroMedic Co. Ltd., Seoul, Korea), and OMOM Capsule Endoscopy® (Jianshan Science and Technology (Group) Co. Ltd., Chongqing, China). With the miniature video camera, light-emitting diode, battery, and signal transmitter all encapsulated in a tiny plastic capsule, VCE provides a noninvasive method of obtaining a luminal view of the small intestine (Figure 11.6). After ingestion, the capsule is propelled along the gastrointestinal tract by peristalsis. It captures images at a frequency of 2–4 frames per second, and the total operating time can be up to 8 hours. The capsule transmits color images to a data collector. The patient wears sensors pads on the abdominal wall which are connected to the data box.

A period of fasting or clear fluid diet is generally required. The use of a bowel preparation before the study improves viewing of the small bowel. Clear liquids are generally allowed 2 hours after capsule ingestion or when the capsule has traversed the pylorus on real time images. The patient can take light meals 4 hours after ingestion of the capsule. Prokinetic agents are sometimes used if the capsule fails to pass beyond the stomach. A capsule delivery system can also be used to deliver the capsule endoscopically in patients with anatomical abnormalities in the upper GI tract or gastroparesis that prevents the capsule from passing into the stomach.

The contraindications for the use of VCE include suspected GI obstruction, strictures or fistula, cardiac pacemakers, and other implanted electromedical devices and swallowing disorders. The patient should also be warned against magnetic resonance imaging after VCE examination until after passage of the capsule has been confirmed. VCE is a well-tolerated and safe procedure. It is associated with a small risk of capsule retention which is defined as having the VCE remain within the digestive tract for a minimum of 2 weeks or requires directed therapy to aid its passage. In a retrospective review of 1291 Korean patients, capsule retention occurred in 2.5% of cases, which were associated with Crohn disease, small bowel tumors (Figure 11.7a and b) and tuberculous enterocolitis (30). In a single center experience of 1000 VCE procedures, capsule retention occurred in 1.4% of patients. Of 14 patients, 11 had NSAID enteropathy near diaphragmatic hiatus (31). Three were due to cancerous obstruction. In another series of 983 VCE examinations in the United States, capsule retention occurred in 5 of 28 (13%) patients with known Crohn disease (Figure 11.8a and b). The incidence was much lower in those with suspected Crohn disease (1 in 64, 1.6%) (32). An agile patency system, developed to predict patients with strictures and to avoid retention, consists of a plastic film encasing a lactose–barium mixture and a small transponder. In patients suspected to have stricture that cannot be demonstrated by other methods, this ingestible and dissolvable capsule will help to determine the functional patency of the gastrointestinal tract. There has been no reported case of capsule retention in patients with normal anatomy.

VCE in OGIB

Pennazio et al. reported a series of 100 consecutive patients with OGIB (33). The diagnostic yield of VCE was the highest among patients with ongoing overt bleeding (92.3%) as compared to occult bleeding alone, with guaiac-positive stools and iron deficiency anemia (44.2%), and the most common findings were angiodysplasia and Crohn disease. VCE has a high positive predictive value of 97% in patients with overt bleeding. Other series reported a diagnostic yield from 42 to 92% (34–39). Some of the series did not distinguish clinical significant lesions from incidental ones. The yield is higher in those with overt bleeding, especially those with active overt bleeding. To improve its diagnostic yield, VCE should be performed as close to the bleeding episodes as possible.

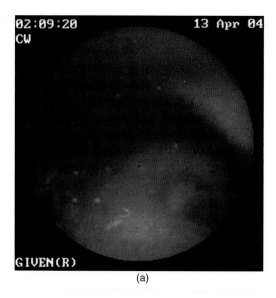

(a)

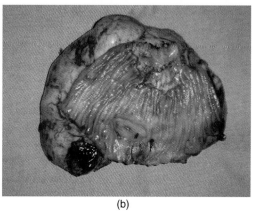

(b)

Figure 11.7 (a) A VCE image of a small bowel stromal tumor with central ulceration. (b) Surgical specimen showing a piece of resected small bowel. The small bowel was opened along its antimesenteric border showing the same ulceration.

Negative VCE

A negative VCE examination is associated with lower rate of recurrent bleeding in the median term and reassures clinicians of a more favorable outcome. In a study of patients after a negative VCE, the rate of recurrent bleeding was only 5.6% after a median follow-up period of 19 months, which was significantly lower than those after a positive VCE (48.4%) (41). In another study from the United Kingdom, Macdonald et al. demonstrated a similar finding (rebleeding rate: 42% in positive VCE versus 11% in negative VCE) (42).

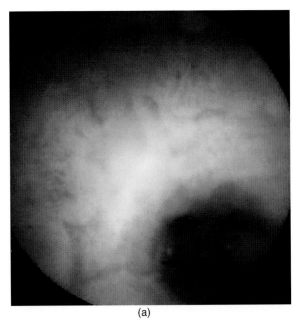

(a)

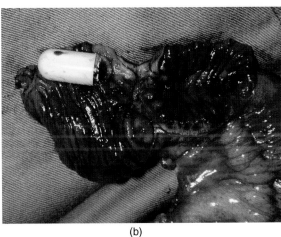

(b)

Figure 11.8 (a) An image of a Crohn stricture as seen by CE. (b) Picture of Crohn stricture with a retained capsule. Also note blood within the small bowel, indicating ongoing bleeding.

False negative VCE examinations

Although uncommon, significant small bowel lesions can be missed by VCE. In a concordance study comparing CE and DBE among 193 patients with OGIB, Marmo et al demonstrated that 7 out of 18 patients with negative VCE had alternative pathologies found by DBE, which include angiodysplasias, ulcers, ulcerated stromal tumour and jejunal diverticula (42). In a small series of 5 patients after negative VCE, significant pathology was found mostly in the proximal small bowel (adenocarcinoma, malignant melanoma, varices, stromal tumor, and Peutz Jegher polyp) (43). Ross et al. reviewed 183 cases who underwent DBE for OGIB. A small bowel mass was identified in 18 patients. Of these patients, 15 had prior VCE. In the series, all 4 cases of adenocarcinoma were missed by VCE (44). The suboptimal performance of VCE in the proximal small bowel, in particular the duodenum and around the periampullary region, is expected. Peristalsis in the proximal small intestine is more vigorous. Without the aid of air insufflation and motion control, lesions behind mucosal folds and nonbleeding lesions can be readily missed.

Second look VCE

If VCE fails to identify the cause of OGIB, a second VCE may be considered. Viazis et al. studied 76 patients after an initial nondiagnostic VCE and subsequently received a second look VCE for a new episode of bleeding and a drop of hemoglobin > 2 g/dl in a follow-up period of 24 months. Thirty-seven of 76 patients had lesions detected on repeat VCE (45). In 20 patients with severe iron deficiency anemia and a nondiagnostic VCE, Bar-Meir et al. repeated VCE and in 7 of them significant findings were seen (46). A second VCE should be considered in patients after a negative initial evaluation if patients should re-bleed.

Deep enteroscopy

When compared to VCE, balloon-assisted enteroscopy not only allows examination of the small bowel but it has the capability of tissue sampling and therapy if indicated. The current techniques include single or double enteroscopy systems and recently enteroscopy using the spirus overtube (Figure 11.9a, b, and c).

Double-Balloon enteroscopy system

The double-balloon enteroscopy (DBE) system (Fujinon EN–450P5/20; Fujinon Inc., Saitama, Japan) contains a video endoscope 8.5 mm in diameter and 200 cm in length, a polyurethane overtube 12.2 mm in diameter and 145 cm in length, a balloon-inflating device, and two soft latex balloons attached at the tips of both the endoscope and the overtube (Figure 11.9). Through its working channel, DBE also enables us to take a biopsy and perform endoscopic interventions (Figure 11.10a and b). By sequential inflation and deflation of the two balloons and passage of the overtube, it pleats the small bowel over the shaft of the enteroscope (Figure 11.11). Usually the examination is performed in two separate sessions –: oral and anal route – although sometimes it is possible to accomplish the whole examination with the oral route only. To ensure completion of total enteroscopy, tattooing at the maximal depth of insertion from one route

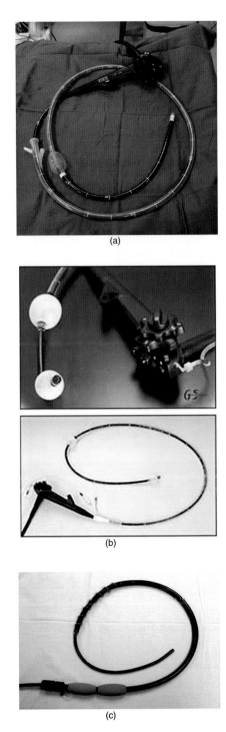

Figure 11.9 A picture of single- and double-balloon enteroscopes and an endoscope with a spiral overtube.

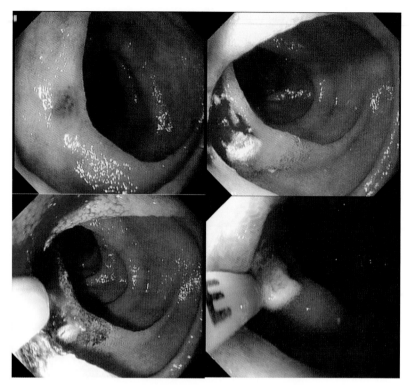

Figure 11.10 A small bowel angiodysplasia treated by argon plasma coagulation during balloon enteroscopy.

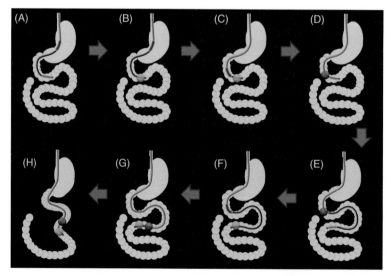

Figure 11.11 Mechanism of DBE. Double Balloon Method. *(Courtesy of Tomonori Yano, Jichi Medical School).*

shall be met by the other route. During the procedure, conscious sedation is often needed in the form of intravenous benzodiazepines or propofol. Carbon dioxide is used to reduce the patient's discomfort.

Yamamoto et al. reported the first large series of 123 patients with use of DBE. Total enteroscopy was attempted in 28 patients with a success rate of 86%. The diagnostic yield was up to 60% (47). Other case series that included more than 600 patients revealed a diagnostic yield ranging from 60 to 90% (48–53). Timing of the DBE is also crucial for its usefulness. In a retrospective review of 10 patients with overt bleeding who underwent emergency DBE, a bleeding source was found in 9 of 10 patients (48).

Complications relating to DBE occur in about 1% of cases. In an US multicenter study of 2478 DBE examinations, major complications occurred in 22 procedures (0.9%) (54). They include pancreatitis possibly due to traction injury on mesentery, bleeding and perforations. Altered anatomy from prior surgeries increases the risk of bowel perforations from DBE. A European multicenter study reported a total of 85 adverse events in 2362 DBE procedures. The rate of complications was higher with therapeutic procedures (4.3%) when compared to that of diagnostic procedures (0.8%) (55).

Similar to other advanced endoscopic procedures, DBE is associated with a learning curve. In an US multicenter study of 237 DBE procedures, the mean time for per oral examination decreased significantly after the first 10 cases coupled with reduced fluoroscopy time (56).

Single-Balloon enteroscopy system

The single-balloon enteroscopy (SBE) system consists of a video enteroscope (XSIF-Q260Y; Olympus Corp., Tokyo, Japan), a sliding tube with balloon (XST-SB1; Olympus Corp., Tokyo, Japan), and a balloon controller (XMAJ–1725; Olympus Corp., Tokyo, Japan). Its specifications are comparable with those of the DBE system from Fujinon, Japan. The videoscope has a working length of 200 cm with an outer diameter of 9.2 mm, but it does not have a balloon on its tip (Figure 11.9). It has a channel diameter of 2.8 mm. The sliding tube is made of silicone, measuring 140 cm in length and 13.2 mm in outer diameter, and an inflatable silicon balloon attached at its tip. The balloon can be inflated up to 5.4 kPa.

The enteroscope is controlled by an endoscopist, and the overtube and balloon controller are operated by an assistant. With the tube fitted onto the enteroscope, enteroscopy is first advanced with the balloon in a deflated condition, either through the oral antegrade route or the anal retrograde route. When the enteroscopy reaches the maximal insertion or small bowel, the balloon is then inflated to fix the tube to the intestinal wall. Both the enteroscope and sliding tube are slowly withdrawn and straightened. Next, the tip of the enteroscope is inserted into the deep part of the intestine and is bent to fix it to the intestine. The sliding tube with the deflated balloon is

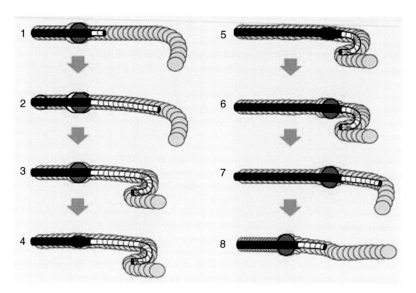

Figure 11.12 Mechanism of SBE.

then moved forward along the enteroscope. This process is repeated until it is no longer able to advance (Figure 11.12).

In a series of 41 patients from Japan (57), the diagnostic yield of SBE was 53.7%. The mean insertion time was 63 ± 20 minutes for the oral approach and 70 ± 19 minutes for the anal approach. Among 24 patients in whom total enteroscopy was attempted, the entire small intestine was explored in 25%. Complications occurred in 2 patients only, with one suspected aspiration pneumonia, and one mucosal tear along a longitudinal ulcer scar requiring endoscopic clipping. Riccioni et al. reported a single center experience of 73 SBE procedures in 70 patients. In 47 patients, a diagnosis was made including 7 small bowel tumors (58). Aktas et al. prospectively studied complications following 166 SBE procedures in 105 patients. One perforation occurred followed a dilatation of a stricture (1 in 21 therapeutic procedures). 16% of patients had hyperamylasemia but none had clinical pancreatitis. SBE appears to be a safe procedure with a rate of complication comparable to that of DBE (59).

Spiral enteroscopy

Akerman et al. reported the first experience in the use of Endo-Ease discovery SB (DSB, Spirus Medical Inc., Stoughton, Mass.) overtube for enteroscopy. A standard video pediatric colonoscope (PCF–140L; Olympus America Inc., Center Valley, Pa) with a working length of 160 cm and an outer diameter of 11.5 mm is used as an enteroscope (60).

DSB is a single use overtube with a working length of 130 cm, an internal diameter of 12.7 mm, and an external diameter of 17.5 mm. The distal 21 cm of the overtube has 5 mm helical spirals. The tube lightly connects to the enteroscope by a lock and rotates independently from the enteroscope. The assembly can be advanced as a unit with the scope locked. The spiral overtube is advanced by rotating the two soft handles below the lock. The scope can be unlocked from the overtube and advanced independently.

In an initial experience of 25 patients, the average depth of insertion was 175 cm beyond the ligament of Treitz and the average time for procedure was 36.5 minutes. There was no major complication except a minor esophageal tear and a sore throat. In a subsequent US multicenter registry (61), 93% of 101 patients with OGIB underwent successful antegrade spiral enteroscopy. The median depth of scope insertion was 250 cm beyond the ligament of Treitz. The diagnostic yield was 65% and commonest abnormality was angioectasia.

Comparative studies of techniques in deep enteroscopy

There have been three randomized studies that compared single- with double-balloon enteroscopy with conflicting results. May et al. randomized 100 patients to receive either single- or double-balloon enteroscopy (62). Complete enteroscopy was possible in two-thirds of patients in the DBE group. The rate of complete enteroscopy was only 22% with the use of a single balloon. Consequently the diagnostic yield with DBE was higher. A randomized trial by Takano et al. (63) reported 0% rate of total enteroscopy with the use of SBE and a rate of 57.1% with DBE. In another multicenter study, Domagk et al. (64) randomized 130 patients (65 in each) to receive either single or double enteroscopy. The mean intubation depth for the per oral route and the per anal route were comparable (258 cm vs. 253 cm and 118 cm vs. 107 cm, respectively). The rate of total enteroscopy was higher with the use of DBE (18 vs. 11%) although the difference did not reach a statistical significance.

There have been few comparative studies between balloon-assisted enteroscopy and enteroscopy using a spiral overtube. In 10 patients, May et al. performed back to back DBE via the oral route and spiral enteroscopy in a randomized fashion (65). DBE consistently reached further beyond the ligament of Treitz (310 cm vs. 250 cm, P = 0.004). In all cases where spiral enteroscopy was followed by DBE, DBE reached a further 100 cm. The mean examination time was, however, shorter with the use of spiral enteroscopy (43 vs. 65 minutes). Frieling et al. prospectively compared anterograde DBE and spiral enteroscopy in 35 patients and found a higher yield with use of DBE (47.1 vs. 33%) (66). In a retrospective cohort study, Khashab et al. compared the performance characteristics of SBE and spiral enteroscopy in 92 patients. The maximum depth of insertion was longer (301 cm vs. 222 cm) and the yield was higher (59.6% vs. 43.4%) with SBE. The examination time was similar between the two. Perforation occurred in one SBE procedure (67).

From these comparative studies, it appears that the rate of complete small bowel examination appear highest with DBE. It takes more time in its preparation, however, and the examination of the small bowel. The choice between these deep enteroscopy techniques often depends on the availability of local expertise. However, as a complete small bowel examination will likely translate into a higher diagnostic yield, most centers will opt for DBE.

Limited data in the literature reassure us that enteroscopic treatment of vascular lesions leads to acceptable median term outcomes. Gerson et al. (68) evaluated 40 patients after endoscopic treatment for AVMs, 17 reported no recurrent bleeding or anemia at 12 months. May et al. (69) followed up 44 patients with angiodyplasias treated by argon plasma coagulation through DBE. During a mean follow-up period of 55 months, mean hemoglobin increased from 7.6 g/dl to 11 g/dl after APC treatment. There was a corresponding decline in blood transfusion requirement. Bleeding, however, recurred in 21 of 44 patients and particularly in those with Osler–Rendu–Weber syndrome.

Table 7.2 summarizes the diagnostic yield of various modalities in small bowel examination of patients with obscure gastroinitestinal bleeding.

Comparative studies

The development of VCE and balloon-assisted enteroscopy has made the evaluation of the small bowel easier. Balloon-assisted enteroscopy also allows therapy to vascular lesions and polyps. Both modalities have made many conventional diagnostic modalities obsolete. Modalities such as mesenteric angiography and CT enterography or enteroclysis are used in specific situations and often complement the use of VCE and BAE.

VCE vs. conventional imaging modalities

VCE allows complete small bowel visualization but lacks the ability to sample mucosa and therapeutic intervention. When compared to most conventional imaging modalities, VCE is superior in its diagnostic yield. In a meta-analysis of 14 prospective studies with 396 patients with OGIB, VCE was superior in detecting clinically significant lesions when compared to push endoscopy (56% and 26%) and small bowel follow-through (47% and 6%, 3 studies with 88 patients). (70)

In a subsequent prospective randomized study (20) that compared VCE to push endoscopy, the initial diagnostic yield was significantly higher with the use of VCE (20 of 40 patients, 50% vs. 9 of 38 patients, 24%). The trial design allowed cross over to the other modality after initial examination. VCE detected an additional 10 lesions (26%) missed by push endoscopy. On the other hand, PE detected 3 lesions (8%) missed by VCE. The finding supports the use of VCE over push enteroscopy as the first line of investigation.

Table 11.2 A summary of studies on various modalities in the diagnosis and management of OGIB.

Imaging modality	First author, year	N	Diagnostic yield	Comments
Second look EGD	Zaman and Katon 1998 (Push enteroscopy)	95	25/39 (64%)	
	Fry et al. 2009 (DBE)	107	26/107 (24.3%)	
	Kitiyakara et al. 2005 (DBE)	140	9/140	
	Tee et al. 2010 (DBE)	179	44/179 (24.6%)	
	Vlachogiannakos et al. 2011 (VCE)	317	11/317 (3.5%)	
Small bowel series and enteroclysis	Moch et al. 1994	128	27, 21% confirmed or high probable lesions	Probably an obsolete imaging modality
	Rex et al. 1989	125	10%	
Radionuclide scan	Voeller et al. 1991	103	85 of 103	Scintigraphy failed to localize bleeding in 85% of patients.
	Howarth et al. 2002	137	70 of 137	Correct location in only 7 of 21 patients with foregut bleeding.
	Brunnler T et al. 2008	92	73%	37% in the small bowel, 25% in the right colon and 4.5% left colon, in 20% no clear localization
Mesenteric angiogram	Kramer et al. 2000	35	29/35	A series on embolization of miscellaneous causes of gastrointestinal bleeding. A high rate of complications (14%) including four intestinal ischemia with fatal outcomes

Continued p.268

Table 11.2 (continued)

Imaging modality	First author, year	N	Diagnostic yield	Comments
	Bloomfield et al. 2000	7	2 of 7	Provocative intra-arterial injection of tolazoline
	Kim et al. 2010	36	12 (11 active extravasation, 1 hypervascular tumor)	Provocative catheter injection of tPA, lower gastrointestinal bleeding only
Push enteroscopy	Peynircioqlu B et al. 2011	42	24 of 45 procedures	Massive bleeding only
	Chak et al. 1998	31	56%	11 of 35 had a source accessible by EGD
	De Leusse et al. 2007	38	9/38, 24%	
	Sidhu et al. 2008	155	30%	
Intraoperative enteroscopy	Schulz and Schmidt 2009		70–100%	
Computer tomography enteroclysis	Khalife 2011	32	11/32 (34%)	
	Jain TP 2007	21	10/21 (47.6%)	
	Voderholzer 2003	22	8/22 (36%)	A series on the diagnosis of Crohn's disease
CT angiography	Ettorre 1997	18	13 of 18	Bleeding sites confirmed at surgery or angiography
	Huprich et al. 2011	22	10/22	High sensitivity in detecting active contrast extravasation

Method	Study	N	Result	Comment
	Yoon et al. 2006	26	21/26 showed contrast extravasation	
	Kennedy et al. 2010	86	22/86 (26%)	86% and 92% positive and negative predictive value
VCE	Estrevez et al. 2006	100 (overt bleeding 48, obscure 52)	68% (33.8% angiodysplasias)	One capsule retention in the series
	Carey et al. 2007	260 (overt bleeding N=126, occult N=134)	53% (clinical significant findings)	Higher yield in overt obscure GIB (60 vs. 46%)
	Saurin et al. 2003	56	92%	
	Viazis et al. 2005	96	62.5%	
	Neu et al. 2005	56	68%	
	Delvaux et al. 2004	44 (22 occult, 22 overt bleeding)	18 (41.9%)	20.8% significance not determined
	Pennazio et al. 2005	100 (57 overt and 43 occult)	92.3% for active overt bleeding, 12.9% for inactive overt bleeding and 44.2% for occult bleedinges	
Double balloon enteroscopy	Monkemuller et al. 2009	10	9 of 10	Retrospective review of emergency DBE in 10 patients with overt bleeding
	Marmo et al 2009	193	59% – 72 (vascular lesions), 30 neoplasia, 12 (ulcers or inflammatory lesions)	Multicenter prospective study
	Arakawa et al. 2009	162	64%	
	Kaffles 2007	60	45 (75%)	Therapy in 34 patients (30 diathermies and 4 polypectomy)
	Sun 2007	152 (135 overt)	115 (75.7%)	
	Manabe 2007	31	23 (74.2%)	
	Hadithi 2006	35	21 (60%)	

In a prospective series of 28 patients with OGIB, CE was shown to be superior to CT angiography or mesenteric angiography (71). These patients were evaluated first by angiography and then with the use of VCE. VCE detected a bleeding source in more patients when compared to either CTA or standard mesenteric angiography (18 of 25, 6 of 25 and 14 of 25, respectively).

In a blinded comparison of VCE to CT enterography in 58 patients (overt bleeding 33, occult bleeding 25) from the Mayo Clinic (27), 16 of 58 patients were found to have a bleeding lesion. CT enterography was more sensitive in depicting these lesions (14 of 16 vs. 6 of 16 with VCE) and identified all of the 9 small bowel tumors in the series. On the other hand, VCE only identified 3 of these tumors.

In a two-center prospective study (72) that compared VCE to intra-operative enteroscopy in 47 patients with OGIB, VCE identified the source of bleeding in 74.4% of patients (100% of patients with active overt bleeding, 67% in those with inactive overt bleeding and obscure bleeding respectively). Using findings at IOE as the standard, VCE compares favorably with positive and negative predictive values of 95% and 86% respectively.

VCE has therefore been consistently shown to be superior in diagnostic yields when compared to PE and other conventional diagnostic modalities, and equal to that of intra-operative enteroscopy in detecting mucosal disease. When the diagnosis of small bowel tumor or a stricture is being considered, CT enterography may prove to be a good alternative.

BAE vs. conventional imaging modalities

Studies have also been conducted to compare DBE with other conventional modalities of investigations. Matsumoto et al. (73) compared antegrade DBE in 27 patients with PE in 91 patients. Length of insertion beyond the ligament of Trietz was longer with DBE (92 vs. 22 cm). More nonbleeding lesions were detected on antegrade DBE (79 vs. 31%) and similar results were found in a German study. DBE was associated with much superior insertion depth (230 cm in DBE vs. 80 cm in push enteroscopy) and diagnostic yield (73% in DBE vs. 44% in push enteroscopy) (74).

VCE vs. BAE

In a meta-analysis of 11 studies (75) that compared CE and DBE, the pooled overall yield for VCE and DBE was 60% and 57% (397 vs. 360 patients respectively). The respective yield for vascular lesions, inflammatory changes and small bowel tumors was similar.

In another meta-analysis of 8 studies (76), the yield of VCE and DBE was similar (170/277 vs. 156/277, OR 1.21). The yield of VCE was significantly higher than DBE performed either per oral or anal route. The yield of VCE was, however, not better to DBE when oral and anal insertion were combined (26/48 vs. 37/48). In a subgroup analysis of patients with OGIB, the yield of VCE was significantly lower than DBE (11/24 vs. 21/24).

VCE is noninvasive, well tolerated, and accepted by patients and safe. It is often preferred to DBE for evaluation of the small bowel. Many advocate a prior VCE as it can reduces the utilization of endoscopy resources and guide route of insertion with DBE if it becomes necessary. DBE is reserved for confirmatory purpose and therapeutic intervention. It can, however, be contended that DBE should be the first modality of choice in small bowel evaluation in patients likely to receive therapy. DBE examination is likely to be more thorough than VCE as the passage of VCE along the GI tract is passive while DBE can be stopped to carefully examine any suspicious lesions and look behind mucosal folds. A DBE first approach may be more appropriate in patients with active overt bleeding who are likely to require endoscopic hemostatic treatment. In a cost-effectiveness model, Gerson et al. (77) compared five different strategies as the initial approach in management of a patient with OGIB. These were PE, IOE, angiography, initial antegrade DBE followed by retrograde DBE in ongoing bleeding, and VCE. Under various assumptions over prevalence of different lesions and costs in their management, an initial DBE is the most cost-effective approach.

Diagnostic approach to patients with OGIB

As discussed in the above sections, VCE is generally comparable with DBE for its diagnostic role in small bowel diseases, but its tolerability and safety make it more acceptable to most patients and clinicians. On the other hand, DBE offers the additional benefit of immediate biopsy and therapeutic capability, which would shorten the time needed for management in OGIB patients. There are several published management algorithms proposed in the literature. These include the American Gastroenterological Association medical position statement, Consensus Statements for small bowel capsule endoscopy by an international panel of experts and, more recently, the Standards of Practice Committee recommendations commissioned by the American Society of Digestive Endoscopy (1, 78, 79). Common to these guidelines, OGIB is categorized into overt or occult bleeding. EGD and colonoscopy are repeated as guided by patients' presentation. VCE has a central or triaging role directing a subsequent imaging technique or therapy. In patients with active overt bleeding, there may be a role of immediate angiography or BAE with a view to offer therapy at the same setting. All other imaging techniques are complementary and should be considered in selected cases. A modified algorithm is presented in Figure 11.13.

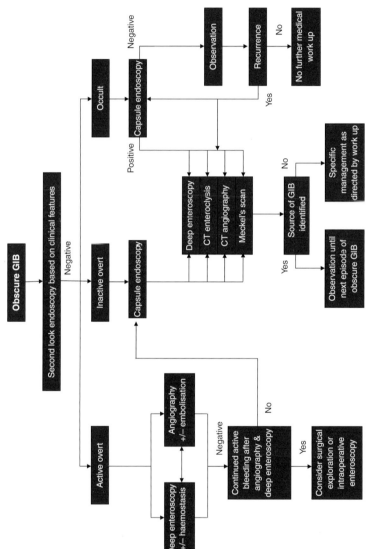

Figure 11.13 A proposed algorithm in the management of patients with obscure GIB.

Overt OGIB

It is useful first to categorize patients with overt bleeding as active and inactive ones. In patients with active overt bleeding, the first goal is to stabilize the patient's haemodynamic state. Once this is achieved, the second objective is to identify and stop the source of bleeding as soon as possible. For patients with clinical features suggestive of upper gastrointestinal bleeding, a repeat EGD is warranted. Investigations for small bowel bleeding should be conducted as soon as possible as diagnostic yield decreases with time. This is because once the bleeding stops, it can be very difficult to identify bleeding from angioectasia, Dieulafoy lesions and small ulcers. VCE is often recommended as the next investigation for OGIB patients after an initial negative EGD due to its high diagnostic yield, safety and excellent patient tolerance. VCE can be helpful in localizing the approximate location of small bowel bleeding to be followed up by deep enteroscopy. However, it should be noted that VCE is time consuming with no therapy possible. Alternatively, mesenteric angiography and deep enteroscopy are appropriate initial investigations for a patient with ongoing active obscure bleeding because both have high diagnostic yield and more importantly, also provide immediate therapeutic intervention should the source of bleeding be identified. Should these investigations fail and the patient continues to have severe active bleeding, exploratory laparotomy and intraoperative enteroscopy may be the last resort.

For patients whose bleeding has stopped spontaneously and hence classified as inactive overt bleeding, there is no urgency for haemostasis and VCE is probably the investigation of choice. VCE is useful both to guide subsequent investigations and stratify the patient's risk of rebleeding. A negative VCE is associated with a better prognosis and fewer episodes of recurrent bleeding but does not preclude the need for further work up. CT enterography or enteroclysis are particularly useful in identifying significant structural lesions such as tumors, strictures and large ulcers. This is especially important among young patients as small tumors remain common in those aged below 50. Elective deep enteroscopy or Meckel's scan should be considered based on the patient's clinical features. These investigations are particularly important in patients contraindicated for the use of VCE such as patients with altered surgical anatomy (e.g. after a gastrectomy and a Roux-en-Y jejunal reconstruction) and in whom a stricture is suspected (e.g. in a young patient with signs of small bowel obstruction and suspected Crohn's disease). All of the above modalities are complementary to each other. Often multiple tests are required before a final diagnosis is made.

Occult OGIB

EGD and colonoscopy are usually repeated in patients with occult bleeding. This is especially relevant in patients with risk factors for upper GI mucosal disease such as users of aspirin or non-steroidal anti-inflammatory drugs. The findings and quality of the index EGD and colonoscopy should be noted. Repeat colonoscopy should be considered if the first examination had suboptimal bowel preparation. During colonoscopy, efforts should be made to intubate and examine terminal ileum.

After a negative EGD and colonoscopy, it is reasonable to consider empirical iron therapy in someone who has had a minor bleed and that bleeding has not been recurrent. In most, VCE is usually recommended as the next investigation. VCE can usually provide clues to subsequent investigations – usually the choice between CT enterography/enteroclysis or BAE depending on nature of lesions found. There have been reports in the literature on the use of hormonal therapy and long acting octreotide in patients with small bowel angiectasias. (80–83) Both have not been investigated extensively or in common use.

Conclusions

The advents of VCE and BAE have significantly improved the management of patients with OGIB. Visualization of entire small bowel is now possible with VCE and BAE. In selected cases, definitive therapy can be instituted with the use of BAE. The improvement in clinical management has been modest. Whether this translates into improved outcome in patients with OGIB is uncertain, as in most cases the bleeding is self-limiting and prognosis is generally favorable. Laine et al. randomized 136 patients with OGIB after negative upper and lower endoscopy and PE to receive VCE and small bowel radiography. The diagnostic yield was higher with VCE (30 vs. 7%). Clinical outcomes of recurrent bleeding, need for intervention, hospitalization and blood transfusion at 12 months follow-up were similar (84). More long-term outcome data following different treatment strategies is required in the literature.

References

1. Raju GS, Gerson L, Das A, Lewis B, American Gastroenterological Association. American Gastroenterological Association (AGA) Institute technical review on obscure gastrointestinal bleeding. Gastroenterology 2007; 133: 1697–717.
2. Braverman IM. Skin signs of gastrointestinal disease. Gastroenterology 2003; 124: 1595–1614.
3. Zaman A, Katon RM. Push enteroscopy for obscure gastrointestinal bleeding yields a high incidence of proximal lesions within reach of a standard endoscope. Gastrointest Endosc 1998; 47: 372–6.
4. Fry LC, Bellutti M, Neumann H, Malfertheiner P, Monkemuller K. Incidence of bleeding lesions within reach of conventional upper and lower endoscopes in patients

undergoing double balloon enteroscopy for obscure gastrointestinal bleeding. Aliment Pharmacol Ther 2009; 29: 342–9.

5. Tee HP, Kaffles AJ. Non small bowel lesions encountered during double-balloon enteroscopy performed for obscure gastrointestinal bleeding. World J Gastroenterol 2010; 21: 1885–9.

6. Kitiyakara T, Selby W. Non small bowel lesions detected by capsule endoscopy in patients with obscure BI bleeding. Gastrointest Endosc 2005; 62: 234–8.

7. Vlachogiannakos J, Papaxoinis K, Viazis N, et al. Bleeding lesions within reach of conventional endoscopy in capsule endoscopy examinations for obscure gastrointestinal bleeding: is repeating endoscopy economically feasible? Dig Dis Sci 2011; 56: 1763–8.

8. Leaper M, Johnston MJ, Barclay M, et al. Reasons for failure to diagnose colorectal carcinoma at colonoscopy. Endoscopy 2004; 36: 499–503.

9. Singh H, Turner D, Xue L, et al. Risk of developing colorectal cancer following a negative colonoscopy examination: evidence for a 10-year interval between colonoscopies. JAMA 2006; 295: 2366–73.

10. Rex DK, Lappas JC, Maglinte DD, Malczewski MC, Kopecky KA, Cockerill EM. Enteroclysis in the evaluation of suspected small intestinal bleeding. Gastroenterology 1989; 97: 58–60.

11. Moch A, Herlinger H, Kochman ML, Levine MS, Rubesin SE, Laufer I. Enteroclysis in the evaluation of obscure gastrointestinal bleeding. Am J Roentgenol 1994; 163: 1381–4.

12. Voeller GR, Bunch G, Britt LG. Use of technetium-labeled red blood cell scintigraphy in the detection and management of gastrointestinal hemorrhage. Surgery 1991; 110: 799–804.

13. Howarth DM, Tang K, Lees W. The clinical utility of nuclear medicine imaging for the detection of occult gastrointestional haemorrhage. Nucl Med Commun 2002; 23: 591–4.

14. Brunnler T, Klebl F, Mundorff S, et al. Significance of scintigraphy for the localisation of obscure gastrointestinal bleedings. World J Gastroenterol 2008; 14: 5015–9.

15. Krämer SC, Görich J, Rilinger N, Siech M, Aschoff AJ, Vogel J, et al. Embolization for gastrointestinal hemorrhages. Eur Radiol 2000; 10: 802–5.

16. Bloomfield RS, Smith TP, Schneider AM, Rockey DC. Provocative angiography in patients with hemorrhage of obscure origin. Am J Gastroenterol 2000; 95: 2807–12.

17. Kim CY, Suhocki PV, Miller MJ Jr, Khan M, Janus G, Smith TP. Provocative mesenteric angiography for lower gastrointestinal hemorrhage: results from a single institution study. J Vasc Interv Radiol 2010; 21: 477–83.

18. Peynircioqlu B, Erkus F, Cil B, Ciftci T, Durhan G, Balkanci F. Mesenteric angiography of patients with gastrointestinal tract hemorrhages: a single center study. Diagn Interv Radiol 2011; 10.4261/1305-3825.DIR.3963-10.1.

19. Chak A, Koehler MK, Sundaram SN, Cooper GS, Canto MI, Sivak MV Jr. Diagnostic and therapeutic impact of push enteroscopy: analysis of factors associated with positive findings. Gastrointest Endosc 1998; 47: 18–22.

20. De Leusse A, Vahedi K, Edery J, Tiah D, Fery-Lemonnier E, Cellier C, Bouhnik Y, Jian R. Capsule endoscopy or push enteroscopy for first line exploration of obscure gastrointestinal bleeding. Gastroenterology 2007; 132: 855–62.

21. Sidhu R, McAlindon ME, Kapur K, Hurlstone DP, Wheeldon MC, Sanders DS. Push enteroscopy in the era of capsule endoscopy. J Clin Gastroenterol 2008; 42: 54–8.

22. Schulz HJ, Schmidt H. Intraoperative enteroscopy. Gastrointest Endosc Clin N Am 2009; 19: 371–9.

23. Khalife S, Soyer P, Alatawi A, Vahedi K, Hamzi L, Dray X, Place V, Marteau P, Boudiaf M. Obscure gastrointestinal bleeding: preliminary comparison of 64-section CT enteroclysis with video capsule endoscopy. Eur Radiol 2011; 21: 79–86.

24. Jain TP, Gulati MS, Makharia GK, Bandhu S, Garg PK. CT enteroclysis in the diagnosis of obscure gastrointestinal bleeding: initial results. Clin Radiol 2007; 62: 660–7.

25. Voderholzer WA, Ortner M, Rogalla P, Beinholzl J, Lochs H. Diagnostic yield of wireless capsule enteroscopy in comparison with computed tomography enteroclysis. Endoscopy 2003; 35: 1009–14.

26. Ettorre GC, Francioso G, Garribba AP, Fracella MR, Greco A, Farchi G. Helical CT angiography in gastrointestinal bleeding of obscure origin. Am J Roentgenol 1997; 168: 727–31.

27. Huprich JE, Fletcher JG, Fidler JL, et al. Prospective blinded comparison of wirelesss capsule endoscopy and multiphase CT enterography in obscure gastrointestinal bleeding. Radiology 2011; 260: 744–51.

28. Yoon W, Jeong YY, Shin SS, Lim HS, Song SG, Jang NG, Kim JK, Kang HK. Acute massive gastrointestinal bleeding: detection and localization with arterial phase multi-detector row helical CT. Radiology 2006; 239: 160–7.

29. Kennedy DW, Laing GJ, Tseng LH, Rosenblum DI, Tamarkin SW. Detection of active gastrointestinal hemorrhage with CT angiography: a 4(1/2) year retrospective review. J Vasc Interv Radiol 2010; 21: 848–55.

30. Cheon JH, Kim YS, Lee IS, Chang DK, Ryu JK, Lee J.K. et al. Can we predict spontaneous capsule passage after retention? A nationwide study to evaluate the incidence and clinical outcomes of capsule retention. Endoscopy 2007; 39: 1046–52.

31. Li F, Gurudu SR, De Petris G, Sharma VK, Shiff AD, Heigh RI, Fleischer DE, Post J, Erickson P, Leighton JA. Retention of the capsule endoscope: a single center experience of 1000 capsule enodscopy procedures. Gastrointest Endosc 2008; 68: 174–80.

32. Cheifetz AS, Kombluth AA, Legnani P, Schmelkin I, Brown A, Lichtiger S, Lewis BS. The risk of retention of the capsule endoscope in patients with known or suspected Crohn's disease. Am J Gastroenterol 2006; 101: 2218–22.

33. Pennazio M, Santucci R, Rondonotti E, Abbiati C, Beccari G, Rossini FP, De Franchis R. Outcome of patients with obscure gastrointestinal bleeding after capsule endoscopy: report of 100 consecutive cases. Gastroenterology 2004; 126: 643–53.

34. Estevez E, Gonzalez-Conde B, Vazquez-Iglesias JL, et al. Diagnostic yield and clinical outcomes after capsule endoscopy in 100 consecutive patients with obscure gastro-intestinal bleeding. Eur J Gastroenterol Hepatol 2006; 18: 881–8. 68%

35. Carey EJ, Leighton JA, Heigh RI, Shiff AD, Sharma VK, Post JK, Fleischer DE. A single center experience of 260 consecutive patients undergoing capsule endoscopy for obscure gastrointestinal bleeding. Am J Gastroenterol 2007; 102: 89–95.

36. Saurin JC, Delvaux M, Vahedi K, Gaudin JL, Villarejo J, Florent C, Gay G, Ponchon T. Clinical impact of capsule endoscopy compared to push enteroscopy: 1 year follow up study. Endoscopy 2005; 37: 318–23.

37. Viazis N, Papaxoinis K, Theodoropoulos I, Sgouros S, Vlachogiannakos J, Pipis P, Markoglou C, Avgerinos A. Impact of capsule endoscopy in obscure small bowel bleeding: defining strict diagnostic criteria for a favorable outcome. Gastrointest Endosc 2005; 63: 712–22.

38. Neu B, Ell C, May A, Schmid E, Riemann JF, Hagenmuller F, Keuchel M, Soehendra N, Seitz U, Meining A, Rosch T. Capsule endoscopy versus standard tests in influencing management of obscure digestive bleeding: results from a German multicenter trial. Am J Gastroenterol 2005; 100: 1736–42.

39. Delvaux M, Fassler I, Gay G. Clinical usefulness of the endoscopic video capsule as the initial intestinal investigation in patients with obscure digestive bleeding: validation of a diagnostic strategy based on the patient outcome after 12 months. Endoscopy 2004; 36: 1067–73.

40. Lai LH, Wong GL, Chow DK, Lau JY, Sung JJ, Leung WK. Long term follow-up of patients with obscure gastrointestinal bleeding after negative capsule endoscopy. Am J Gastroenterol 2006; 101: 1224–8.

41. McDonald J, Porter V, McNamara D. Negative capsule endoscopy in patients with obscure GI bleeding predicts low rebleeding rates. Gastrointest Endosc 2008; 68: 1122–7.

42. Marmo R, Rotondano G, Gasetti T, Manes G, Chilovi F, Sprujevnik T. et al. Degree of concordance between double balloon enteroscopy and capsule endoscopy in obscure gastrointestinal bleeding: a multicenter study. Endoscopy 2009; 41: 587–92.

43. Postgate A, Despott E, Burling D, Gupta A, Phillips R, O'Beirne J, Patch D, Fraser C. Significant small bowel lesions detected by alternative diagnostic modalities after negative capsule endoscopy. Gastrointest Endosc 2008; 68: 1209–14.

44. Ross A, Mehdizadeh S, Tokar J, Leighton JA, Kamal A, Chen A. et al. Double balloon enteroscopy detects small bowel mass lesions missed by capsule endoscopy. Dig Dis Sci 2008; 53: 2140–3.

45. Viazis N, Papaxoinis K, Vlachogiannakos J, Efthymiou A, Theodoropoulos I, Karamanolis DG. Is there a role second look capsule endoscopy in patients with obscure GI Bleeding after a non-diagnostic first test? Gastrointest Endosc 2009; 69: 850–6.

46. Bar-Meir S, Eliakim R, Nadler M, Barkay O, Fireman Z, Scapa E, Chowers Y, Bardan E. Second capsule endoscopy for patients with severe iron deficiency anemia. Gastrointest Endosc 2004; 60: 711–13.

47. Yamamoto H, Kita H, Sunada K, Hayashi Y, Sato H, Yano T, et al. Clinical outcomes of double-balloon endoscopy for the diagnosis and treatment of small-intestinal diseases. Clin Gastroenterol Hepatol 2004; 2: 1010–16.

48. Monkemuller K, Neumann H, Meyer F, Kuhn R, Malfertheiner P, Fry LC. A retrospective analysis of emergency double-balloon enteroscopy for small bowel bleeding. Endoscopy 2009; 1: 587–92.

49. Arakawa D, Ohmiya N, Nakamura M, et al. Outcome after enteroscopy for patients with obscure GI bleeding: diagnostic comparison between double balloon enteroscopy and videocapsule endoscopy. Gastrointest Endosc 2009; 69: 866–74.

50. Kaffles AJ, Siah C, Koo JH. Clinical outcomes after double-balloon enteroscopy in patients with obscure GI bleeding and a positive capsule endoscopy. Gastrointest Endosc 2007; 66: 304–9.

51. Sun B, Rajan E, Cheng S, Shen R, Zhang C, Zhang S, Wu Y, Zhong J. Diagnostic yield and therapeutic impact of double-balloon enteroscopy in a large cohort of patients with obscure gastrointestinal bleeding. Am J Gastroenterol 2006; 101: 2011–15.

52. Manabe N, Tanaka S, Fukumoto A, Nakao M, Kamino D, Chayama K. Double balloon enteroscopy in patients with GI bleeding of obscure origin. Gastrointest Endosc 2006; 64: 135–40.

53. Hadithi M, Heine GD, Jacobs MA, van Bodegraven AA, Mulder GJ. A prospective study comparing video capsule endoscopy with double-balloon enteroscopy in patients with obscure gastrointestinal bleeding. Am J Gastroenterol 2006; 101: 52–7.

54. Gerson LB, Tokar J, Chiorean M, et al. Complications associated with double balloon enteroscopy at nine US centers. Clin Gastroenterol Hepatol 2009; 7: 1177–82.

55. Mensink PBF, Haringsma J, Kucharzik T, et al. Complications of double balloon enteroscopy: a multicenter survey. Endoscopy 2007; 39: 613–5.

56. Mehdizadeh S, Ross A, Gerson L, et al. What is the learning curve associated with double balloon enteroscopy? Technical details and early experience in 6 U. S. tertiary care centers. Gastrointest Endosc 2006; 64: 740–50.

57. Tsuijkawa T, Saitoh Y, Andoh A, Imaeda H, Hata K, Minematsu H. et al. Novel single balloon enteroscopy for diagnosis and treatment of the small intestine: a preliminary experiences. Endoscopy 2008; 40: 11–15.

58. Riccioni ME, Urgesi R, Cianci R, Spada C, Nista EC, Costamagna G. Single balloon push and pull enteroscopy system – does it work? A single center, 3 year experience. Surg Endosc 2011; 25: 3050–6.

59. Aktas H, de Ridder L, Haringsma J, Kuipers EJ, Mensink PB. Complications of single balloon enteroscopy: a prospective evaluation of 166 procedures. Endoscopy 2010; 42: 365–8.

60. Akerman PA, Agrawal D, Chen William et al. Spiral enteroscopy: a novel method of enteroscopy by using the Endo-Ease Discovery SB overtube and a pediatric colonoscope. GI Endosc 2009; 69: 327–332.

61. Morgan D, Upchurch B, Draganov P, Binmoeller KF, Haluszka O, Jonnalagadda S. et al. Spiral enteroscopy: prospective U. S. multicenter study in patients with small bowel disorders. Gastrointest Endosc 2010; 72: 992–8.

62. May A. et al. Prospective multicenter trial comparing push-and-pull enteroscopy with the single- and double-balloon techniques in patients with small bowel disorders. Am J Gastroenterol 2010; 105: 375–81.

63. Takano N, Yamada A, Watabe H, Togo, Yamaji Y, Yoshida H, Kawabe T, Omata M, Koike K. Single balloon versus double balloon endoscopy for achieving total enteroscopy: a randomized controlled trial. Gastrointest Endosc 2011; 73: 734–9.

64. Domagk D, Mensink P, Aktas H, et al. Single- vs. double-balloon enteroscopy in small bowel diagnostics: a randomized multicenter trial. Endoscopy 2011; 43: 472–6.

65. May A, Manner H, Aschmoneit I, Ell C. Prospective, cross over, single center trial comparing oral double balloon enteroscopy and oral spiral enteroscopy in patients with suspected small bowel vascular malformation. Endoscopy 2011; 43: 477–83.

66. Frieling T, et al. Prospective comparison between double-balloon enteroscopy and spiral enteroscopy. Endoscopy 2010; 42: 885–8.

67. Khashab M, Lennon AM, Dunbar K.B. et al. A comparative evaluation of single-balloon enteroscopy and spiral enteroscopy for patients with mid-gut disorders. Gastrointest Endosc 2010; 72: 766–772.

68. Gerson LB, Batenic MA, Newsom SL, Ross A, Semrad CE. Long term outcomes after double balloon enteroscopy for obscure gastrointestinal bleeding. Clin Gastroenterol Hepatol 2009; 7: 664–9.

69. May A, Friesing-Sosnik T, Manner H, Pohl J, Ell C. Long term outcome after argon plasma coagulation of small bowel lesions using double balloon enteroscopy in patients in mid-gastrointestinal bleeding. Endoscopy 2011; May 3. [Epub ahead of print].

70. Triester SL, Leighton JA, Leontiadis GI, Fleischer DE, Hara AK, Heigh RI, et al. A meta-analysis of the yield of capsule endoscopy compared to other diagnostic modalities in patients with obscure gastrointestinal bleeding. Am J Gastroenterol 2005; 100: 2407–18.

71. Saperas E, Dot J, Videla S, Alvarez-Castells A, Perez-Lafuente M, Armengol JR, et al. Capsule endoscopy versus computed tomographic or standard angiography for the diagnosis of obscure gastrointestinal bleeding. Am J Gastroenterol 2007; 102: 731–7.

72. Hartmann D, Schmidt H, Bolz G. et al. A prospective two center study comparing wireless capsule endoscopy with intraoperative enteroscopy in patients with obscure GI bleeding. Gastrointest Endosc 2005; 61: 826–32.

73. Matsumoto T, Moriyama T, Esaki M, Nakamura S, Iida M. Performance of antegrade double-balloon enteroscopy: comparison with push enteroscopy. Gastrointest Endosc 2005; 62: 392–8.

74. May A, Nachbar L, Schneider M, Ell C. Prospective comparison of push enteroscopy and push-and-pull enteroscopy in patients with suspected small-bowel bleeding. Am J Gastroenterol 2006; 101: 2016–24.

75. Chen X, Ran ZH, Tong JL. A meta-analysis of the yield of capsule endoscopy compared to double-balloon enteroscopy in patients with small bowel diseases. World J Gastroenterol 2007; 13: 4372–8.

76. Pasha SF, Leighton JA, Das A, Harrison ME, Decker GA, Fleischer DE, et al. Double-balloon enteroscopy and capsule endoscopy have comparable diagnostic yield in small-bowel disease: a meta-analysis. Clin Gastroenterol Hepatol 2008; 6: 671–6.

77. Gerson L, Kamal A. Cost-effectiveness analysis of management strategies for obscure GI bleeding. Gastrointest Endosc 2008; 68: 920–36.

78. ASGE Standards of Practice Committee. The role of endoscopy in the management of obscure GI bleeding. Gastrointest Endosc 2010; 72: 471–9.

79. Mergener K, Ponchon T, Gralnek I, et al. Literature review and recommendations for clinical application of small bowel capsule endoscopy, based on a panel discussion by international experts. Consensus statements for small bowel capsule endoscopy, 2006–07. Endoscopy 2007; 39: 895–909.

80. van Cutsem E, Rutgeerts P, Vantrappen G. Treatment of bleeding gastrointestinal vascular malformations with oestrogen–progesterone. Lancet 1990; 335: 953–5.

81. Junquera F, Feu F, Papo M, et al. A multicenter, randomized, clinical trial of hormonal therapy in the prevention of rebleeding from gastrointestinal angiodysplasia. Gastroenterology 2001; 121: 1073–9.

82. Rossini FP, Arrigoni A, Pennazio M. Octreotide in the treatment of bleeding due to angiodysplasia of the small intestine. Am J Gastroenterol 1993; 88: 1424–7.

83. Scaglione G, Pietrini, L, Russo F, et al. Long-acting octreotide as rescue therapy in chronic bleeding from gastrointestinal angiodysplasia. Aliment Pharmacol Ther 2007; 26: 935–42.

84. Laine L, Sahota A, Shah A. Does capsule endoscopy improve outcomes in obscure gastrointestinal bleeding? Randomized trial versus small bowel radiography. Gastroenterology 2010; 138: 1673–80.

CHAPTER 12

Design of Clinical Trials in Gastrointestinal Bleeding

Vipul Jairath[1] & Alan N. Barkun[2]

[1]NHS Blood and Transplant and Translational Gastroenterology Unit, John Radcliffe Hospital, Oxford, UK
[2]Division of Gastroenterology, McGill University Health Centre, Montreal General Hospital, Montreal, Canada

Introduction

There are numerous published studies in the literature addressing management of patients with upper gastrointestinal bleeding (UGIB) from a variety of populations. The nature of these studies spans the entire spectrum of epidemiological studies and clinical trials. However, there is A widepread variation in study methodologies and quality, often limiting the internal or external validity of results, or both. For example, meta-analyses of randomized controlled trials (RCTs) of endoscopic therapy for bleeding ulcers have reported that only one-third of studies have a high methodological score (1, 2). In recognition of this, a recent international expert consensus was published in an attempt to provide a methodological framework for the design, performance, analysis, interpretation and communication of randomized clinical trials that assess the management of patients with non-variceal UGIB (3). The aim of this work is to help investigators plan trials of high methodological quality, and to enable health-care professionals to appraise the quality of the reports and results.

In this chapter we critically appraise the methodology of two examples representing two distinct, commonly adopted study designs in UGIB. The first study is an observational database from a large national audit of UGIB conducted in the United Kingdom (UK) in 2007, which has led to a number of recent publications (4–9). The second is an international, multi-center RCT assessing an intravenous proton pump inhibitor for the prevention of recurrent peptic ulcer bleeding (10). We review and contrast the varying methodological assumptions, pitfalls, and implications with regards to the interpretation of results for each.

Gastrointestinal Bleeding, Second Edition. Edited by Joseph J.Y. Sung, Ernst J. Kuipers and Alan N. Barkun. © 2012 Blackwell Publishing Ltd.
Published 2012 by Blackwell Publishing Ltd.

Example of an observational study: the UK comparative audit of upper gastrointestinal bleeding and the use of blood (9)

Observational databases provide descriptive results of "real-life" patient outcomes for UGIB, but by their observational nature, are not conducted with the rigour of that of an RCT. Nevertheless it is recognized that observational databases are useful and important adjuncts to RCTs to determine whether efficacy under the controlled conditions in specialist centres actually translates into effective treatment in routine practice (11).

Methods

What was the research question?
The first large-scale prospective observational study in non-variceal UGIB in the UK took place between 1993 and 1994 (12). This initial study led to the derivation of the Rockall score (13) and to British Society of Gastroenterology (BSG) guidelines in 2002. Non-variceal upper gastrointestinal haemorrhage: guidelines. Gut. 2002 Oct;51 Suppl 4:iv1–6. Given the considerable advances which have occurred over the past two decades in terms of prevention, diagnosis and management of UGIB, the primary objective of the current study was to describe contemporary characteristics, risk factors and endoscopic diagnoses of patients presenting with UGIB throughout the UK, and to ascertain whether patient outcomes had improved since the previous study in 1993–1994 (12). Secondary objectives were to determine the use of red cell transfusion in relation to published guidelines, and to identify associations between early red cell transfusion and clinical outcomes, in recognition of the fact that UGIB accounts for 14% of all red blood cell transfusions in the UK and has been highlighted as a key area for blood conservation strategies (14). The full study report can be found at http://www.bsg.org.uk/clinical/general/uk-upper-gi-bleeding-audit.html.

What was the study design?
This study was a prospective observational study of all patients presenting to hospital with UGIB within a two-month period between May and July 2007. Institutional-level eligibility allowed participation by any UK hospital admitting acute medical or surgical patients. In total, 217 hospitals agreed to take part in the study (84% of all invited). This study provides a "real life" picture of UGIB outcomes throughout the UK from a wide spectrum of University and Non-University hospitals, but could affect data validity by not using dedicated research personnel trained in a standardized fashion.

There were some methodological differences between the current study and the 1993–1994 study which are worth highlighting as they may impact on the ability to make direct comparisons between the two UK studies. The study in 1993–1994, also a prospective observational study examining all presentations with UGIB in four health-care regions in the UK, was carried out in two phases with recommendations made to participating sites between the phases; data-collection was paper based. In contrast, the 2007 study was a true nationwide study with a larger sample size, was carried out in one phase, and used web-based data entry.

Patient population and enrollment criteria

Subtle differences in patient eligibility criteria exist in observational registries of UGIB. In the 2007 study, inclusion criteria were: all adult patients (over age 16) admitted to hospital or who presented as in-patients with symptoms of UGIB; clinical evidence of UGIB on admission, or a history of having experienced such a bleed within ten days prior to the date of admission; and clinical evidence of UGIB whilst in hospital for another reason. Furthermore patients were eligible regardless of whether or not they underwent endoscopy for UGIB, and irrespective of the cause of bleeding (i.e. non-variceal or variceal).

These eligibility criteria differ with those of another national registry highlighting small but clinically important differences in eligibility criteria (Box 12.1): The RUGBE (Registry in patients with Upper Gastrointestinal Bleeding undergoing an Endoscopy) study group from Canada was a patient cohort detailing data from 1,878 consecutive admissions with UGIB from 18 sites over a two-year period ending in 2002 (15–19). This study only included patients presenting with symptoms of UGIB within 24 hours preceding admission, in contrast to the UK study which included patients presenting with symptoms up to ten days prior. This shorter period of inclusion criteria in the RUGBE study compared to the UK study could theoretically select out a subgroup of patients with unequivocal evidence of

---

Box 12.1 Key Differences in Enrollment Criteria Between the UK and RUGBE National Data Registries for UGIB

UK National Audit Data	RUGBE Data
Adults with symptoms of UGIB	Adults with overt UGIB
Symptoms within 10 days of presentation	Symptoms within 24 hours of admission
All cause UGIB	Non-variceal bleeding only
All presentations with UGIB	Patients undergoing endoscopy only
All consecutive admissions over 2 months	Random sample of admissions over a 2 year period

clinically important bleeding. The RUGBE study also only included patients with non-variceal bleeding having undergone endoscopy. The clinical outcomes of patients with variceal and non-variceal UGIB differ as do the clinical features of those patients who do and do not undergo endoscopy; the prognosis is known to be worse for patients with a variceal cause of bleeding as for those too sick to undergo endoscopy. Readers must therefore be cautious when comparing national mortality figures on UGIB, based on such data registries that may have adopted different inclusion criteria.

Subtle differences also exist in the definition of UGIB. The recent international framework for the design of UGIB studies should help to standardize these definitions in an attempt to allow accurate and direct comparison of UGIB studies (3). Table 12.1 compares the clinical characteristics described in the UK study with those recommended by the methodology consensus guideline (even though this group targeted mainly RCTs). Finally, enrollment in the UK cohort was consecutive over two months, while that in the Canadian registry was a random sampling of patients over a 2-year time interval. As a result, selection bias may have more easily been introduced in the latter, while evolution in management strategies and technologies may not have been as broadly captured in the former study.

Table 12.1 Comparison of recommended and actual baseline data recorded.

Recommended baseline characteristics to be recorded in UGIB studies	Actual baseline characteristics recorded in UK Study	Actual baseline characteristics recorded in RUGBE Study
Symptoms/signs	Yes	Yes
Duration of symptoms before presentation	Yes	Yes
Age (mean/median; proportion>65 yrs)	Yes	Yes
Gender	Yes	Yes
Prior UGI Clinical events	Yes	Yes
Major current comorbidities	Yes	Yes
Key medications	Yes	Yes
Hemoglobin	Yes	Yes
MCV/RDW/Iron studies	No	No
Platelets, PT	Yes	Yes
H.Pylori status if ulcer patients	Yes	Yes
Transfusion data	Yes – extensive	Yes
Timing of endoscopy	Yes	Yes
Lesion	Yes	Yes
Location and size of lesions	Yes (location); No (size)	Yes
Stigmata of hemorrhage	Yes	Yes
Risk score	Yes – Rockall score	No

> **Box 12.2** Key Definitions Used in the UK Comparative Study of UGIB and the Use of Blood
>
> **Acute Upper Gastrointestinal Bleeding**
> Hematemesis or passage of melena or other firm clinical or laboratory evidence of acute
>   blood loss from the upper gastrointestinal tract
> **Hematemesis**
> Vomiting of blood or clots
> Coffee ground vomit witnessed by medical or nursing staff
> **Melena**
> Passage of dark or tarry stools or altered blood as witnessed by medical or nursing staff, or
>   discovered on rectal exam
> **Continued bleeding**
> Bleeding for more than 24 hours evidence by high pulse and low blood pressure with no
>   other cause; continued or on-going hematemesis; passage of fresh melena; falling
>   hemoglobin more than can be explained by hemodilution
> **Rebleeding**
> Signs of bleeding as outlined above recurring within 10 days of the last bleed, having been
>   stable for 24 hours in terms of pulse/blood pressure/hemoglobin and the passage of
>   normal stool or old melena
> **All cause mortality**
> Death occurring within the hospital admission

Definition of end-points

In the 2007 UK audit, *a priori* definitions of all outcomes (Box 12.2) were adopted through adaptation of existing definitions in the literature. In most studies of UGIB, whether observational or interventional, rebleeding is often one of the primary end-points. However there are differences in definitions used for this end-point. Rebleeding usually encompasses two components which should be distinguished from one another – persistent bleeding and recurrent bleeding. Persistent bleeding is present at the end of the index endoscopy, i.e. when active bleeding does not stop at the end of the endoscopy. Recurrent bleeding occurs in those patients with successful hemostasis of an actively bleeding lesion at the index endoscopy or in those without initial active bleeding at the time of the endoscopy. In the 2007 UK study, an *a priori* decision was taken to group the definitions of persistent bleeding and recurrent bleeding together to form the composite outcome of "rebleeding." It is often difficult to distinguish between the two and in reality they comprise a spectrum of the same process. Endoscopic confirmation of rebleeding was not a prerequisite for a diagnosis of rebleeding, although some investigators have used endoscopic evidence to confirm rebleeding, usually in the setting of randomized controlled trials (3, 10).

Attention should also be drawn to the definition of all cause mortality. In the present study this was death from any-cause during the hospital admission. Follow-up data beyond hospital discharge was not collected and theoretically deaths may have occurred post-discharge which are unaccounted for. The lack of follow-up data beyond hospital discharge may also influence the reported figures for rebleeding. Although the majority of episodes of rebleeding do occur within 72 hours, recent studies suggest that up to 25% or rebleeding episodes may occur beyond three days (2, 20). In the interpretation of rebleeding and mortality rates, readers should pay attention to the follow-up period as lack of comprehensive post-discharge 30-day follow-up data may underestimate the true incidence of end-points.

Data collection methods

Data entry was performed on-line via a secure dedicated website. Hospital leads were contacted for additional information for incomplete cases and clarification of case data where necessary. However, the study co-ordinating team were unable to independently audit the data entered against actual medical charts. Institutional ethical approval would have been required in the UK to access patient charts and this may have limited both the size of this study and the prompt timescale within which it was conducted. As this study was conducted as an audit process, formal ethical approval for the study conduct was not required.

Recently published large databases examining outcomes in patients with UGIB have used similar (15, 21, 22) or differing data source methodology (23, 24). Indeed, two recent North American publications used large administrative databases (23, 24). Both studies used data from the Nationwide Inpatient Sample, the largest all-payer database of national hospital discharges in the United States, representing a 20% stratified sample of non-federal acute-care hospitals. Although such databases are able to present data from large numbers of patients, they usually cannot provide detailed, disease specific, clinical characteristics and prognostic variables in UGIB e.g. clinical features, risk stratification scores and laboratory results.

Results

Study population

In total 8,939 cases were available for analysis; of these 13% (1,199) were excluded by local hospital leads as they were not deemed to have met the study entry criteria. A further 12% of cases (1090/8939) were submitted without sufficient data and excluded from the final analysis, despite attempts to obtain a full data-set. The main reason given by local hospitals submitting these incomplete cases was time pressure. Indeed, this study was reliant upon the goodwill of busy clinicians to identify and abstract cases at their own pace. In the final study report 6,750 eligible cases (86%) were analysed from 208 hospitals (Fig. 12.1).

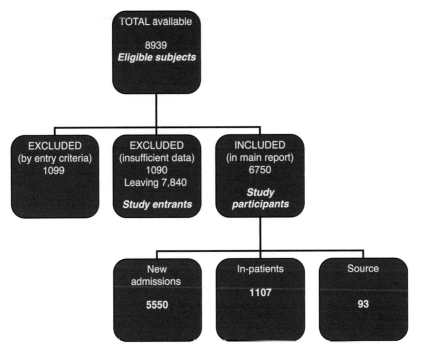

Figure 12.1 Flow chart of included and excluded cases for all UK participating sites.

Internal validity of study

Definitions

The internal validity of a study is usually a measure of how confident we can be that a difference in outcomes between randomized groups can be attributed to an intervention being tested, rather than due to bias, confounding or chance. It is dependent on good design, conduct and analysis of the trial (25, 26). Before we proceed, it is important that we provide a clear explanation of the terms of "bias" and "confounding" commonly used in epidemiological studies. The results of any study, regardless of the nature of the design, can fall under one or more of four mechanisms: bias, confounding, chance or causation. Bias refers to an inaccuracy that is different in magnitude or direction in one of more groups being studied than in the others. It can lead to a measure of association that is exaggerated and can lead to strong associations when there are in fact no true differences in the groups being compared (27). Confounding is the distortion of the association between an exposure and outcomes brought about due to the association of another factor with both outcome and exposure (28, 29). Although the presently described study is an observational study and does not involve the comparison of two different study groups as one would see in a case-control study or randomized controlled trial, basic principles of internal validity still apply.

Could the results be affected by selection bias?

Firstly we should consider the possibility of selection bias in this study. In theory *all* admissions with UGIB who met eligibility criteria over a two-month period in 2007 should have been entered prospectively into the study. Case ascertainment and data abstraction were entirely reliant upon local processes and manpower at each hospital; no additional support or funding was provided. There was considerable variation in the number of cases provided by each hospital and this is likely to have been a reflection of time and manpower limitations. Consequently it is unlikely that *all* cases of UGIB were identified; the final study report comments that the only way to accurately quantify the degree of missing data would be through use of hospital episode statistics. Furthermore it may be that the case ascertainment processes used at a local level selected out a particular subset of patients for inclusion into the study. For example, the pilot study showed that most cases were identified from the endoscopy department rather than from admission wards and emergency departments and this method would preferentially select out those cases who underwent in-patient endoscopy and not those who were discharged or too unwell for endoscopy.

Could the results be affected by observation bias?

A simple but important issue to consider is the possibility of incorrect data entry or mis-coding of data. There is greater possibility for inconsistency in data entry in a large, multi-center study of this nature, where data will be entered by different observers at each site and over more than one occasion. It would not be feasible to review the medical charts of all study participants by checking abstracted data against data recorded in medical charts, however other similar studies have independently audited a certain percentage of abstracted charts (15). In the present study this was not possible as ethical approval for access to patient records by the audit team was not sought. However, great care was taken in the design of questions to reduce the possibility of incorrect data entry. This included mainly the use of multiple choice questions (as opposed to free text entry), a detailed key for each question to clarify the purpose of the question, and a piloting period to ensure clarity. These precautions make it unlikely that there would be any systematic bias in the patient observations made.

Missing data characterization

Finally we should consider the method by which missing data are presented. 12% (1,090/8,939) of study entrants were excluded from the final analyses due to insufficient data, resulting in a total of 6,750 study participants

(Fig. 12.1). In the final study report, data are characterized according to age and gender, comparing differences between the *study entrants* and *study participants*, but other demographic and clinical characteristics are not presented. It is possible that the disease specific characteristics and prognostic variables between these two groups (patients with complete and incomplete data) differ significantly such that it could compromise the internal validity of the study.

External validity of study

Definitions
The external validity of a study refers to the ability to apply the results of a study to a wider population, usually that pertinent to the reader's practice (30). It is important to note that the external validity of a study is only useful if the internal validity is deemed acceptable. Therefore when analysing a study, each attrition moving from the target population to the study participants should be scrutinized to assess whether losses at each point can produce differences in internal validity and, subsequently, external validity.

Can the results be applied to the eligible population?
The results of this study apply to the 6,750 adult patients with UGIB in the final analysis i.e. the study participants. These entrants comprised 76% of the eligible population. Clearly this group make up the majority of the eligible population but, without further details about the clinical and demographic features of excluded patients, readers must consider the possibility of some selection bias. However, considering the breadth of sampling, even in the absence of screening logs of total number of admissions with UGIB at each site, it is reasonable to assume that the results likely apply to the source population.

Can the results be applied to other relevant populations?
The vast majority of all UK hospitals (217/292, 84%) accepting acute medical/surgical admissions took part in this study. It is therefore reasonable to assume that the study results are applicable to UGIB patients cared for throughout the UK. Since UGIB is a multifactorial disease with a number of processes involved in the management of patients, and as a multitude of both patient and provider characteristics may influence the outcome of this condition, we therefore cannot assume complete applicability of these results to other ethnic populations or health care settings.

Summary
The study we have appraised is the largest prospective observational data-set of UGIB ever reported in the UK. It provides detailed clinical characteristics

and outcome data on a large number of UGIB patients from the majority of hospitals throughout the UK. Although there exist some limitations with regards to the internal validity of the data presented, this work provides clinicians with valuable data about current practice and outcomes in UGIB. The framework presented above should enable a critical appraisal of other observational or cohort studies in UGIB.

Example of a randomized controlled trial (RCT): intravenous esomeprazole for prevention of recurrent peptic ulcer bleeding (10)

RCTs exhibit the greatest internal validity of any study design, but at the expense of decreased generalizability and other potential pitfalls. We will review some of these aspects using as example one of the largest RCT in UGIB that was recently published (10).

Methods

What was the research question?

Peptic ulcer bleeding (PUB) accounts for up to 50% of admissions to hospital with UGIB (22, 31). Despite advances in therapeutic endoscopy and critical care, the morbidity and mortality associated with PUB remains significant. After initial stabilization of patients and successful endoscopic hemostasis, profound acid suppression with high dose intravenous (i.v.) proton pump inhibitors (PPIs) has been shown to improve outcomes by clot stabilization at a higher gastric pH (32) and is recommended (16). Results have been conflicting and limitations in study methodology, patient populations and study end-points have limited the external validity and generalizability of published controlled trials of PPIs in this clinical setting (20, 33–36).

This trial was thus undertaken to assess whether high dose intravenous esomeprazole, compared to placebo, significantly reduces peptic ulcer rebleeding after successful endoscopic hemostasis in a high-risk, multi-ethnic population. The intervention tested was the administration of esome prazole 80 mg i.v. as a bolus infusion (over 30 minutes) followed by esomeprazole 8 mg/hr i.v. for 71.5 hours, or placebo 80 mg i.v. as a bolus infusion (over 30 minutes) followed by placebo 8 mg/hr i.v. for 71.5 hours. After completion of i.v. treatment, all patients received oral treatment with oral esomeprazole 40 mg once daily for the ensuing 27 days.

What were the outcome measures?

The primary and secondary outcome measures were explicitly stated *a priori*. The primary endpoint was the rate of clinically significant recurrent peptic

Table 12.2 Diagnostic criteria for clinically significant peptic ulcer rebleeding used in the intravenous esomeprazole for prevention of recurrent peptic ulcer bleeding study (37).

Rebleeding diagnosed by:	Criteria for diagnosis
A. Endoscopy	A1
Initiated by clinical signs of bleeding defined as:	Blood in stomach
One of B1, B2 or B3	A2
Endoscopic verification (i.e. one of A1 or A2)	Verified active bleeding from a peptic ulcer
B. Clinical definition	B1
At least two of B1 and/or B2 and/or B3	Vomiting fresh blood or blood in gastric tube or hematochezia or melena after a normal stool
	B2
	Decrease in hemoglobin >20 g/L (or hematocrit >6%) during 24 hours or an increase in hemoglobin <10 g/L (or hematocrit <3%) despite $\geq$ 2 units of blood having been transfused during 24 hours
	B3
	Unstable circulation systolic blood pressure $\leq$ 90 mm Hg or pulse $\geq$ 110/min (after having had a stable circulation)
	C
C. Hematemesis	Vomiting significant amounts (>200 ml) of fresh red blood, as estimated by the investigator

ulcer bleeding within 72 hours of starting i.v. treatment. The definition of rebleeding in this study was initially made on the basis of hematemesis or other clinical signs in the first instance, and them confirmed by endoscopy. These diagnostic criteria are outlined in Table 12.2 (37). In contrast to some studies, after a clinical suspicion arose, all recurrent bleeding required endoscopic confirmation. Recent international consensus methodology guidelines in RCTs in UGIB should help the standardization of outcome definitions (3).

The secondary outcome measures included clinically significant recurrent bleeding within 7 or 30 days; all cause mortality; a need for emergency surgery to control bleeding; length of hospital stay attributable to rebleeding, and the number of blood units transfused. Furthermore, mortality was divided into all-cause mortality and bleed-related mortality. This is in recognition of the fact that the great majority of cases of UGIB do not in fact die from uncontrollable bleeding, but rather from secondary complications, often reflecting underlying patient comorbidities (4, 38). The use of radiological intervention to control bleeding was not listed as a secondary endpoint; in many countries the low rates of surgical intervention may in part be explained by the increasing use of interventional radiology in instances of failed endoscopic hemostasis. Failing to include this endpoint, may underestimate those cases in which endoscopic hemostasis may have failed.

What was the study design?

The study design was a randomized, double-blind, placebo controlled, parallel group design. Neither the treating clinical team nor the patients were aware of whether the active drug or placebo was used. As in any clinical trial, randomization is a critical factor in controlling for confounding, and it should ideally be performed by personnel not involved in the recruitment or care of the subjects. The whole purpose of randomisation is to ensure that the intervention and placebo group are well matched in terms of potential confounding variables, both known and unknown. In this study randomisation was computer-generated in a central, off-site location, thereby ensuring investigators enrolling patients in no way manipulated patient allocation. Furthermore screening logs were reviewed, and the randomization was carried out by blocks of four (a balanced number of patients allocated to the experimental and control arms was achieved after every four patients randomized). Although it was not explicitly stated in the main (10) or methodological articles (37), we assume that investigators were unaware of block sizes as knowledge of this can inadvertently introduce selection bias in subject recruitment. Stratification of randomization was not deemed necessary in the design of this study, given its size and specific inclusion criteria. Stratification is usually used for small sample sizes as smaller studies have a greater risk of unequal distribution of confounding variables (39). The baseline clinical characteristics reported in the treatment versus placebo group were indeed similar in this study (10), a reflection of the adequacy of randomization. Note that such comparisons are typically carried out without statistical inferential testing, i.e. by only presenting descriptive statistics; it is up to clinicians to decide on the relevance of any observed between group differences that may require adjustment in the analysis.

Several quality control methods were introduced in this study to ensure standardization of endoscopic selection criteria as it is widely recognized that there exists significant inter-observer variability in assessment of endoscopic stigmata of hemorrhage (40, 41). To minimize these and enhance homogenous recruitment and internal validity through standardization of endoscopic outcomes, the study definitions of stigmata were agreed by all principal investigators using both circulation of an educational DVD and face-to-face educational sessions prior to initiation of the study (37). Furthermore, endoscopic lesions were photographed/videotaped and reviewed by a panel of experts comprising the end-points committee. Although patients were not reclassified according to the latter group's opinion,

quantification of their agreement with the investigator's admitting classification was recorded and reported as high (42).

What was the study population?

A key aspect of enabling readers to assess the interpretation of a clinical trial
is clear and transparent methodological reporting. Recognition of the
finding that authors of many studies neglect to provide critical information (43, 44) led to the development of the CONSORT (Consolidated
Standards of Reporting Trials) statement which provides a framework for
diligent and complete reporting of randomized controlled trials (45) and we
encourage readers to refer to this framework when interpreting the results of
a study. The CONSORT statement can be found at http://www.consort-
statement.org where regular updates are also provided. It predominantly
deals with a trial from the point of randomisation onwards, therefore
addressing issues of internal validity, rather than external validity. Most
leading medical journals will only publish the results of trials which have
been registered in advance and reported according to CONSORT criteria.

The inclusion and exclusion criteria for the presently described study are
highlighted in Box 12.3. The study population for any clinical trial can be
divided as outlined in Fig. 12.2. In this study the *target population* was adults
admitted with overt signs of upper gastrointestinal bleeding within 24 hours
of presentation to hospital (new admissions and existing in-patients).
The *source population* was all UGIB patients treated over the study period

---

Box 12.3 Inclusion and Exclusion Criteria

Inclusion criteria	**Major exclusion criteria**
Provision of informed consent	Malignancy or life expectancy <6 months
Male or female ≥18 years of age	Child-Pugh B or C cirrhosis
Upper gastrointestinal bleeding	ASA status >3
(hematemesis, melena or	Severe renal disease
hematochezia) within past 24 hours	Major cardiovascular event at enrollment
One endoscopically confirmed bleeding	or within 3 months prior to study start
gastric or duodenal ulcer ≥5 mm in	Hemorrhagic disorder or need for
diameter	anticoagulation after randomization
Successful hemostasis – achieved by	Multiple bleeding peptic ulcers or
injection therapy and/or heater probe	concomitant bleeding from another
coagulation/electocautery/application	source
of hemoclips	Need for treatment with NSAIDS, aspirin
	or clopidogrel during the first 7 days
	of the study
	Known hypersensitivity to any PPI
	IV administration of a PP>40 mg in the
	24 hours pre-enrollment

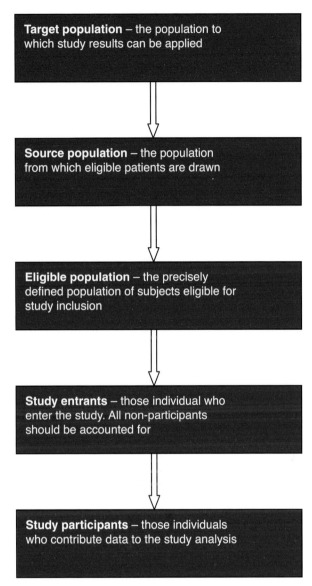

Figure 12.2 Groups of subjects to be considered in the interpretation of a randomized controlled trial.

at the 91 participating institutions in 16 countries. *Eligible subjects* were adults > 18 years of age with confirmed peptic ulcer bleeding at endoscopy from a single gastric or duodenal ulcer showing high risk stigmata, defined as Forrest class Ia, Ib, IIa or IIb (46). *Study entrants* were those eligible subjects who underwent successful endoscopic hemostasis of the offending ulcer and gave informed consent to their participation in the study. Fig. 12.3 provides an outline of the flow of study participants using the CONSORT blueprint.

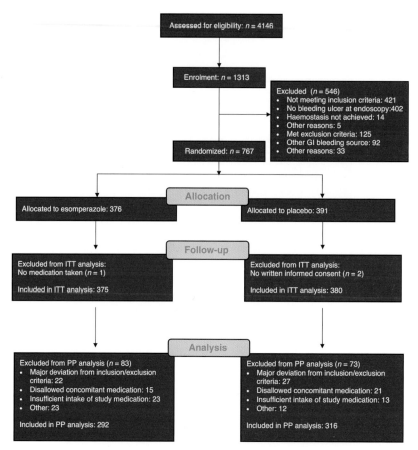

Figure 12.3 Flow of study participants using CONSORT framework.

Of particular interest in this study is the diverse ethnicity of the subject participants. Indeed, previous trials of PPIs for the prevention of peptic ulcer rebleeding have either recruited Asian populations (34, 35, 47) or Western populations (20, 33, 36). However differences between these two ethnic groups are thought to exist in the rate of PPI metabolism, variation in *Helicobacter pylori* prevalence, in gastric parietal cell mass and in disease acuity which may all limit the generalizability of results of PPI trials solely performed in Asian populations (48). The present study, by virtue of its multi-ethnic population, hoped to address such controversies and was the first i.v. PPI study to include such a racially diverse population.

Informed consent was usually obtained before the index endoscopy, but in some cases after the endoscopy (in countries in which no sedation is used at gastroscopy, or if deemed ethically appropriate by the local IRB). This is why almost 50% of patients who were enrolled into the study did not subsequently undergo randomisation, since they ultimately were found not to fulfil the endoscopic selection criteria. This aspect introduces the possibility of selection bias that is best addressed by reviewing clinical characteristics of included and excluded patients, justifying the importance of information obtained from screening logs.

Results

What were the main results?

In terms of the primary outcome, clinically significant recurrent bleeding in the intention to treat analysis within the first 72 hours occurred in 5.9% of patients in the i.v. esomeprazole-treated group and 10.3% of patients in the placebo group (representing an Absolute Risk Reduction of 4.4%, p = 0.026). The investigators had anticipated and accepted that endoscopic therapy would not be completely standardized in a study of this size, and that some patients would be treated with single therapy at endoscopy and others with dual therapy. This is important in terms of interpreting outcomes as dual endoscopic therapy is more effective than epinephrine injection alone in securing hemostasis (49). Therefore the investigators planned an *a priori* analysis of the primary endpoint after adjusting for endoscopic treatment which confirmed the robustness of the primary outcome result. Similarly they anticipated an uneven distribution of ethnicity in participants (87% white, 7% Asian), and therefore a pre-specified analysis by ethnic group was performed confirming similar results in white and Asian patients.

In terms of secondary outcomes, there was a significant reduction in the need for repeat endoscopic therapy, blood transfusion and additional hospital stay attributable to recurrent bleeding in the esomeprazole versus placebo group. There were no significant differences in all cause and bleeding related mortality between the two groups, which is not a surprise considering the sample size required to show such a difference that is more than the planned recruitment as the study was not powered to demonstrate a difference in mortality.

In summary, this international trial found that a 72 hour bolus followed by high dose intravenous esomeprazole infusion administered after endoscopic hemostasis significant decreases rebleeding for up to 30 days compared to the use of placebo.

Internal validity of the study

Was the randomization process adequate?

Randomization does not always guarantee that two groups are comparable with regards to all relevant characteristics. The baseline demographics between the two groups in the present study were for the most part very similar, demonstrating the validity of the randomisation process. There were some between-group differences in endoscopic diagnoses, as discussed above: There were fewer Forrest Class Ia ulcers in the esomeprazole group than in the placebo group (7.5% vs 10.3%). This could have been a potential source of confounding in the study outcomes but this imbalance was not found to bear significant implications as demonstrated by the planned adjustment of the primary endpoint by Forrest Classification.

Could the results be affected by observation bias?

Observation bias is a critical issue in this study. There were strict endoscopic inclusion criteria, each open to inter-observer variation. Each patient had to have a single bleeding gastric or duodenal ulcer, of at least 5mm in diameter, with stigmata of hemorrhage defined as Forrest class Ia/Ib/IIa/IIb, having been successfully treated endoscopically. Careful attention was devoted in the study methodology in order to minimize any potential observation bias. As mentioned, an educational video was developed and distributed (including at a face-to-face meeting) to all investigators prior to the start of the study in an attempt at standardizing the Forrest classification, together with the criteria for endoscopic confirmation of rebleeding. Important components of photographic documentation of bleeding ulcers were thus defined. Furthermore, as also alluded to, the study protocol also required photographic evidence of all ulcers which were centrally reviewed by two experts on the end-points committee blinded to treatment allocation. This meticulous attention and methodology in defining endoscopic appearances resulted in a high degree of concordance between the endpoint committee members and investigators which helped minimize potential observation bias in this study (42). Furthermore the double blind nature of the study protects against systematic observation bias between the two groups, for example, the systematic mis-classification of an ulcer into the incorrect Forrest Classification.

Could the results be affected by confounding?

The principle protection against confounding in this study is the adopted method of randomization, applied to a large number of study entrants, with the correct intention to treat analysis which included all randomly assigned patients who received infusion of the study drug. It would be useful at this point to explore the concept of intention to treat versus pre-protocol analysis of study results: In an ideal parallel group, randomized controlled trial, all participants randomized to an intervention receive the intervention while none in the comparison group do. In practice, this rarely happens; some subjects randomized to the intervention may never receive the intervention due to contra-indications, adverse events, administrative or consent problems and conversely, cross-overs may occur whereby control groups may receive the intervention. The appropriate analysis will compare outcomes in the original patient groups as defined by the randomization process – this is the *intention to treat analysis* and maintains the advantage of the randomized design. Alternately, comparisons may be performed only based upon the subjects who correctly received or not the intervention, a *per protocol* analysis. The latter may not reflect a more "real-life" set of outcomes, and furthermore, any observable difference between treatment groups may be enhanced.

Given the size of the study that was powered to show a clinically relevant difference in the primary end-point, the between-group similarity in base-line characteristics and the reliance on the intention to treat comparison, confounding is unlikely to have any major influence on the results of this trial.

Statistical issues relating to the primary outcome comparison

Could the results be affected by chance variation?

In assessing chance variation we need to assess both whether appropriate tests have been used and whether they have been done at the appropriate time intervals and for an appropriate choice of level of clinical significance. In this study there is a clear study protocol stating the incidence of rebleeding at 3, 7 and 30 days and secondary clinical outcomes at 30 days. Although an interim analysis was performed, this was adjusted for in the final analysis by use of a validated statistical methods.

Is the relationship strong?

In an observational study the value of the strength of a relationship must be defined in relation to possible bias or confounding. In a double blind RCT of this nature, both bias and confounding have been dealt with, so the strength of the relationship relates less to the internal validity of the study. In the current trial, there is a strong treatment effect in terms of the primary outcome of rebleeding at 3 days; indeed, in the intention to treat analysis rebleeding within the first 72 hours occurred in 5.9% in the esomeprazole group and 10.3% in the placebo group (absolute risk reduction (ARR) 4.4%, 95% CI 0.6–8.3, $p = 0.026$). The magnitude of this observed difference makes it unlikely that this difference could be simply due to chance or confounding factors.

Could there be a dose response relationship?

The study was not designed to look for a dose response relationship as fixed bolus and infusion doses of i.v. esomeprazole were used. In trials of other drugs more than one dose or timecourse of treatment is sometimes used to assess dose-response. It may be interesting to determine whether those patients who received the bolus and 72 hour infusion as per protocol, rather than incompletely, had better outcomes. In the per protocol analysis of this study rebleeding occurred in 4.8% of patients in the esomeprazole group and 10.4% of patients in the placebo group (ARR 5.6%, 95% CI 1.5–9.8, p = 0.009).

Is there any specificity within the study?

Consistency is relevant in clinical trials when we wish to know whether the intervention has different effects in different groups of patients. Trials should be specifically designed to answer questions about subgroups of patients. The use of post-hoc analyses looking at subgroups which are defined after the trial has been completed, although common, is open to the problems of comparisons between non-randomized groups. In this paper, subgroup analyses were defined at the start. There were four such analyses. The first was a pre-planned adjustment of the primary endpoint (rebleeding) according to endoscopic treatment received at baseline and *post hoc* analysis (adjustment by endoscopic treatment and Forrest class) which confirmed the benefits attributable to i.v. esomeprazole at day 7 and day 30. The second planned *post hoc* analysis was by ethnic group; 87% of the patients were white and 7% Asian. Both groups showed similar relative reduction in rebleeding at 72 hours. The third planned subgroup analysis, looking at site-specific or country treatment effect, found no difference in the primary variable. Finally the choice of endoscopic tretament did not effect the efficacy of esomeprazole, whether single or dual endoscopic therapy.

In summary, this is a well designed trial with careful methodology and we can be confident about its internal validity. We can dismiss concerns regarding confounding and although we cannot eliminate observation bias, the careful quality control process regarding endoscopic diagnoses minimizes such a possibility.

External validity of study

Can the results be applied to the eligible population?

A significant proportion of patients entering the study did not complete it. In the esomeprazole group 83/376 (22%) did not complete the study. In the placebo group 73/391 (19%) of participants did not complete the study. In a study of 767 patients this is a relatively large number of patients who will have missing outcomes data and probably reflects the difficulties in under-taking a trial of this nature in critically unwell patients, with frequent after regular hours randomization. The main reason for non-completion within each arm was deviation from eligibility criteria and insufficient intake of study medication. Dealing with ineligible subjects who have been included after randomization is a problem. In theory excluding patients after rando-misation can compromise the validity of randomization, but retaining ineligible patients in a study breaches protocol and may affect the internal validity of the main results.

As mentioned in the review of adopted methods, a strong aspect of the study is the use of screening logs that were to track the number of patients assessed for eligibility during the study period (n = 4146), the number enrolled (n = 1313) and the number who were then randomized to treatment (n = 767). Reasons for patients excluded throughout these steps were also provided. Some patients were not eligible as consent was not obtained or there was lack of time. It is possible that those patients from whom consent was not obtained may have had a more severe disease presentation. Since over 50% (767/1313) of those who were enrolled were randomized to treatment it is reasonable to assume that the study results can be applied to the eligible population.

Can the results be applied to the source population?
The source population in this study is comprised of the patients attending these 91 Emergency departments in the 16 participating countries, with specific eligibility criteria, over a two-year period between October 2005 and December 2007. In general, the results of this study are applicable to the source population for all aforementioned reasons.

Can the results be applied to other relevant populations?
We should be cautious in applying these results to other causes of UGIB and to other patients with PUB in whom the naturally history of bleeding may be substantially different; this might include a much older group of patients or those receiving hemodialysis (50). Of particular note is that patients with an ASA (American Society of Anesthesiologists) grade of 4 or 5 were excluded, incorporating patients with severe systemic disease that is a constant threat to life (Grade 4), or moribund patients unlikely to survive (Grade 5). PUB is predominantly a disease of older patients, many of whom may have significant comorbid illnesses. We cannot make assumptions from this study that the reduction in rebleeding after i.v. esomperazole would be as effective in patients with an ASA grade of 4 or 5. The mortality rates found in this study were also lower than those traditionally quoted in other series. This may be a reflection of the fact that patients with ASA grades of 4 and 5 were also excluded from the study.

Are the results consistent with other studies?
Other placebo controlled RCTs assessing PPIs, although mainly single centre studies in Asian populations, have shown improved outcomes in patients with peptic ulcer bleeding (34, 35). This trial therefore adds to the existing literature summarized by recent Cochrane reviews (51–53) as this is the first large

international trial to provide evidence supporting the use of high dose i.v. PPIs as adjunct therapy for patients with high-risk endoscopic peptic ulcers, in what was a principally Causcasian (non-Asian) population. Additional research now requires a determination of optimal PPI dosing and route of administration.

In summary, this study was carried out in 91 Emergency departments in 16 counties and the results should be applicable to patients presenting to those hospitals, in those countries during that time period. The results are likely to be applicable much more widely, excluding the notable exception of patients with ASA scores of 4–5.

Conclusion

We have attempted to review distinct studies of patients with non-variceal UGIB that represent amongst the most commonly adopted study designs (cohort and RCT) while emphasizing the main methodological advantages and limitations attributable to each. Our hope is that this review will permit the reader to expand their knowledge on the management of patients with non-variceal UGIB while acquiring better methodological appreciation that permits a more purposeful critical appraisal of the literature.

References

1. Cook DJ, Guyatt GH, Salena BJ, Laine LA. Endoscopic therapy for acute nonvariceal upper gastrointestinal hemorrhage: a meta-analysis. Gastroenterology 1992;102(1): 139–48.
2. Laine L, McQuaid KR. Endoscopic therapy for bleeding ulcers: an evidence-based approach based on meta-analyses of randomized controlled trials. Clin Gastroenterol Hepatol 2009;7(1):33–47;quiz 1–2.
3. Laine L, Spiegel B, Rostom A, Moayyedi P, Kuipers EJ, Bardou M, et al. Methodology for randomized trials of patients with nonvariceal upper gastrointestinal bleeding: recommendations from an international consensus conference. Am J Gastroenterol 2010;105(3):540–50.
4. Jairath V, Logan R, Hearnshaw S, Travis S, Murphy M, Palmer K. Acute Upper Gastrointestinal Bleeding- Why do patients die? Gastroenterology. [Abstract]. 2010; 138(5;S1):637–8.
5. Jairath V, Logan R, Hearnshaw S, Travis S, Murphy M, Palmer K. Mortality from Acute Upper Gastro-intestinal Bleeding in the UK – Does it display a "Weekend Effect"?. Gastroenterology. [Abstract]. 2010;138(5;S1):21.
6. Jairath VLR, Hearnshaw S, Travis SPLT, Murphy MF, Palmer KR. Can we predict length of stay in patients admitted with Acute Upper Gastrointestinal Bleeding? Gastroenterology. [Abstract]. 2010;138(5;S1):638.
7. Hearnshaw SA, Logan RF, Lowe D, Travis SP, Murphy MF, Palmer KR. Use of endoscopy for management of acute upper gastrointestinal bleeding in the UK: results of a nationwide audit. Gut 2010 Aug;59(8):1022–9.

8. Hearnshaw SA, Logan RF, Palmer KR, Card TR, Travis SP, Murphy MF. Outcomes following early red blood cell transfusion in acute upper gastrointestinal bleeding. Aliment Pharmacol Ther 2010 Jul;32(2):215–24.

9. UK Comparative Audit of Upper Gastrointestinal Bleeding and the Use of Blood. British Society of Gastroenterology. [Accessed at http://www.bsg.org.uk/pdf_word_docs/blood_audit_report_07.pdf]. 2007.

10. Sung JJ, Barkun A, Kuipers EJ, Mossner J, Jensen DM, Stuart R, et al. Intravenous esomeprazole for prevention of recurrent peptic ulcer bleeding: a randomized trial. Ann Intern Med 2009;150(7):455–64.

11. Pocock SJ, Elbourne DR. Randomized trials or observational tribulations? N Engl J Med 2000;342(25):1907–1909.

12. Rockall TA, Logan RF, Devlin HB, Northfield TC. Incidence of and mortality from acute upper gastrointestinal haemorrhage in the United Kingdom. Steering Committee and members of the National Audit of Acute Upper Gastrointestinal Haemorrhage. BMJ 1995;311 (6999):222–6.

13. Rockall TA, Logan RF, Devlin HB, Northfield TC. Risk assessment after acute upper gastrointestinal haemorrhage. Gut 1996 Mar;38(3):316–21.

14. Wallis JP, Wells AW, Chapman CE. Changing indications for red cell transfusion from 2000 to 2004 in the North of England. Transfus Med 2006;16(6):411–7.

15. Barkun A, Sabbah S, Enns R, Armstrong D, Gregor J, Fedorak RN, et al. The Canadian Registry on Nonvariceal Upper Gastrointestinal Bleeding and Endoscopy (RUGBE): Endoscopic hemostasis and proton pump inhibition are associated with improved outcomes in a real-life setting. Am J Gastroenterol 2004;99(7):1238–1246.

16. Bensoussan K, Fallone CA, Barkun AN, Martel M. A sampling of Canadian practice in managing nonvariceal upper gastrointestinal bleeding before recent guideline publication: is there room for improvement? Can J Gastroenterol 2005;19(8):487–95.

17. da Silveira EB, Lam E, Martel M, Bensoussan K, Barkun AN. The importance of process issues as predictors of time to endoscopy in patients with acute upper-GI bleeding using the RUGBE data. Gastrointest Endosc 2006;64(3):299–309.

18. Enns RA, Gagnon YM, Barkun AN, Armstrong D, Gregor JC, Fedorak RN. Validation of the Rockall scoring system for outcomes from non-variceal upper gastrointestinal bleeding in a Canadian setting. World J Gastroenterol 2006;12(48):7779–7785.

19. Muller T, Barkun AN, Martel M. Non-variceal upper GI bleeding in patients already hospitalized for another condition. Am J Gastroenterol 2009;104(2):330–9.

20. Jensen DM, Pace SC, Soffer E, Comer GM. Continuous infusion of pantoprazole versus ranitidine for prevention of ulcer rebleeding: a U.S. multicenter randomized, double-blind study. Am J Gastroenterol 2006;101(9):1991–1999;quiz 2170.

21. Di Fiore F, Lecleire S, Merle V, Herve S, Duhamel C, Dupas JL, et al. Changes in characteristics and outcome of acute upper gastrointestinal haemorrhage: a comparison of epidemiology and practices between 1996 and 2000 in a multicentre French study. Eur J Gastroenterol Hepatol 2005;17(6):641–7.

22. van Leerdam ME, Vreeburg EM, Rauws EA, Geraedts AA, Tijssen JG, Reitsma JB, et al. Acute upper GI bleeding: did anything change? Time trend analysis of incidence and outcome of acute upper GI bleeding between 1993/1994 and 2000. Am J Gastroenterol 2003;98(7):1494–1499.

23. Ananthakrishnan AN, McGinley EL, Saeian K. Outcomes of weekend admissions for upper gastrointestinal hemorrhage: a nationwide analysis. Clin Gastroenterol Hepatol 2009;7(3):296–302e1.

24. Shaheen AA, Kaplan GG, Myers RP. Weekend versus weekday admission and mortality from gastrointestinal hemorrhage caused by peptic ulcer disease. Clin Gastroenterol Hepatol 2009;7(3):303–10.

25. Altman DG, Schulz KF, Moher D, Egger M, Davidoff F, Elbourne D, et al. The revised CONSORT statement for reporting randomized trials: explanation and elaboration. Ann Intern Med 2001;134(8):663–94.

26. Kjaergard LL, Gluud C. Funding, disease area, and internal validity of hepatobiliary randomized clinical trials. Am J Gastroenterol 2002;97(11):2708–2713.

27. Delgado-Rodriguez M, Llorca J. Bias. J Epidemiol Community Health 2004;58 (8):635–41.

28. Morabia A. History of the modern epidemiological concept of confounding. J Epidemiol Community Health 2011 Apr;65(4):297–300.

29. Jager KJ, Zoccali C, Macleod A, Dekker FW. Confounding: what it is and how to deal with it. Kidney Int 2008;73(3):256–60.

30. Rothwell PM. Factors that can affect the external validity of randomised controlled trials. PLoS Clin Trials 2006;1(1):e9.

31. Higham J, Kang JY, Majeed A. Recent trends in admissions and mortality due to peptic ulcer in England: increasing frequency of haemorrhage among older subjects. Gut 2002;50(4):460–4.

32. Netzer P, Gaia C, Sandoz M, Huluk T, Gut A, Halter F, et al. Effect of repeated injection and continuous infusion of omeprazole and ranitidine on intragastric pH over 72 hours. Am J Gastroenterol 1999;94(2):351–7.

33. Hasselgren G, Lind T, Lundell L, Aadland E, Efskind P, Falk A, et al. Continuous intravenous infusion of omeprazole in elderly patients with peptic ulcer bleeding. Results of a placebo-controlled multicenter study. Scand J Gastroenterol 1997;32 (4):328–33.

34. Khuroo MS, Yattoo GN, Javid G, Khan BA, Shah AA, Gulzar GM, et al. A comparison of omeprazole and placebo for bleeding peptic ulcer. N Engl J Med 1997;336 (15):1054–1058.

35. Lau JY, Sung JJ, Lee KK, Yung MY, Wong SK, Wu JC, et al. Effect of intravenous omeprazole on recurrent bleeding after endoscopic treatment of bleeding peptic ulcers. N Engl J Med 2000;343(5):310–16.

36. Schaffalitzky de Muckadell OB, Havelund T, Harling H, Boesby S, Snel P, Vreeburg EM, et al. Effect of omeprazole on the outcome of endoscopically treated bleeding peptic ulcers. Randomized double-blind placebo-controlled multicentre study. Scand J Gastroenterol 1997;32(4):320–7.

37. Sung JJ, Mossner J, Barkun A, Kuipers EJ, Lau J, Jensen D, et al. Intravenous esomeprazole for prevention of peptic ulcer re-bleeding: rationale/design of Peptic Ulcer Bleed study. Aliment Pharmacol Ther 2008;27(8):666–77.

38. Sung JJ, Tsoi KK, Ma TK, Yung MY, Lau JY, Chiu PW. Causes of mortality in patients with peptic ulcer bleeding: a prospective cohort study of 10, 428 cases. Am J Gastroenterol 2010;105(1):84–9.

39. Vickers AJ. How to randomize. J Soc Integr Oncol 2006;4(4):194–8.

40. Laine L, Freeman M, Cohen H. Lack of uniformity in evaluation of endoscopic prognostic features of bleeding ulcers. Gastrointest Endosc 1994;40(4):411–17.

41. Lau JY, Sung JJ, Chan AC, Lai GW, Lau JT, Ng EK, et al. Stigmata of hemorrhage in bleeding peptic ulcers: an interobserver agreement study among international experts. Gastrointest Endosc 1997;46(1):33–6.

42. Jensen D, Ahlbom H, Eklund S, Stuart R, Barkun AN, Kuipers EJ, Mossner J, Lau JY, Sung JJ, Lind T, Kilhamn J Rebleeding risk for oozing peptic ulcer bleeding (PUB) in a large international study- A reassessment based upon a multivariate analysis. Gastrointest Endosc. [Abstract]. 2010;71(5):AB117.

43. Chan AW, Altman DG. Identifying outcome reporting bias in randomised trials on PubMed: review of publications and survey of authors. BMJ 2005 2;330(7494):753.

44. Glasziou P, Meats E, Heneghan C, Shepperd S. What is missing from descriptions of treatment in trials and reviews? BMJ 2008 28;336(7659):1472–1474.

45. Schulz KF, Altman DG, Moher D. CONSORT 2010 statement: updated guidelines for reporting parallel group randomized trials. Ann Intern Med 2010;152(11):726–32.

46. Forrest JA, Finlayson ND, Shearman DJ. Endoscopy in gastrointestinal bleeding. Lancet 1974;2(7877):394–7.

47. Lin HJ, Lo WC, Lee FY, Perng CL, Tseng GY. A prospective randomized comparative trial showing that omeprazole prevents rebleeding in patients with bleeding peptic ulcer after successful endoscopic therapy. Arch Intern Med 1998;158(1):54–8.

48. Leontiadis GI, Sharma VK, Howden CW. Systematic review and meta-analysis: enhanced efficacy of proton-pump inhibitor therapy for peptic ulcer bleeding in Asia – a post hoc analysis from the Cochrane Collaboration. Aliment Pharmacol Ther 2005;21(9):1055–1061.

49. Marmo R, Rotondano G, Piscopo R, Bianco MA, D'Angella R, Cipolletta L. Dual therapy versus monotherapy in the endoscopic treatment of high-risk bleeding ulcers: a meta-analysis of controlled trials. Am J Gastroenterol 2007;102(2):279–89;quiz 469.

50. Cheung J, Yu A, LaBossiere J, Zhu Q, Fedorak RN. Peptic ulcer bleeding outcomes adversely affected by end-stage renal disease. Gastrointest Endosc 2010;71(1):44–9.

51. Leontiadis GI, Sharma VK, Howden CW. Systematic review and meta-analysis of proton pump inhibitor therapy in peptic ulcer bleeding. BMJ 2005;330(7491):568.

52. Leontiadis GI, Sharma VK, Howden CW. Proton pump inhibitor treatment for acute peptic ulcer bleeding. Cochrane Database Syst Rev 2006(1):CD002094.

53. Leontiadis GI, Sharma VK, Howden CW. WITHDRAWN: Proton pump inhibitor treatment for acute peptic ulcer bleeding. Cochrane Database Syst Rev 2010;5: CD002094.

CHAPTER 13

Guidelines and Consensus on Gastrointestinal Bleeding

Alan N. Barkun

Division of Gastroenterology, McGill University Health Centre, Montreal General Hospital,
Montreal, Canada

Introduction

Clinical practice guidelines (CPG) are becoming an ever-increasing part of clinicians' every day practice (1). When done properly, by an expert group allying methodological and unconflicted medical content expertise, a set of consensus recommendations can be instructive, educational, timesaving, and in certain cases may even allow the best available evidence-based practice through rigorous statistical analysis and enlightened informed opinion. Unfortunately, not all guidelines are created equal and many fail to adopt an explicit, transparent, rigorous, and recognized process (2). Such omissions risk leading, at best, to an erroneous interpretation of the literature that may be tainted by a number of deliberate or unrecognized biases, and at worst, to harmful recommendations for patient care. A number of organizations now update their websites with a list of guidelines meeting a standard of quality requirements (for example, www.guidelines. gov). Yet the challenge remains for the practicing physician to be able to properly asses a given set of guidelines, strengths and limitations of its individual recommendations. A number of guidelines have appeared over the last decade, relating to the management of patients with non-variceal upper gastrointestinal bleeding (UGIB) (3–6). An Asian-Pacific initiative was carried out with a full publication that will postdate the writing of this manuscript. This chapter reviews the guideline creating process used at the latest consensus process 2008 Vienna Consensus Meeting on non-variceal Upper Gastrointestinal Bleeding (UGIB) in the hope of providing an improved understanding of this complex process, while reviewing existing criteria to assess the value of proposed consensus recommendations.

Gastrointestinal Bleeding, Second Edition. Edited by Joseph J.Y. Sung, Ernst J. Kuipers and Alan N. Barkun. © 2012 Blackwell Publishing Ltd.
Published 2012 by Blackwell Publishing Ltd.

Defining a need for the creation or updating of guidelines

Defining the need for the guidelines

It is not every management topic that warrants a set of guiding (7). The timing of their appearance also need be considered in the face of evolving existing evidence. Typically, a set of recommendations are useful and therefore needed when significant progress in diagnostics and/or therapeutics in a given area of clinical medicine has emerged - especially if over a short period of time. This was thought to be the case for the management of UGIB in late 2007 when the Vienna Consensus Conference on non-variceal UGIB was planned. First, UGIB remains a common condition (8) that is managed by many clinicians including family practitioners, emergency medicine physicians, intensivists, gastroenterologists, and general surgeons (9, 10). Second, the management of patients with UGIB has significantly evolved since 2003, date of an initial publication of an authoritative Consensus Conference on the topic with a special focus on peptic ulcer bleeding (6). Examples of progress in management have been suggested by audits (9), and have included:

1 Selected aspects of initial resuscitation and risk stratification. Studies have better defined the impact of using risk stratification schemes. There are now, in addition, many randomized clinical trials (RCTs) and observational studies that have assessed specific issues since 2003, including the use of erythromycin (11–13) in providing improved gastric visualization, a more rigorous determination of the role of nasogastric tube lavage (14), and selected aspects of supportive measures (15).

2 A plethora of new RCT and meta-analytical data, sometimes contradictory, on the assessment of different methods of endoscopic hemostasis, including the use of endoscopic clips that has since 2003 gained wide popularity and been the focus of many analyses (16–18). There also now exist additional data on the utility of second-look endoscopy with performance of the largest RCT ever completed on the topic (19), and an updated systematic analysis and meta-analysis that includes the results of this important trial that utilizes contemporary methods of endoscopic hemostasis and pharmacotherapy (20, 21).

3 The publication of additional trials assessing the role of PPI pharmacotherapy following endoscopy, and of multiple meta-analyses on the topic (22–27), with disparate conclusions that remain only partially explained (28). At the source of these disparities lie important issues of timing and dosing of PPI administration that remain unanswered, as well as considerations of generalizability of results from Asian to other populations (29).

4 The publication of many analyses that assess the cost-effectiveness of different strategies including endoscopic (30, 31) and proton pump inhibitors (PPI) administered prior to and following early endoscopic therapy (32–35), as well as recent updated information on costs attributable to upper GI bleeding (36).

5 Recent trial and summary data have suggested no improvement in primary outcomes, but an amelioration of secondary outcomes when administering PPI prior to an early endoscopy (37, 38), with until just recently, few guiding cost analyses or editorials to assist in decision-making (39, 40). Tsoi KKF, Lau JYW, Sung JJY. Cost-effectiveness analysis of high-dose omeprazole infusion before endoscopy for patients with upper-GI bleeding. Gastrointestinal Endoscopy 2008;67:1056–63.

6 The timing and method of optimal diagnosis for *Helicobacter pylori* diagnosis remain unclear and controversial (41, 42).

Other objectives of recommendations may be to address areas not previously tackled by Consensus recommendations. Such a new area in UGIB for the international group was that of secondary prophylaxis for patients taking aspirin (ASA), clopidogrel, traditional non steroidal anti-inflammatory drugs (NSAID), or selective cyloxoygenase-2 (COX-2) inhibitors for which many RCT exist assessing the continued prescribing of these agents with or without a PPI for gastroprotection (43). In this regard, the UGIB guideline update was complementing and building on the recommendations of recent meta-analyses put forth by GI and cardiology societies in the US and Canada (44, 45).

The multidimensional process of guideline development

There exist published blueprints to optimize the methodological process of creating guidelines. Considerations are multiple and complex in order to navigate amidst potential sources of error and bias, while optimizing the yield of the proposed recommendations and planning for their release, dissemination, and even, updating. Box 13.1 provides a modified list of one of these suggested approaches: the AGREE guidelines (www.agreecollaboration.org).

Scope and purpose

The objectives of the Consensus Conference need to be clearly outlined; this step is critical for participants to efficiently and harmoniously decide on the areas to cover and, subsequently, the number of recommendations to put forward. The 2008 Vienna Consensus Conference group decided to focus its attention on patients suspected of bleeding from a non-variceal source, and in particular, for all post-endoscopy recommendations, peptic ulcer bleeding.

Box 13.1 The AGREE Guidelines for Creating Clinical Practice Guidelines

Scope and purpose
- Objectives
- Clinical questions addressed
- Target population defined

Stakeholder involvement
- Guideline-development group includes representative stakeholders
- Target users of the guidelines defined

Rigor of development
- Systematic methods used to search for evidence*
- Criteria for selecting the evidence clearly described*
- Methods used for formulating the recommendations clearly described*
- Health benefits, side effects and risks considered*
- There exist explicit links between recommendations and supporting evidence*
- External review by experts planned
- Procedure for updating guidelines included

Clarity and presentation
- Recommendations are specific and unambiguous.
- Different options for management of the condition presented, if applicable
- Key recommendations easily identifiable
- Application tools to be developed are identified

Applicability
- Potential organizational barriers discussed
- Potential cost implications considered
- Key review criteria for monitoring and audit purposes are discussed

Editorial independence
- Editorial independency
- Conflicts of interest presented and resolved

Additional domains addressed by the consensus meeting
- Future research addressed
- Dissemination of the guidelines discussed

Modified from www.agreecollaboration.org
* See GRADE scoring system in Guyatt et al. (55).

The group therefore set out to develop a tailored update to the 2003 Consensus Conference on the acute management of patients with non-variceal UGIB, based on needs analyses and surveys performed since 2003, using state-of-the-art methodology, and following a sequence of carefully planned steps:

1 Gathering a panel of experts in order to reach consensus on a number of key statements that form the basis for managing patients with

peptic ulcer bleeding (the etiology of most episodes of non-variceal UGIB). These included updates to key recommendations; it was also anticipated that some past recommendations would not be revisited as current evidence did not justify their modification, while new ones would be added, in keeping with evolution in the field as described above (5).

2 Establishing standards of clinical care, based on the presumption of availability of a minimum set of key resources, commensurate with both data from practice as it is carried out coupled to evidence from high-level publications in the literature. The first part of this objective was especially critical in view of the desired international applicability of the guidelines, which was in part assured by a broad international representation of conference participants.

3 Putting forth an evidence-based document that would subsequently allow professional associations (both the ones supporting the initiative and others) to lobby administrative and government bodies to ensure that adequate resources are provided for the optimal delivery of acute care to patients with acute non-variceal UGIB.

4 Identifying areas that require further research.

In addition, the Vienna Conference set out to create documents allowing:

5 Subsequently creating dissemination tools in the form of a slide kit and revised management algorithm (since one had been first published as a result of the 2003 Guidelines (10)) that could facilitate the work of institutions in establishing critical paths, and thus streamlining the management of a majority of patients with acute non-variceal UGIB.

6 Providing a roadmap to facilitate the integration of the produced guidelines such as to optimize their dissemination and implementation (http://www.controlled-trials.com/ISRCTN85537469).

7 Identifying a set of methodological standards for the performance of future randomized clinical trials in this area (46).

8 Determination a list of valid quality indicators that can assist in the subsequent implementation of the guidelines, and auditing the resultant level of quality in the management of patients with non-variceal UGIB (47).

9 Coordinating a possible revision of the Forrest classification based on a reappraisal of published and emerging trial data as they pertain to patients exhibiting selected high-risk endoscopic lesions.

10 Taking this opportunity to embed an Ethics project in the actual guidelines development process, with an aim to improve existing ethics procedures adopted for the development of guidelines by supporting professional associations, while also evaluating current existing standards (http://www.nap.edu/catalog/12598.html).

Stakeholder involvement

The guideline development process requires, optimally, the input of all health care stakeholders to ensure both a valid set of guidelines and facilitate their subsequent uptake. The clinical questions addressed must thus be guided by professionals who take care of the target patient population on a daily basis. In the case of UGIB, these include hospitalists, primary care, emergency room, and intensive care physicians, in addition to specialists (gastroenterologists, general surgeons, and radiologists), as well as nurses, pharmacists, and hospital administrators (48). These also form the target users of the guidelines that may be piloted in some cases, as part of a dissemination strategy. Because of the principally in-hospital, usually brief, nature of an episode of non-variceal UGIB, patients were not included in the guideline development process but their participation in the development of guidelines should, as a rule, be encouraged – especially when dealing with chronic illnesses or conditions where the synchronous production of self-help literature is likely to be useful.

Rigor of development

In addition to the aforementioned group, methodological expertise must be present in the Consensus group in the form of experienced epidemiological researchers in the areas of diagnostic testing, clinical trials, systematic reviews, meta-analyses, administrative databases, and health economics. Key to the validity of the guidelines is indeed the rigor with which the evidence is sought and the corresponding guidelines formulated. This is one area where many guidelines fall short. Systematic methods are required to search for evidence, and appropriate search strings or actual completed meta-analyses are often available, including from the Cochrane Collaboration library. These of course need to be updated and adapted to the different recommendations. The criteria for selecting the evidence need to clearly be described in order to avoid selection bias or missing important information. The corresponding methods used for formulating the recommendations must be clearly outlined (a grading scale, the GRADE system, is discussed in great detail later). In order to further ensure lack of bias and the high quality of produced guidelines, external review by experts must be planned, usually in the form of a corresponding publication in a peer-review journal and at the same time ensure adequate dissemination. Ideally, an explicit procedure for updating guidelines should also be included as part of the final consensus document.

Clarity and presentation

The interpretation of the guidelines is critical and the recommendations must be both specific and unambiguous. Ideally and when clinically indicated, different options for management of the condition, where applicable, should be clearly presented. The authors should also structure the consensus document such that key recommendations are easily identifiable; this may be further facilitated by discussion with the editorial office of the journal publishing the guidelines. The consensus process should ideally also attempt to plan for the development of application tools to favor guideline uptake and dissemination. Examples of these would include the creation of disease-specific algorithms (10), and information documentation for physicians, pharmacists, and patients.

Applicability

Potential organizational barriers need to be discussed or have been studied *a priori* to better understand the needs of the different stakeholders in taking up the guidelines and eventually applying them to their every day practice (48). An example of the composition of discussion groups as part of a need and barriers analysis that were assembled in the preparation of the Vienna Conference guidelines is shown in Table 13.1. The target group should likely be similar to the ones identified in the stakeholder involvement section described above and should not only include primary care and specialty physicians, but also an appropriate selection of allied health professionals tailored to the disease process and delivery of care strategies under consideration (e.g. nurses, pharmacists, dieticians, psychologists, etc.). A better understanding of the potential cost implications resulting from selected recommendations is also required, and the corresponding cost-effectiveness evidence should be included. An effort should be made to target optimization of health care delivery rather than sole cost

Table 13.1 Sample of health-care professionals included in a national needs analysis performed assessing guidelines on the management of patients with non-variceal upper gastrointestinal bleeding.

Profession	Number of participants (n)	Number of provinces (n)
Emergency room physicians	5	2
Intensive care unit physicians	4	2
Gastroenterologists	4	3
Nurses (e.g., Endoscopy, gastroenterology, emergency room . . .)	6	3
Pharmacists and hospital administrators	3	3
Total (n)	**22**	**4**

Canadian provinces that the sample was drawn from included Ontario, Quebec, British Columbia, and Nova Scotia.
Modified from Dupuis et al. (48) with permission from Pulsus Group.

rationalization in order to best guide decision-takers, so that the end-product will be improved patient outcomes with the best use of available resources. Finally, in order to allow for effective monitoring of the impact of the guidelines on patient care with effective and valid auditing, appropriate quality indicators should be developed, adapting the individual recommendations that only provide broad guidance to more specific individual clinical scenarios, and at the same time allowing for deviation from the guidelines, given certain clinical parameters (47). An example of the quality indicators developed as an adjunct to the Vienna Conference recommendations is provided in Box 13.2 (47).

Editorial independence

The CPGs need to be editorially independent from the funding body, with explicit and transparent declarations on this important potential source of bias. In order to best address this issue, the entire guideline creation process, from its inception, should be developed within an established ethical framework, ideally grounded in recognized and valid ethical principles. This requirement is especially needed when the guideline development group includes clinician-experts who often have established relationships with equipment and pharmaceutical manufacturers. It is important to realize, however, that all stakeholders and not just practitioners may bring conflicts to the table, including regulatory agencies and third-party payers (such as Health Maintenance Organizations, insurance companies, and government representatives). The ethical approaches to these complex situations have recently been reviewed by the Institute of Medicine (http://www.nap.edu/catalog/12598.html), as they apply to guideline development. The specific example of the ethical framework and toolbox developed for the Vienna Conference may serve as a partial template for others to carry out further research in this important and often overlooked area. The entire ethical process should be transparent, and may best be overseen by a professional Ethicist, an ad hoc ethics committee comprised of Consensus participants, and assessed through the peer-review process at the time of manuscript submission.

Additional domains addressed by the consensus meeting

Finally, as briefly described above, any set of recommendations must be complemented by a list of future areas requiring research. The timeliness of such a guiding agenda is especially important since it originates as a result of a thorough and hopefully valid evidence-based review of the literature up to the time of the Consensus meeting. There may be very practical reasons why evidence is lacking in a certain dimension of management, however, the importance of such information may outweigh the limitations of trying to address it with a given study. Furthermore, other content areas may have

---

Box 13.2 Examples of quality indicators developed relating to the consensus recommendations on the management of patients with non-variceal upper gastrointestinal bleeding

---

PRE-ENDOSCOPIC INDICATORS
Diagnosis
If patients present with non-variceal UGIB, then they should receive the following tests: complete blood count, levels of electrolytes, blood type, and cross-match at the time of initial evaluation
Risk stratification
If patients present with non-variceal UGIB, then they should have a documentation of risk stratification using one of the previously validated measures as high risk versus low risk for re-bleeding and mortality (e.g., Blatchford or Rockall score) at the time of initial evaluation
Early resuscitation
If patients with non-variceal UGIB exhibit signs of hypovolemia (e.g., pulse >100, systolic blood pressure <100 mmHg; or orthostatic changes), then they should receive crystalloids for fluid resuscitation at the time of initial evaluation.
If patients with non-variceal UGIB have active hematemesis with mental status changes, then they should receive airway protection (i.e., intubation) before upper endoscopy.

ENDOSCOPIC INDICATORS
Diagnosis
If patients present with non-variceal UGIB and do not have contraindications to esophago-gastroduodenoscopy (EGD), then they should receive an EGD within 24 hours of presentation
Risk stratification
If patients present with non-variceal UGIB have an ulcer related bleeding on EGD, then the stigmata of bleeding should be documented in the procedure note for the index endoscopy using a standardized taxonomy (e.g., Forrest classification, NIH Consensus Conference taxonomy)
Endoscopic treatment
If patients have an ulcer related bleeding on EGD, then whether hemostasis was achieved or not should be documented in the procedure note for the index EGD
If patients with ulcer related bleeding have active spurting, oozing, or visible vessel and normal INR (<1.5), then they should receive endoscopic hemostasis using any of the following modalities: hemoclip, combination epinephrine and contact thermal therapy, or combination epinephrine and hemoclip

POST-ENDOSCOPIC INDICATORS
Diagnosis
If patients have non-variceal UGIB from a ≥1 cm gastric ulcer, then they should receive repeat endoscopy within 2–3 months of index endoscopy.
Pharmacological treatment
If patients with ulcer related bleeding have low risk stigmata of bleeding on endoscopy, then they should receive PPI after index endoscopy.
Secondary prophylaxis
If patients have bleeding peptic ulcers and documented *Helicobacter pylori* infection, then they should be treated with a recommended antibiotic combination within 1 month of the positive result
If patients with peptic ulcer bleeding are prescribed aspirin, then they should also receive a proton pump inhibitor.

Modified from Kanwal et al. (47).

been overlooked because of existing beliefs that may or not be grounded in sound evidence. A partial list of areas identified by the Vienna Conference as worthy of future evaluation is listed in Box 13.3 (5).

One of the most frustrating aspects of the guideline development is a phenomenon well-known of knowledge translation specialists that ends up as the Achilles' heel of most sets of recommendations: their implementation and uptake. An example of the difficulty in achieving adequate uptake exists in Canada with the advent of the 2003 international guidelines having resulted in the persistence of significant non-adherence to published recommendations (47, 49). It would also appear that despite the implementation of an intensive, state-of-the art repeated multifaceted tailored educational initiative, the uptake of existing guidelines remains modest (Barkun AN, pers.comm., 2010) with little demonstrable improvement in measurable patient outcomes. Attempts at improving guideline uptake, and even patient outcomes in other therapeutic areas, have met with more success (50). A recent audit of patients with non-variceal UGIB in the

---

Box 13.3 Examples of Areas of Future Research

Pre-endoscopy
- Timing of initial endoscopy in relation to a clinical scale of low vs. high risk (Blatchford, Rockall) and optimal predictive models
- Role of early discharge of very low risk patients (very low Blatchford) without endoscopy vs. early endoscopy or overnight observation until endoscopy

Endoscopic therapy
- Comparative roles of newer endoscopic modalities for hemostasis
- Role of second-look endoscopy in the era of profound acid suppression

PPI and other pharmacological therapy
- Optimal route of administration, dose, and duration of PPI following successful endoscopic hemostasis (direct comparison of oral versus intravenous PPI)
- Role of early switch from intravenous to oral PPI, and optimal dose and duration of PPI therapy following discharge

Classification of stigmata
- Revision of the Forrest 1B (oozing bleeding) classification and clarification of the risk of rebleeding of adherent clots in clinically high and low risk patients
- Standardization and validation of an objective measure to classify stigmata

ASA and NSAID related issues
- Optimal timing of reinstatement of ASA therapy in patients with acute UGIB
- Impact of clopidogrel on endoscopic hemostasis and risk of rebleeding

Economics
- Additional cost-effectiveness analyses to better characterize diagnostic and therapeutic strategies

ASA = acetylsalicylic acid, PPI = proton pump inhibitor, UGIB = upper gastrointestinal bleed. Modified from Barkun et al. (5).

United Kingdom (UK) has suggested an association between the availability of an on-call after-hours endoscopy roster and a strong trend to an improvement in mortality amongst 6750 patients from 208 institutions (51). The difficulty in demonstrating improvements in patient outcomes, especially mortality, in non-variceal UGIB has been addressed in a recent editorial on the topic (52).

Quantifying the strength of the recommendations and corresponding evidence

The GRADE system

Critical to the CPG development process is a systematic, objective and standardized methodology to identify and grade the evidence and the resulting recommendations. A number of systems have been developed and indeed many are modified by CPG creators at times to best serve their needs. Many systems are described elsewhere (7) with no evidence favoring one over another as there exist no data to guide how best to communicate grades of evidence and recommendations. Until sufficient evidence accumulates to demonstrate the superiority of one system over another, concentrating on making recommendations clear and reflective of the evidence is a reasonable approach for most guideline developers (7). The Vienna Consensus Conference on non-variceal UGIB adopted a modified version of the GRADE (Grading of Recommendations, Assessment, Development and Evaluation) system that represents an international effort to standardize the approach to making recommendations (www.gradeworkinggroup.org). The AGREE group defines the quality of evidence as the extent to which one can be confident that an estimate of effect is correct, while the strength of a recommendation indicates the extent to which one can be confident that adherence to the recommendation will do more good than harm (2). AGREE proposes that methods used for formulating the recommendations be clearly described, and include assessments of health benefits, side effects and risks while explicitly linking recommendations and supporting evidence.

Judging the quality of evidence

Judgments about the quality of evidence require assessments of the validity of the results of individual studies for the relevant outcomes. The GRADE system makes sequential judgments about the quality of evidence across studies for each important outcome, which outcomes are critical to a decision, the overall quality of evidence across these critical outcomes, the balance between benefits and harms, and the strength of recommendations.

A systematic review of available evidence should assist in making these judgments, considering four key elements: study design, study quality, consistency, and directness. Details on how to undertake a systematic review (including the possible need for the performance of original meta-analyses) are beyond the scope of this chapter. Study design can be separated into observational, and the highest quality evidence, that of randomized trials (if available). Study quality refers to the study methods and execution, with reviewers using appropriate criteria of assessment. Consistency refers to the similarity of estimates of effect across studies (unexplained inconsistency, for example, would decrease confidence in the estimate of effect). Directness refers to the extent to which the people, interventions, and outcome measures are similar to those of interest (as an example, surrogate outcomes generally provide less direct evidence than those using outcomes that are important to patients).

The GRADE approach initially categorizes evidence based on study design into randomized trials and observational studies (cohort studies, case-control studies, interrupted time series analyses, and controlled before and after studies) (Table 13.2 (2, 53)). Next, the reviewers must consider whether the studies have serious limitations, important inconsistencies in the results, or whether uncertainty about the directness of the evidence is warranted. The following definitions are proposed in grading the quality of the evidence: High = Further research is very unlikely to change our confidence in the estimate of effect; Moderate = Further research is likely to have an important impact on our confidence in the estimate of effect and may change the estimate; Low = Further research is very likely to have an important impact on our confidence in the estimate of effect and is likely to change the estimate; Very low = Any estimate of effect is very uncertain. Considerations that can lower the quality of the evidence include limitations in study quality, imprecise or sparse data, and a high possibility of reporting bias. All these considerations act cumulatively. The same rules should be applied to judgments about the quality of evidence for harms and benefits.

When providing a grade, the lowest quality of evidence for any of the outcomes that are critical to making a decision should provide the basis for rating overall quality of evidence. As much as possible all judgments adopt the values of those who will be affected by adherence to subsequent recommendations.

Assessing the strength of recommendations

Recommendations involve a trade-off between benefits and harms: Does the intervention do more good than harm? Making that trade-off inevitably involves placing, implicitly or explicitly, a relative value on each outcome. GRADE suggests making explicit judgments about the balance between the main health benefits and harms before considering costs, as they apply to

Table 13.2 Criteria for Weighting the Strength of the Recommendation.

Grade of Recommendation/Description	Benefit vs Risk and Burden	Methodological Quality of Supporting Evidence
1A. Strong recommendation, high quality evidence	Benefits clearly outweigh risk and burdens, or vice versa	RCTs without important limitations or overwhelming evidence from observational studies
1B. Strong recommendation, moderate-quality evidence	Benefits clearly outweigh risk and burdens, or vice versa	RCTs with important limitations (inconsistent results, methodological flaws, indirect, or imprecise) or exceptionally strong evidence from observational studies
1C. Strong recommendation, low-quality or very low-quality evidence	Benefits clearly outweigh risk and burdens, or vice versa	Observational studies or case series
Grade of Recommendation/Description	Benefit vs Risk and Burden	Methodological Quality of Supporting Evidence
2A. Weak recommendation, high quality evidence	Benefits closely balanced with risk and burdens	RCTs without important limitations or overwhelming evidence from observational studies
2B. Weak recommendation, moderate-quality evidence	Benefits closely balanced with risk and burdens	RCTs with important limitations (inconsistent results, methodological flaws, indirect, or imprecise) or exceptionally strong evidence from observational studies
2C. Weak recommendation, low-quality or very low-quality evidence	Uncertainty in the estimates of benefits, risks, and burden; benefits, risks, and burden may be closely balanced	Observational studies or case series

Modified from Atkins et al. (2) and Guyatt et al. (53).

specific settings and particular groups of patients (2, 53). The following nomenclature is suggested to assess the different possible trade-off scenarios: Net benefits = the intervention clearly does more good than harm; trade-offs = there are important trade-offs between the benefits and harms; uncertain trade-offs = it is not clear whether the intervention does more good than harm; and no net benefits = the intervention clearly does not do more good than harm. This grading should be based on the trade-offs, taking into account the estimated size of the effect for the main outcomes, the confidence limits around those estimates, the relative value placed on each outcome, the quality of the evidence, and translation of the evidence into practice in a specific setting, taking into consideration important factors that could be expected to modify the size of the expected effects and the uncertainty about baseline risk for the population of interest. GRADE suggests the resulting grading scheme for the recommendations: "Do it" or "don't do it" – indicating a judgment that most well informed people would make; "Probably do it" or "probably don't do it" – indicating a judgment that a majority of well informed people would make but a substantial minority would not. While recognizing the difficulty of making accurate estimates of costs, GRADE also suggests that the incremental costs of healthcare alternatives should be considered explicitly alongside the expected health benefits and harms.

Operational aspects of the CPG development process

Initial steps

Appropriate resources must be secured and realistic timelines adopted for the CPG process to result in high-quality guidelines, especially if carried out by a group of individuals or organizations with limited experience in this area or in the absence of a dedicated methodological team. As in most successful initiatives, a small group of dedicated (and experienced) individuals will need to act as champions of the process from its inception. An example of the different steps and related timetable for the Vienna Conference are shown in Box 13.4. Funding need be secured through an 'at arm's length" process and a preliminary level of interest for targeted stakeholders secured, supported by evidence for the need of the guidelines at this time. It is especially useful that eventual participants be able to predict (as much as possible) the emergence of any critical data during the guideline CPG development process, and that forecasting on the validity of the guidelines at the time of their publication and dissemination be carried out. Initial invitations are then sent out with the explicit aim to secure as participants the most representative and competent group of targeted stakeholders. The scope of the CPGs and the targeted geographic area for

Box 13.4 Different Steps and Related Timetable of the Vienna Conference	
November 2007	Project development
December 2007–January 2008	Project Launch – invitation of WG members
January–May 2008	Develop statements
February–July 2008	Collection of relevant literature
June 2008	First iteration
July–August 2008	Phase 1 of data collection
September–October 2008	Phase 2 of data collection
September 2008	Second iteration
October 2008	Final pre-meeting iteration/vote
October 2008	Consensus Meeting
October 2008–January 2009	Preparation of Consensus document
February–March 2009	Planned submission of Consensus document

eventual dissemination and implementation will also determine whether regional, national or international representation is indicated.

The Delphi technique iterative process

Once selected, the group is then engaged in an iterative process that follows a Delphi technique – a method for structuring a group communication process allowing a group of individuals as a whole to deal with a complex problem (www.is.njit.edu/pubs/delphibook). Further characteristics of this process usually include anonymity (allows change of views without "loss of face"), iteration (a series of rounds with modification of statements, allowing members to change the statements to reflect group opinion), controlled feedback with each round analyzed by a non-voting unbiased central researcher (54). The Vienna Conference assembled 36 participants (including 35 voting members, and one non-voting Chair who led all discussions and was independent of the CPG developing process). Iterative rounds allowed the identification of the areas worthy of recommendations (considering the original 2003 set of CPGs). Initial wording was provided, with a repeat iterative process to wordsmith the statements, with a final round that was supplemented by the evidence reports, prepared by unbiased individuals, to assist in the final grading of both evidence and recommendations by the entire group. Iterative rounds prior to the actual meeting are usually carried out through a transparent, centralized e-mail process with transparent recording of every step.

The head-to-head meeting

At the head-to-head meeting, operational issues on voting are presented to the group. Pre-circulated conflicts of interest are reviewed as are their resolutions. For the Vienna conference, possible methods of resolution

---

Box 13.5 An Example of Selected Instructions to Participants at the Head-to head Meeting of the Vienna Conference

1 Ethics filtering

2 Review statements by subsection

3 Quickly overview of statements with consensus

4 Review and discuss statements with less consensus

5 Presentation of the assigned statements

6 Voting on all statements within a subsection

7 Dissenting minority points will be included in the report

8 Engage in building consensus on matters for which this has not yet been achieved

9 At this stage of the process, only major wordsmithing can be considered

10 Remain in seats during sessions to ensure capture of all discussion and efficiency in voting

11 No side bar conversations, please

12 Make your discussion point briefly and once

13 Respect the chair's queuing of questions and comments

14 Reminder of the objective of the Conference (target patient group).

---

included self-recusal as discussed elsewhere (Barkun AN, pers.comm., 2010). Discussion on the evidence and its grading are reviewed along with the final wording of the given recommendation and its gradings, followed by subsequent anonymous voting using touchpad technology on a six-point Likhert scale (Agree Strongly, Agree Moderately, Just Agree, Just Disagree, Disagree Moderately, Disagree Strongly). Every final statement required 75% approval (some form of agreement) in Vienna in order for the recommendation to be adopted and to move on to the next statement. As group psychology, individual personalities, and their inter-play in the setting of intensive discussions in a limited space are critical for the outcome of the head-to-head meeting, thought needs to be put into seating plan, time allotment to different recommendations, with the inde-pendent Chair fully briefed on such considerations, and a clear *modus operandi* outline explicitly and upfront for the meeting, based on a systematic approach and mutual respect of participants. An example of selected Instructions to participants at the head-to-head meeting is listed in Box 13.5.

Drafting of the document and completion of dissemination initiatives

The drafting of a document follows (ideally within a brief period of time), and is most effectively carried out by a small writing group selected well in advance, with subsequent broad circulation to the group for input, followed by submission for peer-review publication which addresses possible areas of bias as described above. Our group has found it useful to be familiar with the preferences and style adopted by the targeted journal at the outset, prior to the determination of the number of recommendations and well before the first drafting of the manuscript. Satellite initiatives aimed at optimizing diffusion and implementation (as described above) that were prepared in parallel to the CPG development can then proceed along with plans for updating of the guidelines.

Conclusion

CPG development is indeed a complex, multi-stepped trek that requires much knowledge, expertise, and planning to be successful. Although some have suggested this process is best carried out by an independent, specialized group of methodologists, we believe it is optimally patient or people-focused when involving a broad representation of stakeholders possessing both content and methodological expertise, with appropriate rigor and ethical transparence as to ensure a valid, unbiased final product. Readers are encouraged to keep informed on the recommended methods for CPG guideline development which is a rapidly-evolving area, and one critical in this era of medical information overload for patients, allied health care professionals and physicians alike.

References

1. Hayward RS, Guyatt GH, Moore KA, McKibbon KA, Carter AO. Canadian physicians' attitudes about and preferences regarding clinical practice guidelines. Cmaj 1997;156:1715–1723.
2. Atkins D, Best D, Briss PA, et al. Grading quality of evidence and strength of recommendations. BMJ 2004;328:1490.
3. Non-variceal upper gastrointestinal haemorrhage:, guidelines., Gut 2002;51 Suppl 4: iv1–6.
4. Adler DG, Leighton JA, Davila RE, et al. ASGE guideline: The role of endoscopy in acute non-variceal upper-GI hemorrhage. Gastrointest Endosc 2004;60:497–504.
5. Barkun A, Bardou M, Kuipers E, et al. International consensus recommendations on the management of patients with non-variceal upper gastrointestinal bleeding. Ann Int Med 2010;152(2):101–13.
6. Barkun A, Bardou M, Marshall JK. Consensus recommendations for managing patients with nonvariceal upper gastrointestinal bleeding. Ann Intern Med 2003;139:843–57.
7. Palda VA, Davis D, Goldman J. A guide to the Canadian Medical Association handbook on clinical practice guidelines. CMAJ 2007;177:1221–1226.
8. Lanas A, Garcia-Rodriguez LA, Polo-Tomas M, et al. Time trends and impact of upper and lower gastrointestinal bleeding and perforation in clinical practice. Am J Gastroenterol 2009;104:1633–1641.
9. Bensoussan K, Fallone CA, Barkun AN, Martel M. A sampling of Canadian practice in managing nonvariceal upper gastrointestinal bleeding before recent guideline publication: is there room for improvement? Can J Gastroenterol 2005;19:487–95.

10. Barkun A, Fallone CA, Chiba N, et al. A Canadian clinical practice algorithm for the management of patients with nonvariceal upper gastrointestinal bleeding. Canadian Journal of Gastroenterology 2004;18:605–9.

11. Carbonell N, Pauwels A, Serfaty L, Boelle PY, Becquemont L, Poupon R. Erythromycin infusion prior to endoscopy for acute upper gastrointestinal bleeding: a randomized, controlled, double-blind trial. Am J Gastroenterol 2006;101:1211–1215.

12. Coffin B, Pocard M, Panis Y, et al. Erythromycin improves the quality of EGD in patients with acute upper GI bleeding: a randomized controlled study. Gastrointest Endosc 2002;56:174–9.

13. Frossard JL, Spahr L, Queneau PE, et al. Erythromycin intravenous bolus infusion in acute upper gastrointestinal bleeding: a randomized, controlled, double-blind trial. Gastroenterology 2002;123:17–23.

14. Lee SD, Kearney DJ. A randomized controlled trial of gastric lavage prior to endoscopy for acute upper gastrointestinal bleeding. J Clin Gastroenterol 2004;38:861–5.

15. Baradarian R, Ramdhaney S, Chapalamadugu R, et al. Early intensive resuscitation of patients with upper gastrointestinal bleeding decreases mortality. Am J Gastroenterol 2004;99:619–22.

16. Calvet X, Vergara M, Brullet E, Gisbert JP, Campo R. Addition of a second endoscopic treatment following epinephrine injection improves outcome in high-risk bleeding ulcers. Gastroenterology 2004;126:441–50.

17. Marmo R, Rotondano G, Piscopo R, Bianco MA, D'Angella R, Cipolletta L. Dual therapy versus monotherapy in the endoscopic treatment of high-risk bleeding ulcers: a meta-analysis of controlled trials. Am J Gastroenterol 2007;102:279–89.

18. Sung JJ, Tsoi KK, Lai LH, Wu JC, Lau JY. Endoscopic clipping versus injection and thermo-coagulation in the treatment of bleeding non-variceal upper gastrointestinal bleeding: a meta-analysis. Gut 2007 Oct;56(10):1364–73.

19. Chiu PW, Lam CY, Lee SW, et al. Effect of scheduled second therapeutic endoscopy on peptic ulcer rebleeding: a prospective randomised trial. Gut 2003;52:1403–1407.

20. Tsoi KK, Chan HC, Chiu PW, Pau CY, Lau JY, Sung JJ. Second-look endoscopy with thermal coagulation or injections for peptic ulcer bleeding: a meta-analysis. J Gastroenterol Hepatol 2010;25:8–13.

21. Tsoi KK, Chiu PW, Sung JJ. Endoscopy for upper gastrointestinal bleeding: is routine second-look necessary? Nat Rev Gastroenterol Hepatol 2009;6:717–22.

22. Bardou M, Toubouti Y, Benhaberou-Brun D, Rahme E, Barkun AN. Meta-analysis: proton-pump inhibition in high-risk patients with acute peptic ulcer bleeding. Aliment Pharmacol Ther 2005;21:677–86.

23. Leontiadis GI, Sharma VK, Howden CW. Systematic review and meta-analysis of proton pump inhibitor therapy in peptic ulcer bleeding. BMJ. 2005 Mar 12; 330(7491):568.

24. Leontiadis GI, McIntyre L, Sharma VK, Howden CW. Proton pump inhibitor treatment for acute peptic ulcer bleeding. The Cochrane database of systematic reviews 2004: CD002094.

25. Leontiadis GI, Sharma VK, Howden CW. Proton pump inhibitor treatment for acute peptic ulcer bleeding. Cochrane Database Syst Rev 2006: CD002094.

26. Andriulli A, Annese V, Caruso N, et al. Proton-pump inhibitors and outcome of endoscopic hemostasis in bleeding peptic ulcers: a series of meta-analyses. Am J Gastroenterol 2005;100:207–19.

27. Leontiadis GI, Sharma VK, Howden CW. Proton pump inhibitor therapy for peptic ulcer bleeding: Cochrane collaboration meta-analysis of randomized controlled trials. Mayo Clin Proc 2007;82:286–96.

28. Leontiadis GI, Sharma VK, Howden CW. Explaining divergent results of meta-analyses on proton pump inhibitor treatment for ulcer bleeding. Gastroenterology 2005;129:1804–1805.

29. Leontiadis GI, Sharma VK, Howden CW. Systematic review and meta-analysis: enhanced efficacy of proton-pump inhibitor therapy for peptic ulcer bleeding in Asia – a post hoc analysis from the Cochrane Collaboration. Aliment Pharmacol Ther 2005;21:1055–1061.

30. Spiegel BM, Dulai GS, Lim BS, Mann N, Kanwal F, Gralnek IM. The cost-effectiveness and budget impact of intravenous versus oral proton pump inhibitors in peptic ulcer hemorrhage. Clin Gastroenterol Hepatol 2006;4:988–97.

31. Spiegel BM, Ofman JJ, Woods K, Vakil NB. Minimizing recurrent peptic ulcer hemorrhage after endoscopic hemostasis: the cost-effectiveness of competing strategies. Am J Gastroenterol 2003;98:86–97.

32. Enns RA, Gagnon YM, Rioux KP, Levy AR. Cost-effectiveness in Canada of intravenous proton pump inhibitors for all patients presenting with acute upper gastrointestinal bleeding. Aliment Pharmacol Ther 2003;17:225–33.

33. Gagnon YM, Levy AR, Eloubeidi MA, Arguedas MR, Rioux KP, Enns RA. Cost implications of administering intravenous proton pump inhibitors to all patients presenting to the emergency department with peptic ulcer bleeding. Value Health 2003;6:457–65.

34. Barkun AN, Herba K, Adam V, Kennedy W, Fallone CA, Bardou M. High-dose intravenous proton pump inhibition following endoscopic therapy in the acute management of patients with bleeding peptic ulcers in the USA and Canada: a cost-effectiveness analysis. Aliment Pharmacol Ther 2004;19:591–600.

35. Barkun AN, Herba K, Adam V, Kennedy W, Fallone CA, Bardou M. The cost-effectiveness of high-dose oral proton pump inhibition after endoscopy in the acute treatment of peptic ulcer bleeding. Aliment Pharmacol Ther 2004;20:195–202.

36. Adam V, Barkun AN. Estimates of costs of hospital stay for variceal and non variceal upper gastrointestinal bleeding in the United States. Value in Health 2007; *In Press.*

37. Lau JY, Leung WK, Wu JC, et al. Omeprazole before endoscopy in patients with gastrointestinal bleeding. N Engl J Med 2007;356:1631–1640.

38. Dorward S, Sreedharan A, Leontiadis G, Howden C, Moayyedi P, Forman D. Proton pump inhibitor treatment initiated prior to endoscopic diagnosis in upper gastrointestinal bleeding. Cochrane Database Syst Rev 2006:CD005415.

39. Alsabah S, Barkun A, Herba K, Adam V, Kennedy W, Pomier-Layrargues G. The Cost-Effectiveness of Continuous Infusion Intravenous Proton Pump Inhibitors (IV PPI) Administered Prior to Endoscopy in the Treatment of Patients Presenting with Suspected Upper GI Bleeding (UGIB). Gastroenterology 2007;132:A–164.

40. Barkun AN. Should every patient with suspected upper GI bleeding receive a proton pump inhibitor while awaiting endoscopy? Gastrointest Endosc 2008;67:1064–1066.

41. Gisbert J, Khorrami S, Carballo F, Calvet X, Gené E, Dominguez-Muñoz J. H. pylori eradication therapy vs. antisecretory non-eradication therapy (with or without long-term maintenance antisecretory therapy) for the prevention of recurrent bleeding from peptic ulcer (Cochrane Review). In: The Cochrane Library, Issue 2. Chichester, UK: John Wiley & Sons, Ltd; 2004.

42. Laine LA, Nathwani RA, Naritoku W. The effect of GI bleeding on Helicobacter pylori diagnostic testing: a prospective study at the time of bleeding and 1 month later. Gastrointest Endosc 2005;62:853–9.

43. Lanas A, Hunt R. Prevention of anti-inflammatory drug-induced gastrointestinal damage: benefits and risks of therapeutic strategies. Ann Med 2006;38:415–28.

44. Bhatt DL, Scheiman J, Abraham NS, et al. ACCF/ACG/AHA 2008 expert consensus document on reducing the gastrointestinal risks of antiplatelet therapy and NSAID use. Am J Gastroenterol 2008;103:2890–2907.

45. Rostom A, Moayyedi P, Hunt R. Canadian consensus guidelines on long-term nonsteroidal anti-inflammatory drug therapy and the need for gastroprotection: benefits versus risks. Aliment Pharmacol Ther 2009;29:481–96.

46. Laine L, Spiegel B, Rostom A, et al. Methodology for randomized trials of patients with nonvariceal upper gastrointestinal bleeding: recommendations from an international consensus conference. Am J Gastroenterol 2010;105:540–50.

47. Kanwal F, Barkun A, Asch S, et al. Measuring quality of care in patients with nonvariceal upper gastrointestinal hemorrhage: development of an explicit quality indicator set. Am J Gastroenterol 2010;105(8):1710–1718.

48. Dupuis M, Hayes SM, Dawes M, Hawes I, Murray S, AN. B. Barriers to the implementation of practice guidelines in managing patients with non-variceal upper gastrointestinal bleeding: A qualitative approach. Can J Gastroenterol. 2010;24(5):289–96.

49. Barkun A, Gasco A, Jewell D, Nevin K, and the REASON Study Investigators. Management of Nonvariceal Upper GI Bleeding (NVUGIB) After Guideline Publication: The Reason Study. Can J Gastroenterol. 2006;20:80A #7.

50. Davis DA, Taylor-Vaisey A. Translating guidelines into practice. A systematic review of theoretic concepts, practical experience and research evidence in the adoption of clinical practice guidelines. Cmaj 1997;157:408–16.

51. Hearnshaw SA, Logan RF, Lowe D, Travis SP, Murphy MF, Palmer KR. Use of endoscopy for management of acute upper gastrointestinal bleeding in the UK: results of a nationwide audit. Gut. 2010 Aug;59(8):1022–9.

52. Barkun AN. Emergency endoscopy cover: cost and benefits? Gut. 2010 Aug; 59(8):1012–4.

53. Guyatt G, Cook D, Jaeschke R, Pauker S, Schunemann H. Grades of recommendation for antithrombotic agents: American College of Chest Physicians Evidence-Based Clinical Practice Guidelines (8th Edition). Chest 2008;133(6 Suppl):123S–31S.

54. Vakil N, van Zanten SV, Kahrilas P, Dent J, Jones R. The Montreal definition and classification of gastroesophageal reflux disease: a global evidence-based consensus. Am J Gastroenterol 2006;101:1900–1920;quiz 43.

55. Guyatt GH, Oxman AD, Schünemann HJ, Tugwell P, Knottnerus A. GRADE guidelines. Journal of Clinical Epidemiology. J Clin Epidemiol. 2011;64(4):380–2. Epub 2010 Dec. 24.

Index

Gastrointestinal Bleeding, Second Edition. Edited by Joseph J.Y. Sung, Ernst J. Kuipers
and Alan N. Barkun. © 2012 Blackwell Publishing Ltd.
Published 2012 by Blackwell Publishing Ltd.